EMDR Solutions

EMDR Solutions

Pathways to Healing

Robin Shapiro, Editor

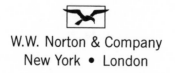

W.W. Norton & Company
New York • London

For information about permission to reproduce
selections from this book, write to
Permissions, W. W. Norton & Company, Inc.,
500 Fifth Avenue, New York, NY 10110

Production Manager: Leeann Graham
Manufacturing by R. R. Donnelley, Harrisonburg

Library of Congress Cataloging-in-Publication Data

EMDR solutions : pathways to healing / Robin Shapiro, editor.
    p. ; cm.
  "A Norton professional book."
  Includes bibliographical references and index.
  ISBN 0-393-70467-X
1. Eye movement desensitization and reprocessing. 2. Post traumatic
stress disorder—Treatment. 3. Neuropsychiatry. I. Shapiro, Robin,
1952–

RC489.E98E467 2005
616.85'210651—dc22   2005040526

W. W. Norton & Company, Inc., 500 Fifth Avenue, New York, N.Y. 10110
www.wwnorton.com

W. W. Norton & Company Ltd., Castle House, 75/76 Wells St., London W1T 3QT

3 5 7 9 0 8 6 4 2

To my mother, Elly Welt, with love and respect,
who, by her example, taught me to write

To Francine Shapiro, creator of EMDR,
who taught us to heal

Contents

Contributors

JAMES W. COLE, Ed.D., is a psychologist in private practice in Ellensburg, Washington. He is an EMDRIA-Approved Consultant and has presented workshops with Robert Tinker and Sandra Wilson on the use of EMDR with phantom pain. He has written seven books. The last two include forewords by Desmond M. Tutu and The Dalai Lama respectively.

ROY KIESSLING, L.I.S.W., Senior HAP (Humanitarian Assistance Program) EMDR Trainer and EMDRIA Approved Consultant, has a private practice in Cincinnati, Ohio. He provides telephone consultation and advanced EMDR specialty workshops throughout the United States. As a volunteer Trainer for EMDR-HAP, he has conducted EMDR trainings for mental health professionals throughout the United States, in the Middle East, and in Russia.

MAUREEN KITCHUR, M.S.W., is in private practice in Calgary, Canada, where she runs couples therapy groups and trains and consults to North American therapists. She has treated sexual and homicide offenders and clients with complex posttraumatic stress disorder (PTSD). She has published articles on the treatment of child sexual abuse and the Strategic Developmental Model for EMDR.

JIM KNIPE, Ph.D., has been a psychologist in independent practice since 1994. He is currently the Colorado Springs regional coordinator for the EMDR International Association and an instructor at the Colorado School of Professional Psychology. Since 1995, he has been involved in humanitarian EMDR training projects in Oklahoma City, Turkey, Indonesia, and the Middle East. In addition, he has written on the use of EMDR with complex cases.

ULRICH F. LANIUS, Ph.D., is a psychologist in private practice in Vancouver, British Columbia, specializing in the treatment of traumatic stress syndromes. He is a facilitator for the EMDR Institute and an EMDRIA Approved Consultant. He has presented nationally and internationally on the neurobiology of attachment and dissociation, as well as on the use of EMDR in populations with dissociative disorders. He has recently coauthored a paper on hyperarousal and dissociation in PTSD in *Psychopharmacology Bulletin.*

CAROLE LOVELL, M.S.W., Psy.D., founded and directs the Personal Growth and Learning Center in Cookeville, Tennessee. She has worked as a clinician, consultant, manager, and teacher. She supervises graduate students from several universities and teaches in the University of Tennessee Extended Education Program.

ARNOLD (A. J.) POPKY, Ph.D., is an addiction specialist and consultant conducting trainings and workshops nationwide. Certified in Ericksonian hypnosis and EMDR, Dr. Popky has been involved in EMDR programs since its inception, including as a presenter for the EMDR Institute, EMDRIA, and as a primary clinical contributor in the EMDR Research Project at the Mental Research Institute (MRI) in Palo Alto, California. He is a coauthor of the integrative *EMDR Chemical Dependency Treatment Manual* distributed by the EMDR Humanitarian Assistance Programs.

SUSAN SCHULHERR, L.C.S.W., has a private practice in psychotherapy in New York City. She has presented to a variety of professional and general audiences on issues of weight, eating and eating disorders. Her article, "The Binge-Diet Cycle: Shedding New Light, Finding New Exits," appeared in the fall 1998 issue of *Eating Disorders.*

ANDREW SEUBERT, L.P.C., N.C.C., is the codirector of ClearPath Healing Arts Center in Corning, New York. He is a licensed psychotherapist and a trained music therapist and has extensive training in Gestalt therapy. He works with couples, trauma, eating disorders, dually diagnosed (MH/MR) adults, integrating spirituality and psychotherapy.

He has written several articles about therapeutic approaches with mental health/mentally retarded people.

ROBIN SHAPIRO, L.I.C.S.W., an EMDRIA-Approved Trainer and Consultant, maintains a private practice in Seattle. She teaches the EMDR Weekly Class, Parts One and Two, and has presented at regional and international EMDRIA conferences. In the 2003 *Seattle Magazine,* her peers voted her one of Seattle's Top Doctors for Women.

ROBERT H. TINKER, Ph.D., is a psychologist in private practice in Colorado Springs. He has trained therapists around the world on the use of EMDR with children. With Sandra Wilson, he is coauthor of *Through the Eyes of a Child: EMDR with Children.*

ELIZABETH TURNER, L.I.C.S.W., is an EMDRIA-Approved Consultant and Trainer on Bainbridge Island, Washington. In her private practice, her specialties include working with children, adolescents and adults, people with chronic illness and pain, and people with attachment issues.

JOANNE H. TWOMBLY, L.C.S.W., an EMDRIA-Approved Consultant, has presented at EMDRIA regional and international conferences and has a private practice in Waltham, Massachusetts. She is past president of the New England Society for the Study of Dissociation.

SANDRA A. WILSON, Ph.D., is executive director and founder of the Spencer Curtis Foundation in Colorado Springs, which conducts research and humanitarian treatment outcome studies of EMDR with special populations. Her research has been published in the *Journal of Consulting* and *Clinical Psychology.* With Robert Tinker, she is coauthor of *Through the Eyes of a Child: EMDR with Children.*

Most of the writers are available for consultation and to teach workshops. You can find their contact information at http://www.emdrsolutions .com.

Acknowledgments

Thank you to all the writers, who gave freely of their innovations and the time to make them into chapters, while struggling through multiple versions, reformatting, and computer miscommunications. Clinicians will be using the contents of your work to ameliorate suffering. We have made a book to be proud of.

Thanks to the clients who continue to teach us all how to do therapy. You have cocreated every innovation in our chapters.

Thank you, Elly Welt, my mother, for teaching me to write and edit. Thanks for going over every word, comma, and many-claused sentence, twice. Thanks for arguing with me, with such good humor, over the rules of punctuation. And thanks for letting me, on occasion, win.

Thanks to Deborah Malmud, my editor at Norton, for believing in the book, despite that "Norton isn't doing more anthologies," and to Andrea Costella and Michael McGandy for answering my many questions in many e-mails.

Thanks to Elizabeth Turner, a former journalist and current therapist, for her editing assistance.

Thanks to Joan Golston for getting me thinking about this book. David Calof and his long-running consult group were great supports, as were the friends I used to see before I started writing. Thanks to all the people who ever said, "You should write a book." I did.

What can I say to my husband, Doug Plummer? Let me count the roles: photographer, computer systems administrator, transcriber (of the interview with Sandra Wilson), Web site manager (emdrsolutions. com), chef, differentiated container of my crankiness and occasional ranting, hand-holder, playmate, cheerleader, and my beloved. Your presence continues to be a blessing in my life.

EMDR Solutions

Introduction

Robin Shapiro

As a clinician, I exult in the moments when transformation occurs: the trauma fades from frightening reality to mere memory; the need to distract from life with substances or dissociation changes to the will and the way to get on with living fully; or the chronic, unbearable pain disappears. Since 1993, eye movement desensitization and reprocessing (EMDR) has allowed me to give my clients thousands of these moments. In my twelve years of practice before EMDR, I helped clients learn to tolerate the effects of trauma. Francine Shapiro's EMDR (2001) gave me the tool to make the trauma go away.

The Standard Protocol of EMDR works to reduce or eliminate the effects of trauma. The American Psychological Association said so when they decided to offer credit for EMDR courses. The Department of Veterans' Affairs and Department of Defense (2004) both said so when they placed EMDR in the highest possible category as an effective treatment for posttraumatic stress disorder (PTSD). At least 16 peer-reviewed research studies say so, too (Maxfield and Hyer, 2002). There are more than 40,000 active users of EMDR, effectively treating hundreds of thousands of clients in over 80 countries worldwide.

So what is left to say about EMDR?

Plenty!

Since Francine Shapiro created the Standard Protocol, she and her students have been finding ways to enhance all its phases for maximum effect on myriad clinical problems and populations. Each year, presenters at regional and international EMDR conferences, workshops, and classes introduce at least a hundred new pathways to healing. As an EMDR consultant, instructor, and clinician, I'm always looking for elegant solutions to clinical problems. This book contains sixteen of my favorite EMDR solutions with step-by-step instructions for using them with your clients. Whether you read the book cover-to-cover or peruse the one chapter that speaks to your client population, you will be adding to your EMDR toolbox.

THE CHAPTERS

Maureen Kitchur's Strategic Developmental Model is a meta-model for EMDR practice that encompasses all of the phases of the Standard Protocol. Using Ericksonian utilization language and attachment-enhancing practices to motivate and contain her clients, she has created a clear order for EMDR processing, a way to process wordless, implicit experience, and the best intake system that I've ever used.

Roy Kiessling gives his take on Resource Development, a Preparation Phase procedure useful for externally or internally disorganized clients. His hierarchy of resource installation strategies is easy to learn and very helpful for clients in crisis. I especially like the way he turns resources into Cognitive Interweaves.

EMDR therapists keep finding ways to use this powerful tool with different kinds of clients and clinical issues. Joanne Twombly and Ulrich Lanius teach two very different preparations for doing EMDR with people with dissociative disorders. Many of Twombly's techniques are derived from hypnosis and ego-state work. Lanius shows how to use medication to allow EMDR to work with dissociated clients. Robert Tinker and Sandra Wilson have continued to develop a very effective treatment for phantom limb pain. Much of their protocol focuses on the History-Taking and Preparation Phases of EMDR. Susan Schulherr takes on the Binge/Starve cycle from History Taking through Installation. Andrew Seubert teaches the language and procedures necessary to use the Protocol in working with mentally retarded clients. I point out useful targets for people with anxiety disorders.

In 1993, when I took the EMDR Level I training from Francine Shapiro, she said that EMDR could be used with any other treatment modality. Many people have taken her at her word. Elizabeth Turner fluidly engages children with art therapy, play therapy, and storytelling in all phases of EMDR. Carole Lovell unites dialectical behavior therapy, EMDR, and EMDR offshoots for effective therapy groups for women with borderline personality disorder. I bring together narrative therapy questions and object relations theory to target culturally and generationally transmitted issues. Later, I talk about using EMDR with differentiation-based couples therapy. Jim Cole uses a reenactment tool from guided imagery for a quick and painless way to remove discreet trauma and pain.

Some of us have created variations on the EMDR theme. A. J. Popky and Jim Knipe turn the Subjective Units of Distress Scale (SUDS) on its head by targeting inappropriate positive affect. Popky shares his DeTUR protocol with its Level of Urge to Use (LOUU) for the treatment of addictions and compulsive behavior. Knipe clears lovesickness, procrastination, avoidance, and codependence using the Level of Urge to Avoid (LOUA). I write about the Two-Hand Interweave, a simple exercise of discernment, often used in the Preparation Phase.

USING *EMDR SOLUTIONS*

This book is a manual for doing EMDR with diverse client populations. If you took both parts of the EMDR training and have experience and knowledge of a specified client population, you should be able to use the procedures with few problems. If you aren't schooled in EMDR (full trainings run from 34 to 54 hours), get the training before you mess up your clients with this powerful psychotherapy! If you know what you're doing, know your client well, and remember that the therapeutic relationship must be strong before you try any technique, you will find uses for many of the solutions in this book.

You might think about reading about your specialties and skipping the rest of the chapters. I hope you read them all. There are gems in every chapter. I don't want any of you to miss Andrew Seubert's four *M*'s of representational resources—Memories, Mirrors, Models, iMaginings—just because you don't think you need to know about working with mentally disabled people. Tinker and Wilson's Phantom Limb Pain Protocol can be used for many kinds of pain. You may not work with groups, but if you have even one borderline client, read

Lovell's chapter. In it, you'll find a hundred things to do with your client. Even if you're not working with a binge-eater, you might be able to adapt Schulherr's protocol to a client with another cycling compulsive behavior. Start each chapter; skim through the ones that don't seem to fit your clients. Even if you never see kids, do not miss the dog story at the end of Turner's chapter. It will heal *your* separation anxiety!

Here's how this material works for me: I use Kitchur's Strategic Development Model including Ericksonian language, the genogram, attachment-enhancing procedures, and, if necessary, First Order Processing, on nearly every client (except the rare car-accident-client-with-no-prior-trauma). Every attachment-impaired client receives at least three resources: first, a Safe Place that includes a mythic or supernatural mother/nanny/angel/bodhisattva/immortal dog/caretaker; second, the circle of people and beings that have ever loved (and not hurt) the client; and third, Kiessling's Conference Room of Resources. I use Kiessling's simpler resources with people who are having trouble getting through their days. My Two-Hand Interweave pops into several sessions each week to help clients delineate between feeling states or choices. If I'm working with substance or behavioral addictions or compulsions, I measure and target the client's "urge to use" with Popky's DeTUR protocol. With procrastinators, it's Knipe's "urge to avoid." At an "Introduction to EMDR" class, I spent 10 minutes using the LOUA protocol to cure 35 Employee Assistant Program (EAP) therapists of paperwork avoidance. Several of them signed up for EMDR training on the spot. I've used the Phantom Limb Pain Protocol on all kinds of chronic pain. It works like a charm. Living in Seattle, I've been sending borderline people to Marsha Linehan's dialectical behavior therapy groups for years, while I provided containment, resource building, and trauma processing in individual sessions. It was delightful to see that Lovell had combined all those functions into one treatment. When the trauma is huge, but singular, and the client has no affect tolerance, I've been using Cole's Reenactment Protocol. I love the part when the client begins to giggle. I use many of Twombly's tools for working with dissociative people. This fall, I'm trading an EMDR training with a psychiatrist for his collaboration in using Lanius's opiate-inhibitor treatment with one of my more dissociative clients. Schuller's binge/diet procedures are new to me—I can't wait for the next binger to walk in my door!

RESEARCH CONSIDERATIONS

EMDR's Standard Protocol has stood the test of peer-reviewed research and hundreds of thousands of individual clinical experiences. EMDR's full protocol is empirically validated when used on PTSD. Many chapters in *EMDR Solutions* focus on trauma targets and thus conform to the research. Some of the uses in this book must be labeled experimental. When the writers point EMDR toward a non-trauma target, it may work very well or even be the most efficacious use of EMDR in a specific circumstance. However, only Lanius's Opiate Inhibitors, Popky's DeTUR Protocol, and Tinker and Wilson's Phantom Limb Pain chapters are backed up by systematic case evaluations. Even those don't have the weight of peer-reviewed research. Any readers who would like to do research on any of the topics should talk to the writers.

CASE HISTORIES

Every case history in *EMDR Solutions* is either a composite or is here with the client's permission. Only one name and story remained unchanged because the client wanted it that way. All other names and life circumstances are changed in order to preserve anonymity.

CHAPTER CONVENTIONS

What the therapist says or should say to a client is in italics, with no quotation marks. Occasionally, italics are used for other emphases, and I'll leave it to you to know the difference. Common EMDR terms are capitalized, especially those referring to a step of the Standard Protocol. If you've forgotten some of the terms, there's a glossary near the end of this book.

THE EIGHT-PHASE PROTOCOL OF EMDR

EMDR is an eight-phase approach with protocols that attend to three prongs—past events that set the foundation for pathology, current situations that cause disturbance, and future templates for appropriate future action.

- Phase One: Client History includes client readiness, client safety factors, and dissociation screening. Targets are identified to address past, present, and future.
- Phase Two: Preparation, includes creating a bond with the client, setting expectations, creating a safe place and testing the eye movements or Dual Attention Stimulus (DAS)
- Phase Three: Assessment, includes selecting the picture that represents the target, identifying the Negative Cognition (NC), developing a Positive Cognition (PC), rating the Validity of Cognition (VoC or VOC), naming the emotion, estimating the Subjective Units of Disturbance (SUD or SUDS) and Identifying Body Sensations.
- Phase Four: Desensitization includes reprocessing the memory, using DAS, according to standardized protocols.
- Phase Five: Installing the Positive Cognition, while holding the memory in mind
- Phase Six: Body Scan, searching for any bodily disturbance
- Phase Seven: Closure, includes homework to monitor changes, expectations, and, if needed, bringing the client to a state of emotional equilibrium
- Phase Eight: Reevaluation includes checking in at the next session to see if the client requires new processing for the previous target or associated material.

ATTRIBUTION

Francine Shapiro created and named EMDR, the Standard Protocol, and most of the common EMDR terms. Assume attribution to her and her invention in every chapter. Her definitive guide to EMDR is *Eye Movement Desensitization and Reprocessing: Basic Principles, Protocols and Procedures* (2nd ed., 2001). If you are an EMDR clinician and you haven't read it, go get it now!

REFERENCES

Department of Veterans' Affairs & Department of Defense (2004). *VA/DoD clinical practice guideline for the management of post-traumatic stress.* Washington, DC: author.

Maxfield, L., & Hyer, L. A. (2002). The relationship between efficacy and methodology in studies investigating EMDR treatment of PTSD. *Journal of Clinical Psychology, 58,* 23–41.

Shapiro, F. (1993, October.) *EMDR Level I training. EMDR Institute.* Seattle, WA:

Shapiro, F. (2001). *Eye movement desensitization and reprocessing: Basic principles, protocols and procedures* (2nd ed.). New York: Guilford Press.

Chapter 1

The Strategic Developmental Model for EMDR

Maureen Kitchur

THE STRATEGIC DEVELOPMENTAL MODEL (SDM) FOR EMDR ORIGINATED in Canada in 1996. It is a model that was born out of desperation in the face of the overwhelming treatment needs of severe- and multiple-trauma victims, forensic clients, and short-term funded high-risk individuals. It is an efficient and comprehensive method for maximally delivering the benefits of EMDR to high-needs clients before their therapy might be prematurely interrupted by the realities of funding or of a multiproblem life. Such a method, I felt, would need to effectively facilitate rapid engagement and address or circumvent the fear, hostility, anxiety, and resistance that so often undermine or sabotage therapy with high-need and high-risk populations. Clinical experience also suggested the importance of having some systematic manner of assessing and treating the often multiple fundamental underlying causes of pathology and symptomatology in order to assist these high-risk and high-need clients to break the cycles and patterns that likely would repeat in their lives. I hypothesized that any process or strategies that might facilitate healing in these ways could also be anticipated to optimize therapeutic outcome for high-functioning clients and diverse client populations.

CORE PRINCIPLES

Many high-risk, high-needs, mandated or forensic clients share a common pattern of unresolved early-life negative experiences (from infancy through adolescence in many clients). These experiences include neglect, abandonment, abuse, and other types of losses and traumas. Current psychobiology research (including research in attachment, child development, and child and adult trauma) suggests that such negative experience impacts on both the developing brain and the mature brain (Fox, Calkins, & Bell, 1994; Schore, 1994, 1996). Negative experience can impact limbic and cortical structures that thereafter modulate perceptual, emotional, and behavioral processes. Suboptimal life experiences can thus affect the developmental process for an individual, impeding the ability to address and complete fundamental tasks at various developmental stages and compromising the achievement of maturational milestones throughout the life cycle. These developmental wounds lie at the heart of immature, anxious or fearful clients and those labeled "resistant" or "defensive."

Such suboptimal early-life experiences are not confined to a few limited segments of the population but are often hidden in the presentation of many apparently high-functioning individuals. As such, it is reasonable to suggest that some of the perplexing, intractable, and chronic symptomatology seen in our more cooperative, self-referred, and advantaged clients are also a reflection of developmental injuries. These considerations have yielded a core assumption in the SDM: unless there is solid evidence to the contrary, clinicians would be wise to assume that virtually all clients carry with them some degree of developmental fixation or stuckness. Furthermore, the SDM advances a fundamental proposition that wherever possible and appropriate, effective psychotherapy should not simply alleviate a presenting problem, but should facilitate developmental recapitulation or catch-up. Based on this, the SDM provides an overall strategy for addressing developmental deficits or fixation in order to bring healing to issues that underlie current symptomatology. Therefore, rather than working from a symptom base, the starting point of the presenting problem, or a list of the 10 most disturbing memories (Shapiro, 1995), the SDM proposes that clinicians first identify and chronologically treat with EMDR all the nodal events in an individual's life that are likely to have impeded developmental progress. In contrast to a simple chronological targeting of traumas, this developmentally oriented treatment process often effectively clears the developmental path, resulting in faster or more comprehensive resolution of all other targets and presenting problems. This process results in psychologically older clients whose primary and secondary symptoms often tend to shrink or disappear before being directly targeted.

While clinical practice suggests the importance of facilitating developmental healing through comprehensive clearing of a client's history, it is equally clear that work of such scope can only be accomplished if a client is maximally comfortable and engaged. The SDM therefore interweaves strategic structure, techniques, and language with a developmental orientation at every stage of therapy. The nature of these strategies is at the heart of the second core principle of the SDM: therapeutic strategy is not simply in the service of accomplishing a developmental agenda; rather, therapeutic strategy in the SDM must foster or serve an attuned relationship with the client. It is ultimately the attuned relationship that is reparative, and it is only in the context of that relationship that a therapeutic agenda or strategy can be safe and effective. (The concept of therapeutic attunement is discussed more fully later in this chapter.)

The term *strategic*, when used in the SDM, refers to a wide variety of structures, processes, techniques, and language that are employed to efficiently produce a climate of safety, engage cooperation, minimize resistance, relapse, and regression, and to facilitate developmental catch-up. These structures, processes, techniques, and language are strategic in the sense that they are designed and employed for these specific purposes and are directed toward achieving a goal of efficient and comprehensive healing. They include some elements of the Strategic therapies of the 1970s and 1980s (Bandler & Grinder, 1982; Haley, 1976; Watzalawick, Weakland, & Fisch, 1974), such as "reframing" information to manage resistance and organizing a brief and efficient solution to a clinical problem, but the strategic techniques of the SDM differ considerably in tone and focus from those of the Strategic school of the 1970s and 1980s, and to some degree those of the 1990s. Specifically, the SDM avoids focussing on "the problem" or on symptoms. It does not look for cycles or sequences to illuminate the nature of a problem experienced by an individual. Rather, it seeks to interrupt the problem by resolving the developmental conditions that have been perpetuating the problem and the symptoms. While the SDM employs strategic language to bypass resistance and facilitate rapid progress, it chooses language that is specifically designed to strengthen ego, impute resourcefulness, and honor the individual. In contrast to the Strategic school of the 1970s and 1980s, it is a central strategy of the SDM to lead clients to heightened levels of self-esteem and a sense of integrity or wholeness, without using strategies that might depersonalize, mystify, or confuse the client. These therapeutic outcomes of self-esteem, integrity, and wholeness are seen as equally important to the resolution of "the problem." All techniques and processes of the SDM are therefore designed to persuade and empower while resolving the conditions contributing to the problem.

In practical terms, the strategic nature of the SDM is reflected in its very structure. The developmentally sequenced treatment process, in addition to its capacity to resolve material contributing to current dysfunction, is itself highly strategic in terms of its ability to create safety and minimize resistance, dissociation, regression, and relapse; the developmental sequencing of work (which can be structured quite flexibly) does not require a client's young ego states to engage in the work of later life stages. As a result, in Strategic Developmental therapy, it is safer for all ego states to show up to a session because the therapeutic tasks of each stage of therapy are age appropriate, and younger ego states have the opportunity to be healed before the individual is engaged in later adult trauma work. Dissociation is less needed as a protective coping strategy when young ego states are not asked to participate in therapeutic work that belongs to a later developmental stage. This sequencing strategy of the SDM, when done within the context of a warm and nurturing therapeutic style, usually elicits rapid and deep engagement in populations that are typically resistant to or afraid of therapy. The SDM has often obviated the need for lengthy resource installation or ego strengthening in ego-compromised clients such as severe-sexual-abuse survivors and multiple-childhood-trauma survivors.

MAJOR COMPONENTS

To facilitate the safety and developmental recapitulation intrinsic in the SDM, the clinician should follow a set of clear steps and guidelines from the first moment of client contact. First, the SDM encourages deliberate utilization of transference to facilitate reparative attachment and it encourages deep attunement between client and therapist. Based on current knowledge from the fields of attachment and neurobiology, when attunement and attachment occur within a developmentally sequenced information processing model, developmental recapitulation is potentiated.

Second, the SDM provides clinicians with a structured, directive history-taking and assessment format that quickly yields a developmental hypothesis or template, from which it becomes possible to formulate a macro therapy plan that addresses virtually all the experiences and developmental interruptions contributory to pathology or dysfunction in a client's life.

Third, the SDM provides highly sensitive, facilitative, flexible language that assures clients of their safety and rapidly engages both the client's conscious and unconscious resources and cooperation, effectively creating a "healing trance." The strategies and language of the SDM facilitate a relaxed and focussed state of mind and behavior characterized by some traditional trance phenomena, but direct all trance behavior toward a profound belief in the inevitability of healing. (For example, attention is "coned," refocussed or redistributed onto the imminence and predictability of healing. The individual is "de-focussed" from the problem or symptom and begins to suspend usual planning functions. Symptom-maintaining attitudes and behaviors lapse. The client's heightened ability for fantasy production allows the client to envision a positive outcome with a relaxed and somewhat detached curiosity, paradoxically leading to the manifestation of that outcome. A reduction in reality testing and a tolerance for persistent reality distortion allow the client to suspend the limiting beliefs that have prevented change. An increased suggestibility allows the client to align with the therapist's confident vision of healing.)

Fourth, the SDM offers considerable flexibility in targeting strategies to meet the needs of diverse populations, including (but not limited to) children, adolescents (cooperative or hostile), mandated or wary adults, recent trauma victims, and entrenched PTSD victims, physically ill clients, and those with repressed memory, fragmentary memory, or amnesia.

THERAPEUTIC ATTUNEMENT AND NEUROBIOLOGICAL RECAPITULATION

Perhaps the most important thing about the SDM is that while it encourages therapists to be directive and structuring, it requires them at the same time to be flexible, sensitive, and nurturing. It is through an interplay of developmentally sequenced targeting and therapeutic attunement that the therapist has an opportunity to apply the powerful effects of EMDR accelerated information processing in a manner that can facilitate profound developmental recapitulation and recovery. An attuned therapeutic relationship is at the heart of the SDM, and in fact, the SDM cannot be safely used without such a relationship being in place.

What is this thing called attunement? Attunement or "affective attunement" consists of momentary alignments of one person's internal state with that of another person's, allowing each to "get" what the other is feeling. This has been observed between parents and babies, and it's known that this "getting" of an infant's state makes secure attachment possible for them (Ainsworth et al., 1978). When attunement occurs, both brains involved "coregulate" (Hofer, 1984). This coregulation "hardwires" the infant brain, making it more able to self-regulate (Schore, 1994).

Affective attunement is so necessary in parent-child relationships that when it is lacking, attachment is compromised and limbic and cortical structures don't develop optimally. Children exposed to abusive and abnormal environments are more vulnerable to developing abnormal neural circuits and to acting out accordingly (Joseph, 1992, 1996). If the right-brain template for affect regulation and a healthy sense of self don't get a chance to develop well, psychopathology can later develop (Joseph, 1992, 1996; Schore, 1994). A lack of early attunement because of abuse and trauma can compromise the function of the amygdala and hippocampus in the brain (Joseph, 1996; van der Kolk, 1996).

Encouragingly, studies suggest that the brain "is exceedingly plastic and is capable of undergoing tremendous functional reorganization . . . within a few years, months or even weeks of a single individual's lifetime" (Joseph, 1996, p. 663). Schore's studies (1996, 1997) suggest that the orbitofrontal cortex (whose neurophysiological mechanisms integrate social relationships, emotional regulation, and self-knowledge) remains plastic throughout life, and is able to develop beyond childhood.

It has been proposed that psychotherapy affords a powerful context within which recapitulatory experiences of attunement can engender the attachment experiences that facilitate healthy psychological development (Siegel, 1999). When we establish a nurturing, safe relationship and structure therapy with a developmental focus, we foster more mature object relations in developmentally delayed clients. By being consistent and trustworthy, keeping commitments, being punctual, being unconditionally accepting, and maintaining boundaries while at the same time being warm, caring, and available, we teach trust and model good ego boundaries. When we are "real" with clients, model a range of affects, and facilitate and sometimes induce affect, we have a fertile environment in which to teach affect recognition and promote affect development. When we model complete comfort with intense affect, coach clients to express and articulate emotion, and teach self-soothing strategies as well as problem-solving and communication strategies, then we may facilitate the affect regulation that truly is, as Allan Schore terms it, the foundation for the origin of the self (Schore, 1994).

The SDM proposes that the attuned relationship is the necessary context within which therapeutic strategy facilitates developmental healing. As effective parents have long known, well-attuned nurturing and strategic language, pacing and use of self can create deep connections and powerfully support growth and behavior change. Indeed, just as in a healthy parent-child relationship, when the caregiver's posture, facial expression, and vocal timbre, pitch, melody, amplitude, and rate of speech are sensitively adjusted within the communication feedback loop between the caregiver and the client, the client hears and internalizes both the message and the meta message conveyed prosodically, and potential exists for neurobiological repair and growth. These attuned experiences tap into the right brain structures that mediate affect regulation. When we engage in attunement behaviors such as these, we are likely to engender positive corrective attachment.

Simple things like warm caring eye contact between EMDR sets have the potential to deepen the client's internal experience of being "known" and, thus, sense of self. (Our eyes, if you will, hold up a mirror to our clients.) A therapist's body language, attention to proximity, and use of touch (where appropriate) can have profound effects on a client's internal experience, including on the electrical activity of the brain (McCraty, Atkinson, Tomasion, & Tiller, 1998).

Body language, proximity, and use of touch can be used to pace a client and to lead. For example, closer proximity, a "soft" posture, gentle voice, and warm touch of a client's hand or shoulder (where appropriate) can effectively engage, encourage, and empower a developmentally young client. As clients make treatment gains, the therapist can adjust physical boundaries, tone of voice, and facial expression to send a meta-message about the client's emerging maturity and competence.

When these types of attunement and attachment occur within a developmentally sequenced information processing model, there are profound implications, both psychological and neurobiological, for the developmental recapitulation that ensues. Clients are not only assisted toward more functional and adaptive information processing, but, given the plasticity of the brain, nurturing attunement from the therapist during developmentally sequenced information processing may facilitate in the client a new right-brain template for self-regulation and, thus, sense of self. The client is cleared out, caught up, and ready to self-manage with newly internalized and self-generating structures—in short, a healthy independent adult, regardless of "age" at the start of therapy.

HISTORY TAKING AND ASSESSMENT FORMAT

An attuned relationship of course takes time to develop. Nonetheless, our effectively conveyed intent to create a safe and sensitive environment can allow us to move into history-taking and assessment fairly quickly with most clients. In fact, the starting point in the SDM with virtually all clients is the taking of a comprehensive history, using the genogram format, usually in the very first session. Clinical discretion may, of course, dictate that stabilization is first accomplished with some clients, such as those who are severely fragmented or dissociative, highly ego-compromised, or in acute grief from a very recent loss. Sessions are typically 75 minutes in length, and weekly when possible. I use a genogram-mapping format similar to that described in McGoldrick and Gerson (1985, 1999; see Figure 1.1). Strategic, Ericksonian (hypnotic) language is employed to introduce this and all other aspects of the Strategic Developmental therapy process. I tell clients, *In order to obtain the best possible information that will allow me to map out a treatment plan to address all of the issues you'd like to have resolved, I have a history-taking process I'd like to take you through today. I'm even going to ask you my "nosy, snoopy questions" that I ask everyone, and all of this information will assist me in making real sense today of the issues you'd like to unload (or heal). Many of the questions will only require brief answers today because one of the things that I think you'll like about being in therapy here is that the toughest stuff is only discussed in detail on the days that we actually use EMDR to heal it. By the way, I'm going to tell you all about EMDR in your next session so that you'll have a deep understanding of how and why we can clear the experiences that underlie many of the issues and symptoms you've brought with you today.* This introduction is carefully geared to accomplish several purposes: it seeds the notion that

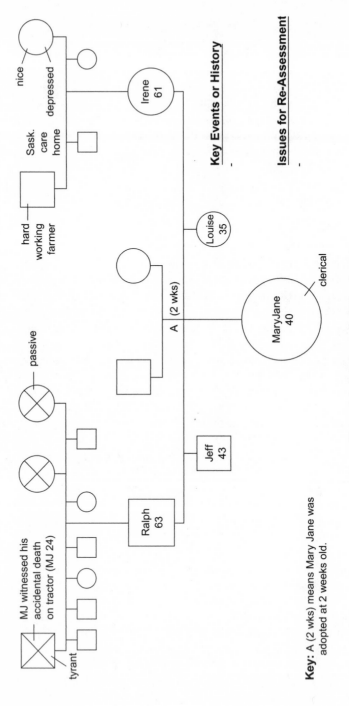

Key: A (2 wks) means Mary Jane was adopted at 2 weeks old.

Figure 1.1 Genogram 1 of Mary Jane

comprehensive healing may be possible,* it normalizes the sharing of deep personal information at an early stage of therapy, it imputes to the client an innate and expectable capacity for self-regulation during the sharing of information, it foreshadows a structured treatment plan, and it suggests a causal and potentially interruptible link between that experience and current functioning.

The following information-gathering processes are structured to move smoothly and efficiently from basic demographic details through family systems, family dynamics, and large and small *t* trauma experiences to contextual information such as medical and therapy history. The flow of questions is intended to assist clients to see the unfolding of their own history in a larger context, and to therefore facilitate comfortable disclosure of their deepest issues and therapy goals. In order to accomplish this, the following categories of questions are generally asked, in approximately the order below, during the genogram process, or they are interwoven in the first two or three sessions (whichever is most appropriate for the client and length of appointment). Clinical discretion must be exercised in the selection and use of assessment questions with each individual client. Clinicians may wish to supplement the categories of enquiry below for specific client populations.

I. Basic Demographic Details and Structure

Basic demographic details and structure of the individual's family back to grandparents' generation and forward to include client's children (stepchildren or adopted children). This is obtained through genogram mapping (see Figure 1.1).

II. Family Systems and Family Dynamics Questions

These questions are asked in a neutral and curious manner. These introduce a consciousness of intergenerational relationship styles and patterns. As the questions unfold, the focus is intended to narrow gradually and comfortably from grandparents on to the client, so that the client is able to comfortably (i.e., without guilt or blame) reflect on

---

*The American Psychological Association (APA) states that you may not tell a client that a particular intervention will be successful, even an APA-approved therapy like EMDR.

the family patterns or reactions to family patterns that the client has carried into adult life and relationships. A typical hierarchy of these questions is as follows (although the questions would naturally be modified to fit the experience of adopted children, or children who grew up in foster care or with relatives or with stepparents):

1. *What do you know about your dad's family? Where was he in the birth order? What was it like for him to grow up in his family?*
2. *What was his parents' marriage like? Do you know how they parented their kids? Do you know how the kids got along?*
3. *How do you think that shaped your dad? What do you think he brought with him out of his family?*
4. Same questions re: mom. (Of course, the questions can begin with mom if preferred).
5. Same questions re: stepmom(s) or stepdad(s) if required.
6. *So, with your dad/stepdad coming from that background, and mom/stepmom from hers, each of them fully formed people, what kind of marriage(s) did they create? How did their individual "stuff" interact with each other's?* (The use of the phrase "fully formed people" is intended to seed for members of couples that they, too, came to their relationship as individuals with a distinct history and set of issues, independent of whatever issues, history or baggage their spouse might also bring. Later they will be assisted to see that those issues are ones that they, and they alone, are responsible for, regardless of the spouse's issues.)
7. *How has their relationship changed over the years? (Was it different during different phases of child rearing or during different economic periods in the family or while you lived close to or far away from particular relatives?)*
8. *How do you think your parents' backgrounds shaped the way they parented you and your sibs?*
9. *What was it like for you to be the oldest? (middle? youngest? a twin? only girl? only boy? only child? only stepchild? only adopted child? only biracial child?)*
10. *Were you and your sibs all parented the same or were there differences? Was anyone picked on or favored?*
11. *Did anyone carry an unfair load in your family in any way?* ("Unfair" lets the client know that you will be sensitive to justice issues.)

12. *How do you think that set of experience shaped who you are now? What do you think you brought with you out of your family?*
13. *How do you think that has helped shape your choice of partners? (friends? work? or the lack of partners, friends, work in your life?)*
14. *How do you think all of that has helped shape the way you parent your children? (your delay/speed in having children? your decision not to have children?)*
15. *Probably without you fully realizing it, your history has naturally influenced many of the patterns, habits, decisions, and behaviors you are living with today, as an individual or as a member of a couple. There are just a few more things I need to ask you so we can decide which parts of your history need healing to free you up to live in a more satisfying way.*

(For additional systemically oriented optional assessment questions to assist in gathering information about attachment, emotions, anger, gender, sexuality, romantic love, or culture, clinicians may refer to De-Maria, Weeks, & Hof, 1999).

III. Developmentally Interruptive Experiences

As clients reply to the above questions, they often reveal their developmentally interruptive experiences. The clinician may, however, need to introduce specific questions to ensure that all such events are identified and noted on the genogram.

At this point, the clinician can proceed with what are smilingly referred to as the *"nosy, snoopy questions."* Use clinical discretion in the selection and timing of these questions. It is recommended that the client be guided to give brief answers where possible.

A typical introduction of the "nosy, snoopy questions" is as follows: *Great, we've got a lot of the information we'll need to map out a good treatment plan. I just have a few more nosy, snoopy questions that I ask everybody. These are questions about some of the tougher things you've lived through, or that you know have happened in your family, but fortunately I only need brief answers to these questions today—just a few words or sentences will tell me what we need to note on our genogram for future healing.* The clinician then adopts a rather matter-of-fact, curious, and neutral tone of enquiry and responds to replies with a compassionate yet focused attitude, conveying the meta message that *we are simply identifying targets for healing, we can maintain a healthy detachment.* The therapist's style needs to be such that it models safety, nurturing, and, most important, self-regulation. Clients can experience that, indeed, difficult material can be touched on, and the therapist's model of emotional equilibrium can be followed and even gradually internalized. Modeling and initiating this well-regulated survey of difficult material seeds an even more powerful unspoken message for the client: *When we address each of these issues with EMDR you will already have some experience of how to self-regulate. You are learning, just through a genogram enquiry, both how to be with your trauma and how to be detached from it at the same time. You are a reporter of your own experience, and together we can approach it in a safe yet direct way without your having to either dissociate from it or drown in it.*

Give appropriate comfort if a question provokes a deeply emotional response, but generally the pace set is one that allows the following questions to be answered in a single session (e.g., *I'm so sorry that happened to you. You don't need to give me the details right now. I'll ask you more about it on the day that we're going to heal it* (patting client's arm, offering a tissue). *Let me just note what you've told me on your genogram and we'll move on to our next question, okay? . . . Thank you, I really appreciate your hanging in with me as we identify what needs to be healed.*).

Questions can include, and are not limited to:

- Witness or victim of domestic violence; physical, sexual, or emotional abuse
- Alcohol or substance problems in the family or caregivers
- Neglect or abandonment; separations (apprehensions, foster care, adoption, hospitalization)
- Separation or divorce; traumatic losses; scapegoating; serious accidents or injuries
- Medical conditions or surgeries
- Pregnancy traumas (in grandmothers, mother, sisters if relevant, or self) including multiple births, abortions, miscarriages, sudden infant death syndrome (SIDS), infertility, or birth defects
- Untimely moves or job losses; immigration
- Incarcerations; disasters (floods, fires, etc.); victim or witness to crime
- Peer or school traumas; learning disabilities
- Religious trauma or abuse

Abuse and violent relationships are depicted on the genogram by means of an arrow from the perpetrator to the victim. The type of abuse (physical, emotional, verbal, or sexual), the client's approximate age(s) at the time(s) of the trauma, and the general frequency of the abuse are noted along the arrow. See Figure 1.2. Other information obtained in this section is noted on the genogram beside the client or key individuals involved, or may be listed as "Key Events" on a separate list or section of the genogram. See Figure 1.2.

IV. Contextual Information

Contextual information is gathered, including:

- Relevant medical history
- Therapy history
- Substance history and current usage
- Medication history and current medications, including nutritional supplements, herbs, vitamins
- Nutrition (especially important for mood-disordered and eating-disordered clients, but also for those with somatic complaints and body-image issues)

This information is usually too lengthy to be noted on the genogram but is often listed on an attached page, so that the open genogram, which sits on the desk for client and therapist to refer to in every session, is a complete summary of the information that influences the client's functioning.

V. Other Clinical Assessment as Needed

Exercise clinical judgment and discretion about the extent of assessment required for a thorough understanding of particular presenting clinical problems, such as substance problems, sexual addictions, eating disorders, dissociative tendencies, anger management problems, depression, and severe borderline personality. Obtain sufficient comprehensive information in order to ensure safety of the client and the community before proceeding with other stages and process of the SDM. Related to this, client safety factors must be assessed before memory processing can commence. Clients must have a reasonable social support

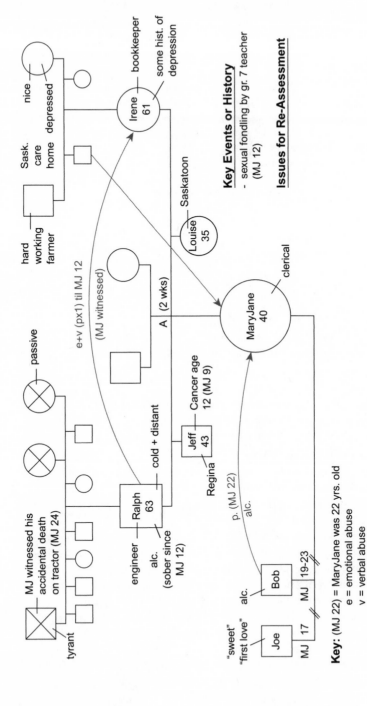

Figure 1.2 Genogram 2 of Mary Jane

system and sufficient physical health and ego strength to ensure that they can remain stable during the course of treatment (see Shapiro, 1995, Chapter 4).

When a reasonably comprehensive history has been gathered, and client safety (and community risk, where applicable) has been addressed, EMDR targets can be identified and prioritized in preparation for memory processing (see additional guidelines later in this chapter for prioritizing targets with ego-compromised, resistant, wary, anxious, or mandated clients). However, before addressing the target-setting and treatment phases of the SDM, a closer look at the strategic language of the SDM is in order.

STRATEGIC, ERICKSONSIAN (HYPNOTIC) LANGUAGE

At least 7 essential language strategies are employed throughout all stages of the SDM to relax clients, facilitate comfortable disclosure, foster cooperation and trust, and deepen clients' sense of their natural ability to heal. Without strategic language, the structure and rapid pacing of the chronological developmental clearing process could feel overly directive and even intimidating. The major types of strategic language include immediate seeding of the expectation of comprehensive healing or problem resolution; reframing of almost everything as helpful toward the goal of healing; utilization of whatever the client brings (Erickson & Rossi, 1989; Haley, 1993); normalization of all of a client's experiences and feelings; de-focussing from the problem and refocussing attention on healing; use of confident and celebratory language; and description of therapy as having specific, clear, and finite stages. These strategies of the SDM allow language to be used to excite clients about the probability and imminence of natural change, so that their conscious and unconscious resources are quickly mobilized to facilitate the healing process. This makes the therapist's job easier!

The first major language strategy, the immediate seeding of an expectation of comprehensive healing,* is accomplished by means of statements that create anticipation and foster curiosity. For example, in the target mapping stage, the clinician may remark, *Let's decide the order in*

---

*Again, be aware that the APA rules say that you must not promise a cure.

which we're going to resolve things or *When we've finished abuse issues, we'll address . . .* or *It will be fun to discover the specific positive changes you'll notice.* At various points throughout therapy, the clinician may interweave comments such as *As you dump off (or unload or notice) those feelings shrink . . .* or *When your healing is almost done . . .* These statements send a powerful early message that therapy can be expected to proceed through somewhat predictable phases and stages, that healing is to be expected at each step, that progress will be tangible, that outcome will be the result of a collaborative process, and that the process will move toward an end point.

The second major language strategy involves reframing of almost everything as helpful toward the goal of healing. For example, fearful reactions and deep emotions are compassionately responded to with a comforting touch or gesture, and then are often observed to be an indicator that *"your stuff* or *your experience" is so accessible. These feelings will really allow us to move directly toward healing.* After a pause (and perhaps more comfort), the therapist may use the reframe as a springboard to move further, by saying, *Shall we go further and see what else is ready to be unloaded?* In the face of this reframing (which must be sensitively done), clients often attach a new meaning to, and thus have less fear of, their own intense feeling states. And as affect regulation is thus facilitated, so too are developmental "catch-up" and psychologically older clients. Reframing is also used in the SDM to manage resistance. When a resistant client, for example, sits very far away, the therapist comments, *I'm glad you'll be good at letting me know your preferences.* Reframing, of course, can also be used to change the meaning a client attaches to a symptom (but it must be well timed and sensitive, e.g., *So your body chose to store all that fear and powerlessness in your digestive system! Of course, since it didn't have anywhere else to put it! Now your ulcer (or acid reflux or irritable bowel) makes sense!* Reframing can also change the meaning a client attaches to their entire history. Wolinsky (1991) has referred to the "trances people live." A well-constructed reframe can entirely shift the trance a client lives in, e.g., *So you have been a warrior through all those events in your family! It's really awe-inspiring to hear how you have used your energy to fight back and never give up!*

The third language strategy, utilization, is a technique adopted from the work of hypnosis legend Milton Erickson (1980). He pointed out that a therapist must pace a client before being able to lead a client. Utilization involves a subtle and indirect embracing of a client's perspectives, attitudes, fears or resistance in order to lead the client to a new conclusion, all while still speaking their language. Utilization makes use of both conscious and unconscious material offered by the client. It involves the therapist's attunement to the behaviors that reveal conscious or unconscious needs for pacing, safety, and structure in the client. For example, a client comes in and, unconsciously delaying therapy, tells a long, irrelevant story. The therapist, rather than redirecting the client or asking what the client is trying to say or to avoid, utilizes the whole story or a point in the story as a springboard, link, bridge, or framework to move in closer to an area of therapeutic focus. The therapist may even tell a story back to the client. It is subtly done, so that no "shift" is perceived by the client. The therapist typically uses language, tone of voice, and pacing that are deeply relaxing or "hypnotic," and the client's attention gradually narrows or "cones down" so that the client is engaged in a therapeutic way without having to acknowledge a shift. Many clinicians untrained in clinical hypnosis have a natural aptitude for utilization. However, given that utilization is a hypnotic technique, those who wish to implement it in the SDM would find this easiest by obtaining training in Ericksonian hypnosis.

The fourth language strategy is to normalize clients' experiences and feelings, for example, use "we" language, as in *When we come from families where there's been a lot of tough stuff* . . . Also, make frequent nonidentifying mention of similar experiences, thoughts, and feelings of other clients, except with narcissistic clients. (It's like being in group therapy in absentia.) And, where possible, maximize or "double" the effect of those normalizing statements by linking them to imminent healing. For example, *You know, a woman I worked with recently noticed exactly those same feelings as she was in the latter stage of her healing on that issue.*

In the SDM, a fifth language strategy consists of a deeply implied assumption conveyed to the client that the client has all the positive internal resources—however deeply buried, undeveloped, or uknown— needed to live successfully, even in forensic clients and severe multi-problem clients. The focus of therapy, therefore, is primarily on healing the developmental interruptions and traumatic experiences that have blocked access to those resources. Unless dealing with highly fragmented or ego-compromised clients, positive resources themselves are often not usually installed early in therapy because the unconscious or meta message would be that the client lacked them. Rather, clients are told that when *we reach the second phase of therapy (fine tuning), it will be clear whether any existing skills require strengthening or whether any 'extra' new skills are needed, and we'll simply build them in at that point.* The paradoxical effect of this strategy is that early on, many clients begin to take for granted internal resources they did not know they possessed and begin to manifest them quite steadily throughout therapy. Clinical discretion must, of course, be used to determine which clients require resource installation for stabilization before and during EMDR targeting. Another way in which the SDM de-focuses from the problem is by using strategic language to repeatedly refer to symptoms in a distancing, past-tense manner. This tends to reduce client "ownership" of attachment to symptoms, and allows "self" to be newly defined (and gradually experienced) outside the parameters or limits of the illness or symptom. For example, clinicians can refer to "those" fibromyalgia symptoms, rather than "your" fibromyalgia symptoms, and can gradually shift to past tense when referring to current symptoms (e.g., *"the depression you described when you first came to see me"*).

The sixth language strategy is the judicious use of confident and celebratory language, in order to facilitate a positive expectancy set. Obviously, discretion must be used, and only realistic expectations fostered. It can be helpful to educate clients about the many relevant applications of EMDR that have been successfully used around the world and to share nonidentifying information about the mastery and healing experiences of clients you have worked with. It can be helpful to identify for clients your own areas of expertise. At the same time, however, clinical judgement must be used to ensure that clients who have a need to work slowly, or who have a need to please, do not perceive an implicit demand. For such clients, language may need to be adjusted accordingly to ensure that no performance expectation is construed from these positive statements. For example, it may be helpful to gently comment, *And I've been so delighted to see how my clients have progressed, each one at his or her own speed.* This allows the unconscious to choose the most important part of the message to be retained.

The seventh major language strategy involves the provision of an implicit and explicit sense that therapy involves clear, generally predictable phases of work (Core Targeting from the Developmental Baseline followed by Re-Assessment and "Fine-Tuning"), generally predictable progress, and positive outcomes. The phase-oriented and progressive structure of the therapeutic model tends to deepen the sense of the inevitability of healing, and it keeps clients focussed and engaged in doing the work necessary to reach the "fine-tuning" phase. Clients are given a sense that therapy is a finite process that produces outcome, a perspective that maintains the healing trance and keeps both conscious and unconscious resources accessible at all times.

In summary, the seven language strategies of the SDM, when used in combination, ensure that clients experience the directive structure of the developmental targeting process to be sensitive, empathic, and rapidly empowering.

ESTABLISHING THE TARGET LIST

After basic demographic and family-relationship-trauma-medical information is gathered, all major EMDR targets are numbered on the genogram in the chronological, developmental order in which they occurred (including non-family-related EMDR targets listed at the side of the genogram) (see Figure 1.3). This is the "Developmental Baseline." I explain to clients that, for the most part, the first phase of therapy will consist of clearing these "core" events that subtly or overtly have tended to compromise the client's coping resources and left them more vulnerable to subsequent negative experience or trauma or illness. I further explain that as these core targets are cleared, they are likely to notice other presenting problems and symptoms shrinking or disappearing. Indeed, much of clients' presenting symptomatology, and even some of what might traditionally be considered "targets" are placed on an Issues for Re-Assessment List. I explain that at the end of Phase 1, *we'll check to see how much is left on the Re-Assessment List, and depending on what remains, we'll do some fine-tuning.*

THE RE-ASSESSMENT LIST

The assessment processes of the SDM typically result in a fairly comprehensive list of potential targets. However, once developmental and trauma targets have been formally identified and numbered, the client is encouraged to cast an even wider net and identify all the troubling symptoms and current issues that they may wish to have resolved, even those that they think are too minor, too chronic, too big, or too embarrassing to address. This is often done by means of the statement, *I want to make a list with you now of all the things you wish were*

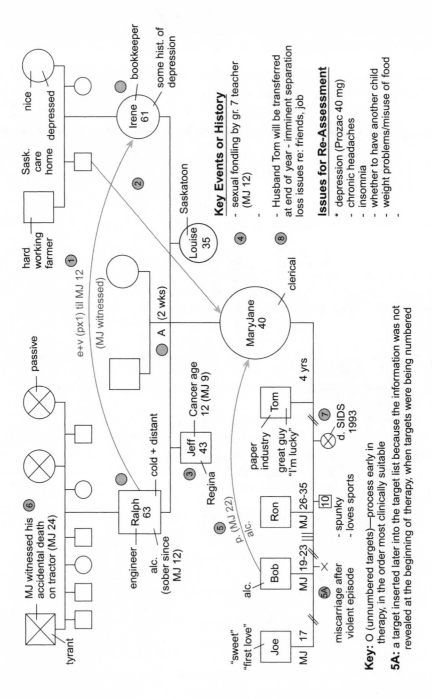

Key Events or History

- sexual fondling by gr. 7 teacher (MJ 12)

-

- Husband Tom will be transferred at end of year - imminent separation loss issues re: friends, job

Issues for Re-Assessment

* depression (Prozac 40 mg)
- chronic headaches
- insomnia
- whether to have another child
- weight problems/misuse of food
-

Key: O (unnumbered targets)—process early in therapy, in the order most clinically suitable

5A: a target inserted later into the target list because the information was not revealed at the beginning of therapy, when targets were being numbered

Figure 1.3 Order of Processing

*gone or were functioning better in your life. Effective therapy can often
shrink or wipe out a number of the traits or conditions you've given up on or
feel embarrassed about. It can make a big difference in some of the physical
ailments you've believed could only be changed by medical intervention. It
can help change habits, behavior patterns, and relationship patterns. Think
about what you'd like to include on this list. When we've done your core targeting, we can take a look at this list and see what has shrunk or disappeared.
We can then do some fine-tuning, depending upon how much time we have,
to get these things into the best possible shape. What would you like to put on
this list?*

Unless a client is presenting with a very recent trauma that may
need to be processed early in therapy, most of the primary and secondary clinical issues identified by the client and therapist can be placed
on the Re-Assessment List. Most are best left unaddressed until
Core Targets from the Developmental Baseline are cleared. Even some
recent major traumas are best placed on the Re-Assessment List,
because in some individuals they clear more easily and quickly if
not "anchored" by old material. However, clinical judgement must
be exercised when deciding which issues may be placed on the Re-
Assessment List. The structuring of the treatment plan must always fit
the needs of individual clients for comfort and stability. As well, clinical discretion is required as to frequency of monitoring the issues and
symptoms that are placed on the Re-Assessment List. Some issues and
symptoms might require attention parallel to Core Developmental
Baseline Targeting in order to ensure safety and stability.

Typical clinical issues and symptoms that can usually be placed on
the Re-Assessment List include, but are not limited to

- Anxiety
- Lack of assertiveness
- Anger and anger management issues (depending upon severity
  and risk to others)
- Bruxism (tooth-grinding) (but should be monitored by a dentist)
- Low to moderate depression, and even most forms of severe de-
  pression as long as they have been medically assessed and sup-
  ported with medication if needed
- Difficulty making decisions
- Low self-esteem
- Intimacy and trust issues

- Headaches and migraines (provided they have been medically assessed)
- Skin conditions: acne, eczema, hives (In the meantime, ensure the client is on a healthy diet that includes daily essential fatty acids and omega 3 and 6 oils such as flax, primrose, borage, and fish oils.)
- Allergies
- Procrastination
- Sleep problems (insomnia, nightmares, some sleepwalking) (monitor medically where appropriate)
- Weight and body image (in the meantime, ensure client is on a diet that includes a balance of protein, complex carbohydrates, fresh fruits and vegetables, essential fatty acids, and water, in order to balance blood sugar and maintain neurotransmitters for cognitive and mood function)

A number of typical major presenting problems can usually be placed on the Re-Assessment List (provided that those of a medical nature have been medically assessed and that the problem does not require immediate attention). These include, but are not limited to

- Chronic fatigue
- Fibromyalgia
- Severe, acute, or chronic depression
- Female sexual dysfunctions:

  - Dyspareunia (painful intercourse, usually involving inadequate lubrication)
  - Vaginisimus (painful intercourse, usually involving vaginal clenching)
  - Vulvar vestibulitis (tenderness, pain, and redness, usually preventing intercourse)
  - Vulvodynia (chronic vulvar burning, stinging, irritation, or rawness)

- Male sexual dysfunctions: premature ejaculation, impotence
- Marital problems or relationship problems
- Obsessive-compulsive symptoms

- Panic
- Phobias
- Sexual addictions (including chronic use of pornography, chronic masturbation, cruising for prostitutes, calling 1-900 sex lines, visiting peep shows, downloading porn from the Internet). (These must be carefully and frequently monitored for risk to others and may require some parallel cognitive-behavioral intervention, such as Relapse Prevention [Marlatt & Gordon, 1980]. In some cases, where available, a specialized treatment program is the best option or is the best adjunct to EMDR treatment.)
- Substance abuse. (This also must be carefully assessed and frequently monitored, and may require parallel processing using an addictions protocol for EMDR such as the DeTUR model [see Chapter 7], or relapse prevention.)

As clients are assisted to identify and list the foregoing Re-Assessment Issues, there is often a shift in their perception about the scope of change that may be possible in their lives. It is through this process that some clients (even forensic or mandated ones) frequently disclose for the first time shameful secrets they have been carrying (e.g., a fetish, a compulsive behavior such as hoarding or chronic masturbation, or having perpetrated sibling incest). It would appear that as the expectation of healing or problem resolution (indeed, the imminence and inevitability of it) is reinforced throughout the first few sessions, clients begin to see therapy as an opportunity for a thorough housecleaning and they themselves expand the focus beyond the referring complaint. (This is often the first tangible evidence in the first session that clients' unconscious cooperation has been enlisted, that is, that they have entered a healing trance.)

FLEXIBILITY IN TARGETING

As noted earlier, the chronologically identified developmental targets are the Developmental Baseline from which the therapist works. Targets are usually processed in the order in which they occurred in the client's life, but the sequencing can be adjusted to allow for four equally weighted priorities: developmental catch-up, minimization of resistance, safety, and efficiency.

Deviations from the Developmental Baseline may be needed to ensure that the therapy plan is highly sensitive to individual need. For example, individuals who have experienced recent trauma (i.e., within the last two months) frequently need to process that trauma immediately. Mandated, resistant clients (such as parolees) or ego-compromised clients may need to process a small, low Subjective Units of Distress Scale (SUDS) target first to gain comfort. Adolescents may need to be given the opportunity to decide upon the initial order of targeting in order to bypass resistance and enhance a sense of competence and healthy control for them. I sometimes draft a "laundry list" (i.e., target list) with the adolescent, and suggest that *we should put on it the things you wish people would get off your back about.*

Whereas tailoring the therapeutic pace and intensity for the client may necessitate departures from the Developmental Baseline, a return to baseline targeting (i.e., chronological, developmentally sequenced targeting) usually follows any such departures. This maintains the clarity, direction, structure, predictability, and safety that maximize client cooperation and healing. At all times, clinical discretion must be exercised to meet client needs for safety. The SDM must not be implemented like a cookie cutter. Therapists require a wide range of assessment and intervention skills to safely guide clients to healing, and the developmental and chronological processes of the SDM are not a substitute for clinical judgment. After stabilization, targeting of very recent trauma if needed, starting with a low SUDS target to gain comfort, clinicians can begin targeting childhood traumas and family-of-origin experience with the Standard Protocol. Where possible, clinicians should target the parental relationship(s) the client was exposed to, as well as the client's relationship with each individual parent over time. The family may be described as the "crucible" within which an individual's personality forms. It is frequently the case that clients do not always recognize the ways in which their familial relationship experience has set them up for styles of relating, communicating, and coping (including illness) that are less than optimal in adult life. Individuals may not identify these familial relationships as needing clinical attention unless there are obvious traumas attached to one or more members of their family. Setting up and checking on these targets can be efficiently done with EMDR, since if no negatively charged material emerges, therapist and client can move on to other identified targets.

Middle-childhood targets (defined as approximately ages 4–11) are generally addressed first. Known, identified traumas from this time period are targeted, and so are concrete, tangible negative memories of family-of-origin relationships. When these targets are clear, or reduced as low as possible at this point in therapy, the therapist may wish to check on and process suspected or identified preverbal or early childhood targets. These targets must often be cleared before middle- and later-childhood issues will fully resolve. They are done out of order for the simple reason that nonverbal, fragmentary early-childhood targets often involve deep somatic processing, powerful affect, and little of the cognitive or left-brain processes that typify standard EMDR processing. In this type of early-life targeting, clients are in touch with very early ego states. They may be highly vulnerable and least able to verbally articulate their needs. Early-life nonverbal fragmentary memories are processed only after middle-childhood targeting. In that way clients can safely be prepared since they have a foundation of EMDR experience. By doing the processing in this order, the clinician can have a solid sense of a client's processing style and a context within which to evaluate the client's responses. Guidelines for processing these types of memories can be found in "First Order Processing," an appendix to this chapter.

Where clinician and client do not see the need to check on early-life targets after middle-childhood targeting, they may proceed to adolescent targets, then to adult targets, including identified traumas and family-of-origin relationships. In some cases, adolescent and adult targeting reveals more fully the need to address early-life targets (i.e., where adolescent targets or adult targets do not resolve to a SUDS of 0 or 1, they may be "anchored" by early-life material). There are several reliable clues, however, that can assist in determining whether early-life targets would be wise to address before moving on to adolescent and adult targets. Clients who present with chronic, generalized, undifferentiated somatic complaints, self-regulatory problems (anger or rage problems, addictions, acute chronic depression), or intimacy and trust problems are often carrying the hallmarks of developmental interruption. (See Clarke and Dawson [1998], for detailed lists of the hallmarks of developmental delay at every life stage up to adulthood.) These problems are often underpinned by "attachment wounds," or deficits in the hardwiring of the right front cortex and limbic system that result from interruptions or compromises in parent-child bonding during infancy and early childhood.

It must be emphasized that where evidence exists of attachment wounds, clinicians must proceed with caution. Severe attachment wounds may also be clues to the presence of personality disorders, including narcissistic, borderline, antisocial, and dissociative identity disorders. These disorders typically require lengthy treatment and demand a high level of skill and sophistication in the therapist. EMDR may or may not be appropriate in the treatment plan of individuals with these disorders, and clinicians should seek appropriate consultation.

Developmentally oriented targeting, though conceptualized as phase oriented, is in fact an organic process, and clinicians should be prepared to be guided by emerging material. As long as the client has a solid foundation in the therapeutic process and therapeutic relationship and is ego-ready, it may be wise to follow emerging early-childhood nonverbal fragmentary material even if not all middle-childhood targets have been addressed. Similarly, a client may need to move ahead to finish off emerging material about later experiences with mother or father and then return to developmental baseline targeting. The main idea is to avoid a multiplicity of open, unfinished targets, for which they may not be ego-ready, and to provide clients with an opportunity to target phases of their experience in a somewhat orderly fashion, leading to a sense of finishing off the past.

Childhood and adolescent targeting can be a short or long process, depending upon whether there are important sibling relationships to address, and whether there are multiple peer, school, and extended-family targets to explore. Clinical discretion is required, since it is very important for clients to have a definite sense of forward movement in a reasonable amount of time and at a pace they can financially afford. Some sibling, peer, school, and extended-family targets can be grouped to create as much efficiency as possible (e.g., *the worst of your experiences with your sisters, the most unkind peer from your junior high years, the most sexually inappropriate of your uncles*). This type of targeting can create a generalized treatment effect on associated targets. Where it does not, this type of selected targeting in childhood and adolescence can contribute to sufficient developmental readiness enabling a client to move on and achieve some reasonable progress on later necessary targets within the time frame and budget to which they are limited.

TARGETING OPTIONS AND STRATEGIES

The SDM requires both flexibility and clinical depth on the part of the clinician in order to be able to safely and effectively meet the challenges and complexities of developmentally oriented treatment.

I developed First Order Processing to access and safely process early-life nonverbal fragmentary or amnesic experience. With the SDM, targeting options are available for clients of varying levels of ego readiness.

When preparing to address early life, nonverbal, or fragmentary material, it is essential that a clinician have basic understanding of memory development. It is important to understand that clients may present with amnesia for some of the most important events in their history. For example, individuals may have a fully or partially repressed (or dissociative) memory of an emotionally traumatic experience, or they may present with amnesia (memory that is recorded primarily in right-brain, nonlinguistic form). Amnesia can occur for at least two reasons:

1. Normal childhood amnesia results from the fact that in children ages of 6–10, the corpus callosum is not fully developed in the brain, and the right and left hemispheres operate more independently of each other than they will at later stages of development. As a consequence, much social-emotional experience is stored in nonverbal form in the right hemisphere, never making its way into left-brain digital (verbal) form.
2. Traumatic experience can so overwhelm or damage the limbic nuclei (amygdala and hippocampus) that the hippocampus is later unable to retrieve memory of the experience. The memory remains in nonverbal form, encoded in the right brain and somatosensory systems of the body.

I developed First Order Processing for targeting early-life, nonverbal, fragmentary, or amnesic material. It is a set of clinical strategies that can be used for early-childhood material, and at any point along the Developmental Baseline where a client presents with incomplete memory of experience suspected to be important in their development. See the Appendix at the end of this chapter.

The order and pacing of targeting must be sensitive to a client's ego strength and readiness. Some clients will require a short or lengthy period of resource installation before targeting can begin. High-functioning clients may require none. Highly skilled and experienced clinicians who are deeply attuned to their clients, and who can convey safety to their clients through multiple levels of communication, may find that no resource installation is necessary because, in the words of one therapist, "the Model and the therapist act as the container for the client" (R. Shapiro, personal communication, December 15, 1998).

The following guidelines are intended to assist in establishing the order of targeting.

1. For clients who have reasonable ego strength, and are coopera-tive both within and between sessions (and after sufficient client stability has been ascertained), developmental catch-up can usually set the agenda (unless a recent trauma requires im-mediate attention). Targets can usually be processed in this order:

    i.   Middle- and later-childhood targets (family-of-origin, peer, small and large "t" traumas),

    ii. Preverbal or fragmentary childhood targets if needed (using first-order-processing guidelines),

    iii. Adolescent and adult targets.

    This general progression through the Developmental Baseline can be flexed if required, dependent upon whether intervening events or crises require attention, or if the client has limited time or energy due to an impending holiday, exam, or family event.

2. In situations where the therapist's skill, experience level, or fa-cility with meta-communication is less strong, a wide range of resource and strengthening strategies can be used to prepare for targeting. With clients who require a greater sense of safety or greater ego strength, but who otherwise are cooperative and have sufficient social support and stability, there are at least 2 ways to prepare for developmentally oriented targeting.

    i.   Ego strengthening and safety work (using EMDR positive installations or hypnosis)
    OR
    ii. Process a mini-target or off-topic target (a recent or old small event that is likely to have a lower SUDS

and is not related to one of the core developmental
or trauma targets).

Then, if client is sufficiently prepared, begin to address targets from the Developmental Baseline as in #1 above. Alternatively, if you still wish to proceed slowly, you can choose a later
target if it's a "stand-alone" type of target and reasonably small
or of lower intensity. When appropriate, move into Developmental Baseline targeting, and be prepared to flex the targeting
agenda where required, as noted in #1 above.

An additional way to pace clients who have increased needs
for safety or ego strength (before leading them further through
developmental targeting) is to alternate EMDR sessions with
skills training or ego-strengthening exercises appropriate to the
developmental level at which they are working.

3. Clients who are mandated, resistant, wary, or otherwise guarded
   may benefit from the suggestions in #2 above only after the es-
   tablishment of the therapeutic relationship and after ensuring
   that all safety factors are in place.

4. For clients who have dissociative identity disorder (DID), or
   dissociative disorder not otherwise specified (DDNOS), the
   current lack of controlled research on the SDM necessitates
   caution and judicious application. While clinical reports have
   indicated that the model has been successfully utilized with
   DID, it may not be suitable for all DID clients. It is recommended that clinicians have substantial experience and expertise in working with DID clients and at least a year's experience
   with the SDM with general clinical populations before applying it to DID clients.

CASE EXAMPLE

Monique was 29 years old when she presented with posttraumatic
stress disorder (PTSD) after having been held hostage in a bank robbery the year before. A single mother of three children, ages 7, 8, and
10, Monique was experiencing profoundly disturbed sleep due to a
persistent auditory hallucination of an alarm bell ringing. (The alarm

had gone off in the bank and rang for the duration of her 4-hour ordeal.) Monique was using a common sleeping medication prescribed by her family physician and was experiencing no relief for her insomnia. She was also on an antidepressant to combat persistent anxiety and hopelessness. She had seen a psychologist for 3–4 months and reported no improvement.

The genogram mapping of Monique's history in her first session revealed that she was the middle of five children and had been physically and sexually abused in her family "from as early as I can remember" until she left home in her teens. Her parents' relationship was characterized by chronic violence, and she had an older brother whose mental illness had impacted severely on the family while she was growing up.

Monique was a resourceful young woman and had put herself through a postsecondary diploma program in a technical field while raising her firstborn. Monique had had only a brief involvement with the father of that child, and he was not involved with her or her son after the boy's birth. Monique's two younger daughters were the product of her relationship with a violent alcoholic. Monique and her children had escaped to a women's shelter when she was 25, and she did not return to the relationship. Approximately 5 weeks after this history was obtained, Monique revealed that she had also been involved in a protracted struggle to obtain child support from the children's father.

Monique had maintained ties with her mother and three sisters, but they lived at such a distance that they were not able to be of significant assistance in her posttrauma period. She had two close girlfriends who were supportive. Monique reported a good relationship with her children and perceived herself to be a competent mother. She reported no concerns about her children, other than wanting them "to have their mother back." The man she had been dating at the time of the trauma, and who had remained involved for several months, had grown distant as Monique's symptoms intensified, and she feared that she would lose this relationship, confirming her fear that "I'm a loser with men."

I explained the SDM to Monique in her first session, telling her, *Based on all the information you've given me, I'd like to make a target list with you, and use EMDR to heal things most likely in the chronological order in which they've happened to you. I've found that if we heal the underlying early experiences that shaped who you are and how you cope, then when we turn our attention to later issues like the bank holdup and man troubles, they usually resolve pretty straightforwardly. I also find that when we heal things*

pretty much in the order they happened, people discover a lot of new inner re-
sources along the way, and they find that many areas of their lives start work-
ing better, even if we haven't had a chance yet to focus directly on those areas.
This process allows us to work toward making your whole life better, not just
resolving a few isolated pieces of your experience.

Our target list will include the obvious bad experiences you've had, like the
bank, and your ex-husband, and I usually include our experiences in the fam-
ilies we grew up in. What we were exposed to in our families sets us up to ei-
ther cope well or less well with life's challenges, so checking on and healing
those experiences actually makes all the rest of our work go faster.

Monique's targets were then identified and enumerated in the
chronological order in which they had occurred. They were as follows:

1. Her parents' violent relationship
2. Her physical abuse
3. Her sexual abuse
4. Her older brother
5. Her relationship with the alcoholic father of her two younger children
5A. Her struggle to obtain child support. (We called this 5A because it was a target identified after we had already begun EMDR processing, and we simply inserted it into our target list.)
6. Being held hostage at the bank
7. Her disintegrating relationship with her boyfriend.

I explained to Monique that we would also make a list of the symptoms and life issues that she would like to see change in by the end of
therapy. I told her, *Many of these issues will resolve on their own as a conse-*
quence of our EMDR on your targets, but we want to list everything you'd
like to have working better in your life. Then, once we've done our major tar-
gets, we can see what's disappeared, what's better, and if there's anything left
we'd like to fine-tune.

Monique and I then drafted her Re-Assessment List, and on it we
placed

1. Auditory hallucinations
2. Anxiety
3. Hopelessness

4. Insomnia
5. Her judgment, choices, and behaviors with adult males.

I explained to Monique that we may or may not need to target #7, her disintegrating relationship with her boyfriend, since it was highly possible that the natural changes in her resulting from resolution of her other targets would produce a very positive "spillover" effect onto that relationship. We could of course pay some attention to that issue parallel to our other healing work, but I recommended that Monique inform her boyfriend about the healing she would be doing and suggest to him a reassessment of their relationship toward the end of her EMDR.

Since Monique had moderate stability and social supports, and reasonably good ego strength, resource installation consisted only of installing a relaxing image, anchored by a physiological self-cue. (I had Monique tuck her thumb inside the palm of her hand while we used gentle tapping on her knees, as she focused on her relaxing image, the corresponding emotions and physical sensations, and a pleasant cue word associated with the image.)

(I do not refer to this installation as a "Safe Place" because to do so can convey a meta-message that the other "places we go" in therapy are not safe; rather, I emphasize that the therapy room and everything we do there is safe, and the client may use the self-cue in the office or outside it to access a state of relaxation.)

We considered starting targeting by focusing on childhood material, as I normally do in the SDM, but we decided to address the bank trauma first, since it was producing such debilitating symptoms. I had earlier told Monique, *If for any reason we decide that we should get any particular target resolved first, no matter when it happened, we can start with that one. We can figure out, for example, if it makes sense for us to start with the bank holdup.* As we focused on the target image in the bank, however, Monique suddenly announced, "There's no way I'm going there!" I reminded Monique that I could do what I usually did in the SDM, which would be to target older underlying material first because it so often anchors current trauma symptoms. (My thinking was that, in her case, early experiences of powerlessness had likely anchored the powerlessness she had experienced as a hostage, and she would likely be less fearful of the bank target if she approached it with a foundation of childhood healing in place.) She replied, "I'd rather go there first than think about what happened at that bank!"

We therefore prepared to do a fairly standard SDM handling of her targets, and I explained to her, *I usually process some of your negative experiences from middle childhood first, to give you a sense of how EMDR will begin to heal those events and relationships. If we need to, we'll do a special process* (First Order Processing) *to heal infancy and early-childhood experiences. And then usually we can move straight ahead from there and clear out adolescent and adult material. We can stop at any point along the way if important things crop up in your current life that we want to take care of. And we can make room for new discoveries, forgotten issues, or new targets along the way if we need to. The process is kind of front-end-loaded, in that I think you'll find your family and childhood targets can take a fair amount of energy. The payoff is that your later targets won't be as anchored as they have been, and they often fall like dominoes.*

We began EMDR processing using the Standard Protocol, focusing on tangible memories of her parents' relationship from her middle childhood (ages 4 to 11). I explained to Monique, *You know, I usually get people to focus on childhood images from their parents' relationship because our parents' relationship shapes us in so many ways. It's often the first place we get exposed to relationship styles, communication patterns, anger management, and problem-solving skills. It's kind of a 'crucible.' It's the place where we can internalize unhelpful coping models, and if it's a troubled relationship, it can distract our parents from attaching to us. So by getting this material cleaned out, we can help to lay a new foundation to build on.*

I then asked her to focus on a remembered image of her parents' relationship from when she was somewhere between age 4 and 11, *a time or situation when they were really struggling and you remember it was hard for you. It might be a single event, or it could be a picture representative of a dynamic that repeated over and over between them.* She chose a picture of the family sitting at the kitchen table, her parents in cold silence, "mad at each other as usual." Processing of this memory led to several related incidents over several years, and to specific memories of each individual parent's behaviors as well. We spent 3 weeks on those memories and were able to reduce their valence to a SUDS of 2. We then focused on target #2 (physical abuse) and in 2 weeks were able to reduce it to a SUDS of 3. We targeted #3 (sexual abuse) and in 2 weeks were able to reduce it to a SUDS of 3. Monique was pleasantly surprised by the reduced intensity of these targets.

However, in order to fully clear these targets, we decided to use First Order Processing since Monique felt her exposure to violence and abuse stretched back "as far as I remember." Since of course Monique had no memory of her early childhood, we had her focus on a photo of her parents from her early childhood, in which her mother stood rigidly beside her father, both with stony faces. I simply asked Monique, *As you look at this photo of your parents, knowing you were a little girl at the time, I just want you to scan your body and tell me what you're feeling.* Monique experienced tension in her jaws and slight nausea as she concentrated on the photo, rating them with a SUDS of 8. We then processed these somatic symptoms as per First Order Processing guidelines. The symptoms intensified, the tension moving into her forehead (the orbitofrontal lobe area of the brain), then into her temples and the back of her neck. The nausea came and went. She experienced weakness in her arms, followed by tingling. The tension in her jaw reappeared briefly, then resolved. The tingling spread to her lower limbs, and an "electric" sensation crawled along the top of her scalp and crown of her head. Throughout her processing, I had Monique remain silent during bilateral stimulation and to talk only in between sets, explaining, *We want to allow your right brain to access what it needs to.* After each set, I reassured her in a gentle voice, using statements like, *Good for you . . . that's good . . . just notice . . .* or *It's so interesting how your body is expressing what happened . . .* or *What a thorough job your body is doing, dumping off what it's had to hold.* At the end of the session, Monique reported feeling "lighter" and "bigger." When reviewing the photo, she remarked, "That's weird, but I want to laugh when I see those sourpuss faces!" Her SUDS was 0.

In her next session, she had the same reaction to the photo. We then addressed remainders of her physical abuse by having her think about a wooden spoon she vaguely associated with early-childhood physical punishment. She had selected it because "it reminds me of the house we lived in til I was five, and when I think of it I feel really tense and I feel like crying." We processed this memory fragment and these somatic symptoms as per First Order Processing guidelines. Partway through, as Monique was experiencing tingling in her buttocks, she began to feel tension in her inner thighs then a heavy pressure on her chest, and then she began gagging. It appeared that we had "tripped" into her sexual abuse. I reassured her. *Your body has a wisdom all its own, and these symptoms are likely coming up at the same time because your memory has stored these experiences in the same file drawer—they're likely from the same time period or they're all leftovers from experiences when you felt powerless. Your body knows how to deal with these somatic memories, now that we've given it safety and permission to do so. So just notice these sensations, knowing that your body has chosen to heal what's causing them.* We processed as far as time permitted, selecting as our temporary stopping point a moment when the pressure and gagging had abated. I reassured Monique. *Your body knows how to hold whatever's left, and it may or may not want to process a little more on its own this week. If it does, you may get a bit of restless sleep, or you may have some fluctuating mood states. If you do, just know that your brain and body are in charge and are healing at the pace that is right for you.* Monique was assisted to shift to her relaxing place, and when she reported feeling relaxed enough to terminate the session, she was given self-care instructions, told she could call me if needed, and we scheduled her next appointment for 1 week later.

Monique reported that during the week after that session, she experienced a few days of on-and-off sensation in her buttocks and thighs and a tension in her throat. She assumed it was, as I had suggested: *The body wanting to dump off just a little more*, so she didn't worry about it. We resumed processing of her early-childhood abuse, having her focus again on the image of the wooden spoon. Her body quickly reactivated the chest pressure and gagging, and we processed through (using First Order Processing) until her body felt clear and comfortable. Remeasurement of the spoon image produced a SUDS of 0. We also checked our progress by having Monique focus on remembered images of her sexual-abuse perpetrator. She smiled and said, "I see him blowing away like a dust ball!" Her SUDS was 0. We were fortunate that Monique's early childhood sexual and physical abuse processed together in an interwoven way, but this is a fairly common phenomenon once First Order Processing is started. We could have focused on each type of abuse separately (as we had begun to), but ended up not needing to.

We returned to check Monique's middle-childhood memories of her physical and sexual abuse. I told her, *Now that we've healed as much early experience as we can get our hands on, let's check back to where we left off with your conscious memories of childhood abuse.* We focused on the target images and her SUDS were 0. Her body felt clear and comfortable. This is a good example of how processing of early childhood experience can produce a generalized treatment effect on later targets, even ones that had refused to budge below SUDS of 2 or 3. Having "cleared the foundation," we were now ready to proceed to target #4, her older brother, using the Standard Protocol. We did three sessions on this issue. The following week, Monique reported that while she still had auditory hallucinations and poor sleep, she thought it was "weird" that she seemed to have fewer anxiety attacks and less hopelessness. We proceeded to target #5, her relationship with the father of her younger children. Then two sessions later we targeted #5A, her struggle for child support, both using Standard Protocol.

Two weeks later Monique said, "Let's get that stupid robbery done," and we proceeded to target #6, being held hostage. Monique's relative lack of fear and, indeed, even determination to approach the target illustrate the empowerment that typically ensues from clearing earlier material that has often anchored and underlaid current PTSD presentations. We required only one session to clear her hostage experience, using Standard Protocol, to a SUDS of 0.

We had a 2½-week break due to schedule conflicts, but it was a break that would have been worth scheduling even had we not had to because at this point Monique was in an excellent position to rest and to enjoy her progress. When she returned, she reported that "the bell stopped ringing!" that she'd had several good sleeps, and she didn't feel as stressed out. She also reported that she'd had "a pretty decent conversation" with her boyfriend. While she felt a mild optimism about the relationship, which surprised her, she stated that she'd like to work on the hurt she still felt from his distancing behavior. We therefore targeted #7. Monique's processing of this issue, using Standard Protocol, quickly generalized to item #5 on her Re-Assessment List (her judgment, choices, and behaviors with adult males), and she reviewed in detail her high school dating history, the anxiety that had paralyzed her around males, and her choice of adult partners ("What was I thinking?"). We spent four sessions on these interrelated issues. She resolved to a SUDS of 1 regarding her current boyfriend, explaining, "I have to see how it turns out." Her new cognition regarding men was, "I can be as successful with men as any other woman," and she reported a Validity of Cognition Scale (VOC) of 6 about this belief.

I saw Monique for a progress review 2 weeks later. She reported that all treatment gains had been maintained. She had begun to reduce her sleeping medication and her antidepressant after consulting with her doctor, with the goal of going off them completely. At this point, we were ready to move into "fine-tuning." I saw Monique every other week to monitor her transition off medications and to assist her in developing more effective relationship skills with her boyfriend. During this period, she brought her children in to a family session, so that they could be supported to talk about how the past year had been for them. We did not identify a need for the children to be seen individually beyond the family session. Monique maintained her treatment gains upon follow-up, successfully went off all medication, and reported that she felt like she was living a new life "all because of a bank robbery!"

COUPLES

The SDM, when implemented with couples, facilitates a very different type of relationship repair than that offered within traditional couples counseling. Controlled outcome studies of traditional therapy reveal that following treatment, only 50% of couples significantly improve. Of those, 30–40% relapse within 2 years (Atkinson, 1999). Why is this so? What we know about the impact of unresolved trauma on development suggests that when two unhealed individuals come together, there may not be the emotional and cognitive structures in place to assist those individuals in making use of cognitive or behavioral interventions. Where wounds occurred in early childhood, individuals may be easily triggered to "limbic rage" with each other, may lack the capacity to empathize, or may cope by means of inappropriate or even addictive self-soothing strategies. Where wounds occurred at any stage of childhood or adolescence, individuals may not have achieved the developmental milestones that are an essential foundation for mature interaction. Therapy is set up to fail if it is essentially being conducted with the competing child or adolescent ego states of each individual.

The SDM can be applied to couples therapy by addressing each individual's developmental "stuckness" before attempting to implement cognitive and behavioral strategies with the couple. Several variations of this process are possible, but the starting point is the same for all couples. A couple is seen together for the first appointment. Most appointments are 1½–2 hours. Minimal information is taken during the telephone referral to avoid any sense of alliance that would imbalance the first session. I explain on the telephone that the first and possibly second session will consist of taking individual histories and then a brief couples history. The perspective obtained from the individual histories will allow a preliminary hypothesis to be offered regarding the reasons for the marital difficulties, and a treatment plan will be proposed.

At the first session, I take a joint genogram, usually minus many of the "nosy, snoopy questions." If, however, the openness and voluntary offerings of the couple make it possible to comfortably ask about abuse and substance histories, and about previous partners, for example, then these issues will be covered as part of the initial joint interview. The preamble to this interview, and a refrain throughout the interview, is often that *we are looking to find how your family-of-origin history and experiences, in spite of everybody's best intentions, may have left you with some unfair burdens that set you up for difficulties in adult life. As we review your individual histories, it will be easy to see the kinds of experiences that may have undermined your individual well-being or resources before you ever entered an intimate adult relationship, and may have slanted your understanding of what you could expect in that relationship. As we identify these things, we really are identifying for ourselves a list of "targets" or issues that we'd like to heal, so that those experiences no longer create a set of triggers or a "filter" that interferes with your relationship. The more healed you are as individuals, the better position you will be in to know what you need to do about your relationship.*

Of course, in some situations, this framework may not be made explicit at the front end. As the therapist attunes to each member of the couple in the opening minutes of the first session, careful decisions are made about what language and pacing will suit the clients. A laid-back, low-activity approach may be the most effective with some hostile or fearful clients, as the therapist looks for the clues and opportunities to "utilize" (per Erickson) the framework offered by the client(s).

Pacing the client is always necessary in order to be able to lead the client, and in a strategic approach the therapeutic model must serve the client, not the other way around. As the clients are well-paced, the conceptual framework of the SDM can be gradually introduced, either explicitly as "a means of organizing our work," or implicitly if that is strategically preferable.

With respect to outcome, it is of course never assumed that the couple will choose to remain together, since individual healing can reveal deep flaws and fundamental incompatibility in any relationship (marital or otherwise). However, I emphasize for the couple that *we will structure a treatment plan that gets each of you as strong and healthy as possible. A marriage (or relationship) is only as strong as the two individuals in it. Once we have some of that healed foundation in place, we'll be able to address your couple issues in a way that will go more smoothly for you. You won't react to each other through the same old individual filters, and you'll have a deeper sense of self that will allow you to remain grounded and resilient as I teach you new ways of interacting.*

By the end of the second session, the therapist and the clients typically make a decision about how therapy will proceed. When time and finances permit, each member of the couple is seen individually in parallel fashion (usually weekly). Occasional conjoint sessions may punctuate this process when home life is highly conflictual and stabilization is needed (for example, if an extramarital affair has recently been revealed) or if the couple needs to be educated, informed, or coached about how to respond to each other's healing or changing behaviors. When sufficient gains are in place, regular conjoint sessions can be held to begin repair of the dyadic dynamic. Both individuals should ideally have completed virtually all of their family-of-origin and childhood material before the regular couple repair sessions begin. It is not essential that all individual targets be complete at this point. Some isolated targets such as accidents or injuries—depending upon the type—may not interfere if they are as yet unresolved. Similarly, many adult targets may not need to be complete before couple repair can effectively begin. Conjoint sessions can be conducted using a variety of modalities. Cognitive-behavioral interventions, solution-focused strategies, communications and problem-solving training, and sexual therapies are typically more efficient and effective at this point.

Many variations of this basic model may be required, depending upon the characteristics of the couple. Where finances are extremely limited, or where each member of the couple is high-needs, each member of the couple may be seen in staggered fashion (e.g., 4 weeks for her, 4 weeks for him, punctuated by stabilizing couple sessions as needed, followed by 4 weeks for her, 4 weeks for him, followed by a break). The goal is to assist each member of the couple to clear as many developmentally interruptive experiences as possible in order to be able to "show up as an adult" to conjoint sessions.

Boundaries may need to be explicitly set for the couple's interaction at home during their individual healing and during the phase of conjoint couple repair. If they are highly conflictual or otherwise enmeshed, the couple may be instructed to create space for themselves by remaining largely in separate areas of the house, or even one or the other staying with friends or relatives, or at the cabin for a period of time. The couple is generally able to cooperate with these boundaries once they see that their enmeshment can sabotage their own individual healing or the possibility of any constructive couple work.

Highly conflicted couples may also require a format that allows for more frequent in-office management of their interaction, parallel to their individual sessions. As this type of process unfolds, however, they are generally able to see that the expediting of their individual work will make such sessions less necessary, and they often are willing to cooperate to move toward a faster resolution.

In situations where a large differential exists in the maturity levels of each member of the couple, it is preferable to see the more compromised member first for their individual healing, in order to help that client get "caught up," before commencing the more mature partner's healing process. Failure to do so can result in an increased differential between the couple and can set the couple up for fragmentation.

Couples are strongly advised to postpone decisions about ending the relationship until both have healed and until they have had their first real opportunity to interact as healed adults. Comprehensive healing can dramatically change what was seen as possible. Couples can see each other in a brand-new light and build a new dynamic that is radically different from their earlier one.

Alternatively, if it would be better for a couple to end their relationship, doing so from a place of deep healing allows them to manage the process optimally, and it ensures that they are prepared to function well in future relationships. Finally, if there are children involved, the couple is more able to cooperate in making constructive decisions for the family if they are operating from a healed foundation. They will also better withstand the rigors of single parenting or shared parenting (and model mature behavior for their children) if they have healed to a place of maturity.

CONCLUSION

The SDM for EMDR was devised to respond to developmentally compromised individuals and couples whose interruptive life experiences and traumas interfered with their ability to make effective use of therapy or to profit maximally from standard EMDR. The SDM provides strategic methods for expediting the completion of interrupted development while resolving all identified EMDR targets. The SDM is based on the premise that the application of accelerated information processing within a developmental framework and an attuned therapeutic relationship have potential to trigger neurobiological repair. A carefully paced and sensitively structured developmentally oriented healing process results in clients who self-regulate and self-manage more effectively, who have a more developed and healthy sense of self, who have healthier abilities to interact and relate, and who, in short, are more adult. The SDM for EMDR has application with diverse and challenging populations. Clinicians trained in this model have applied it with short-term or long-term funded clients, in complex and multiple trauma, with high-risk, forensic, addicted, and chronically ill clients. The SDM has equal application with high-functioning adolescents and adults, individuals and couples. Many EMDR clinicians have used it to resolve their own issues.

APPENDIX: FIRST ORDER PROCESSING

First Order Processing is a set of clinical strategies that has evolved to meet needs in the following situations:

- Dissociated experiences, memories of unpleasant and emotionally traumatic experiences that would otherwise be overwhelming to the conscious mind.
- Implicit memories [sometimes referred to as amnesia], memories that were recorded primarily in right-brain or nonlinguistic form, either because

  - of the natural immaturity of the child's corpus callosum and consequent hemispheric lateralization at the time of the experience (i.e., under age 6–10)
  - the experience was emotionally so traumatizing that it overwhelmed or damaged the limbic nuclei, resulting in later failure of the hippocampus to retrieve it

- Incomplete or partial memory that may be dissociation, implicit memory, or a recollection of one or more parts of the behavior, affect, sensation, or knowledge (BASK) that make up all of experience (Braun, 1988).
- To facilitate processing more easily in stable clients who have profound fear of focussing on trauma memories or fear of remembering repressed material.

First Order Processing facilitates the accessing of primary material in its virginal state. With the exception of "flashbulb memory," most memory is processed as it is stored and therefore is, to some degree, distorted in both the storage and recall process. First Order Processing allows clients to access traumatic and early social-emotional memory material stored mostly in the right brain in close-to-original form (i.e., in somatosensory form, which is nonlinguistic) and to process it nonlinguistically and mostly noncognitively. For many clients, this has allowed comprehensive clearing of material that has not been available or amenable to standard methods of processing. It facilitates more comfortable processing for many fearful clients and is an excellent way to process primary material without cognitive interference in clients who cognitively block or undermine their own processing. The following are the steps for First Order Processing:

1. Complete the genogram process of the SDM with the client and establish the Developmental Baseline (the chronological list of trauma targets and developmentally significant targets).
2. Determine whether the client requires any low-SUDS targeting to establish comfort or off-topic targeting to facilitate engagement and bypass resistance.
3. Process any fully remembered childhood targets between ages 6 and 10, using standard processing. This will allow the client to have some experience of EMDR, to complete some targets, and, therefore, to have a sense of comfort and accomplishment. It also allows the clinician to gain a sense of the client's processing style, both in session and between sessions. This essential information provides a context within which to make sense of the body-oriented processing that predominates in First Order Processing.
4. Next, work with whatever childhood memory fragment is available, using the following steps:
    (a) Ask for the details of what the client remembers (*not* what they've been told, and *not* what they think happened). Be wary of full, complex narratives. These are not memories laid down by the child, as the child's brain was too immature to create complex verbal memories. A genuine childhood memory fragment will focus on a sensory detail such as a sound, smell, or simple picture, (e.g., "It was a sunny room, I remember hardwood floors. That's all. I just get this terrible feeling. I think I was about two." OR
    (b) If the client has no sensory memory fragment, but it is reasonably certain that an event occurred (e.g., other family members substantiate that the individual was indeed in a fire or kidnapped, or the client remembers details before and after the

alleged incident), ask the client to bring in a photograph from that time period (of the client or of any other individual believed to have been involved in the experience or of the place where it is believed to have happened).

If no photograph is available, an artifact from the period may suffice (e.g., a stuffed toy, a baby mug). The rationale for this use of photographs or artifacts is based on the encoding specificity principle (Tulving, 1983), which states that when something is experienced only or repeatedly within the same context, the context becomes part of the memory trace. Therefore, cues most suited for triggering these memories are those that are most similar to these memories. The more the cue matches or complements information contained in the memory, the greater the likelihood of accessing it.

THEN

(c) While the client is focussed on the sensory fragment or on the photograph or artifact, the clinician asks for the feeling being experienced and a SUDS score. For some clients, that question invites an adult perspective or triggers related adult cognitions, which involve left-brain functions, not actually a part of the right-brain stored material being sought. This can profoundly interfere with accessing dissociated or implicit material. In order to circumvent this problem ask:

(i) *With your eyes gently closed, please scan your body, head to toe, inside and out, and let me know what you are noticing in your body.*

(ii) *If 0 is no disturbing or upsetting feelings, and 10 is the most disturbance or upset you could feel, what number is that feeling in your stomach or chest or jaw?*

(d) Have the client focus on the client's body, and begin processing. Eye movements are *not* recommended during this processing. It is important that the client be able to go deeply into somatosensory memory, undistracted by adult visual cues such as the therapist's face, fingers, or office surroundings. I recommend a gentle tactile stimulus (tapping) or auditory tones.

(e) In between sets, ask the clients what they are getting in their body. As right-brain or somatosensory material is accessed, clients tend to process mostly nonlinguistically. Affect and sound are expressed, but verbalizations are typically fragmentary and childlike. Validate whatever the clients are getting, then redirect to the body. If clients are gently and repeatedly assisted to continue noticing their body processing, they tend to process straightforwardly through to comprehensive clearing.

Be wary of complex memory or cognition expressed during this type of processing, as they tend to be indicators of left-brain (i.e., adult) functioning. The authentic emergence of memory into left-brain (i.e., into language) will usually sound something like: "Oh, now I remember" or "I think he had a green jacket." An overactive adult cognitive self, on the other hand, tends to verbalize statements like: "You know, he was always such a controller . . . I've always thought he did that to my sister, too." With clients whose adult cognitive self tends to interfere in their somatosensory processing, and thus impedes accessing of material hidden in the right brain, simply respond to their cognitive statements by redirecting them to the body: *And as you notice that thought, Mary-Jane, what do you get in your body? Ah! Now just follow that feeling in your chest/jaw/etc.*

5. If no memory fragments are available, but clients hold a strong belief that something traumatic happened to them at an approximate age, and clinical indicators would tend to support the possibility, use body-oriented processing to investigate. Ask the clients to:

    (a) *Focus on what you feel in your body when you are aware of your belief that something unpleasant happened to you when you were about X years old. What do you notice? Where do you notice it?*

    (b) *If 0 is no disturbing or upsetting feelings, and 10 is the highest disturbance or upset you could have, what number is that feeling in your chest/leg/pelvis/etc.?*

    Process as above (d) and (e).

6. Because First Order Processing techniques are body-oriented, some clients (especially therapists!) may find that their "helpful" adult self (or other ego states) have a need to be active by interpreting or trying to make sense of what their body experiences in each set. When that happens, simply ask the client to send that observer self over to the sidelines to be with you (therapist) and to observe with you, *while the body does what it knows it needs to do.* Repeat these instructions as needed, with language such as: *Your body and brain are so wise; they know exactly what needs to*

*be cleared out of your body, and in exactly what order. Just go ahead
and notice as they do their job. They will actually do it better if we just
observe. . . . Good . . . that's right . . . just noticing . . .*

7. If clients are directed to focus on the body, with supportive language linking whatever is happening to imminent healing, they
tend to process comprehensively in from one to four sessions.

8. Sometimes processing is incomplete at the end of a session (i.e.,
there is still considerable body sensation or affect, and SUDS
are not down to 0 or 1). When that happens, advise the client
that the material will be safely stored in "the vault" of the right
brain until next session because the body has long known how
to do that. It is wise to then close down the session with a relaxation exercise. This can be preferable to doing anything cognitive, as it may invite left-brain interpretation of processing,
which at this point is not helpful.

9. Clearing of the material can be assessed in the following ways:
(a) When asked to refocus on the fragment of memory, photograph, artifact, or belief that something happened, clients report that the SUDS are down to 0 or 1, and the body feels clear
and comfortable.
(b) Clients spontaneously report unexpected comfort, resourcefulness, or resilience in their day-to-day life in situations
that would normally have produced discomfort. Some examples: client suddenly notices that she did not flinch this week
when touched by her partner in a particular way; client notices
that at a family gathering she felt comfortable for the first time
around a particular uncle; client notices that this week she did
not have the usual back or neck stiffness or that her usual pre-
menstrual symptoms have failed to appear; client notices that
she is not feeling intimidated by adult males as she previously
always did; client "suddenly" had an urge to write to her suspected perpetrator; a client reports that she had an urge to drive
by her childhood home or to the site of a suspected trauma and
felt absolutely fine while there.
(c) Targeting of later developmental targets does not produce
the same range and intensity of physical symptoms that manifested in middle-childhood targets and in the First Order Processing of dissociated material.
(d) All of the above are maintained.

10.   The utilization of a particular memory fragment, photograph, artifact, or belief about experienced trauma, coupled with body processing, often appears to have served as a spring-board backward to very early life material that otherwise cannot be accessed in a controlled and safe way. This type of processing appears to clear the somatosensory or right-brain "vaults" of negative memory, without involving the left-brain processes, which have been known to contribute to inaccurate memories.

11.   At the end of the session in which a client reports a clear and comfortable body and a SUDS of 0 or 1 (preferably 0), it is safe (and important) to engage the cognitive. All healthy individuals need a balanced inner narrative—it is a crucial part of self-hood. Here is a gentle, empowering way to assist the client to put the remembered (or suspected) event into cognitive perspective while maintaining the healing trance:

After remeasuring the target, ask: *Now that you've had a chance to unload that experience, as you leave it behind, what do you want to know and believe about yourself and your life today and for the rest of your life?* If needed, assist the client to generate one or more positive statements about herself relative to the experience. Assistance is often not needed, as the client now spontaneously verbalizes the positive cognition (PC) that was deliberately not elicited at the beginning of this work. (The left brain is thus in cooperation with the right brain at the conclusion of this process.)

Install the PCs with gentle, hypnotic tones and gentle tapping or other Dual Attention Stimulation (DAS).

12.   Proceed with any other childhood targets that involve dissociated or implicit memory. Usually, the process triggered by First Order Processing directs itself so effectively that all interlinked childhood right-brain material has cleared at this point. The client is often ready at this point to proceed with Baseline Targeting (i.e., into adolescence and beyond). Be prepared to be surprised at how quickly these later targets clear, since they are generally no longer anchored by early material.

REFERENCES

Ainsworth, M. D. S., Blehar, M. C., Waters, E., & Wall, S. (1978). *Patterns of attachment: A psychological study of the strange situation.* Hillsdale, NJ: Erlbaum.

Atkinson, B. (1999). The emotional imperative psychotherapists cannot afford to ignore. *Family Therapy Networker,* July/August, 60.

Bandler, R., & Grinder, J. (1982). *Reframing: Neuro-linguistic programming and the transformation of meaning.* Moab, UT: Real People Press.

Braun, B. (1988). The BASK model of dissociation. *Dissociation, 1,* 4–23.

Clarke, J. I., & Dawson, C. (1998). *Growing up again: Parenting ourselves, parenting our children* (2nd ed.). Center City, MN: Hazelden.

DeMaria, R., Weeks, G., & Hof, L. (1999). *Focused genograms: Intergenerational assessment of individuals, couples and families.* Philadelphia: Brunner Mazel.

Erickson, M. H. (1980). *The nature of hypnosis and suggestion.* The collected papers of Milton H. *Erickson on hypnosis,* vol. 1. New York: Irvington.

Erickson, M. H., & Rossi, E. L. (1989). *The February man: Evolving consciousness and identity in hypnotherapy.* New York: Brunner Mazel.

Fox, N. A., Calkins, S. D., & Bell, M. A. (1994). Neural plasticity and development in the first two years of life: Evidence from cognitive and socioemotional domains of research. *Development and Psychopathology, 6,* 677–696.

Haley, J. (1976). *Problem-solving therapy: New strategies for effective family therapy.* New York: Harper and Row.

Haley, J. (1993). *Uncommon therapy: The psychiatric techniques of Milton H. Erickson, M.D.* New York: Norton.

Hofer, M. A. (1984). Relationships as regulators: A psychobiologic perspective on bereavement. *Psychosomatic Medicine, 46,* 183–197.

Joseph, R. (1992). *The right brain and the unconscious.* New York: Plenum.

Joseph, R. (1996). *Neuropsychiatry, neuropsychology and clinical neuroscience* (2nd ed.). Baltimore, MD: Williams and Wilkins.

Marlatt, G. A., and Gordon, J. (1980). *Relapse prevention.* New York: Guilford Press.

McCraty, R., Atkinson, M., Tomasion, D., & Tiller, W. A. (1998). The electricity of touch: Detection and measurement of cardiac energy exchange between people. In K. H. Pribram & J. King (Eds.), *Brain and values: Is a biological science of values possible?* (pp. 359–379). Hillsdale, NJ: Erlbaum.

McGoldrick, M., & Gerson, R. (1985). *Genograms in family assessment.* New York: Norton.

McGoldrick, M., & Gerson, R. (1999). *Genograms: Assessment and intervention* (2nd edition). New York: Norton.

Schore, A. N. (1994). *Affect regulation and the origin of the self: The neurobiology of emotional development.* Hillsdale, NJ: Erlbaum.

Schore, A. N. (1996). The experience-dependent maturation of a regulatory system in the orbital prefrontal cortex and the origin of developmental psychopathology. *Development and Psychopathology, 8,* 59–87.

Schore, A. N. (1997). Early organization of the nonlinear right brain and development of a predisposition to psychiatric disorders. *Development and Psychopathology, 9,* 595–631.

Shapiro, F. (1995). *Eye movement desensitization and reprocessing: Basic principles, protocols and procedures.* New York: Guilford Press.

Siegel, D. J. (1999). *The developing mind: Toward a neurobiology of interpersonal experience.* New York: Guilford Press.

Tulving, E. (1983). *Elements of Episodic Memory.* Oxford, UK: Oxford University Press.

Watzlawick, P., Weakland, J., & Fisch, R. (1974). *Change: The principles of problem formation and problem resolution.* New York: Norton.

Wolinsky, S. (1991). *Trances people live.* Falls Village, CT: Bramble.

Chapter 2

Integrating Resource Development Strategies into Your EMDR Practice

Roy Kiessling

As EMDR BECAME MORE ACCEPTED WITHIN THE PSYCHOTHERAPY COMmunity and more clinicians became trained, a greater number of clients with diagnoses other than posttraumatic stress disorder (PTSD) were introduced to it. As a result, it became apparent that some of these more difficult, complex clients were not immediately ready for EMDR targeting and reprocessing. Many were either too unstable, had affect tolerance issues, or lacked the ego strengths to withstand the potential rigors of target desensitization. Others lacked needed coping skills, lacked the ability to recognize that they have the tools available to address their issues, or were fearful of addressing their traumatic experiences. Resource Development and Installation (RDI) strategies were developed and, over time, have been accepted within the EMDR community as valuable solutions for these challenging clients.

DEFINITIONS AND CASE EXAMPLES

In this chapter, resources are any coping skills clients have that help them deal with or manage stress. These coping skills include the ability to access and use Safe/Calm Places, imaginary containers, inner strengths, or skills and traditional stress management skills such as deep breathing, progressive muscle relaxation, meditation, and yoga. With this definition in mind, let's take a moment to look at the history of resource utilization in EMDR.

EMDR Reprocessing refers to the Standard EMDR Protocol's Phases 3 through 6 (Assessment, Desensitization, Installation, Body Scan, Closure, and Reevaluation). I assume that Phases 7 and 8 are being done every session whether the sessions are used for developing and installing resources or to target reprocessing.

All case examples in this chapter are abbreviated compilations of numerous cases.

HISTORY

Francine Shapiro first introduced resources into EMDR protocols when she developed and utilized the Safe/Calm Place exercise as part of the Preparation Phase of the Standard 8 Phases of EMDR (Shapiro, 1995). Subsequent RDI strategies have remained essentially the same as her Safe Place exercise. Andrew Leeds, an EMDR Institute Senior Trainer, was the second major contributor to the EMDR community's awareness of resources through his presentations at the EMDR International Association (EMDRIA) Conference (Leeds, 1997). Andrew Leeds and Debra Korn published the first single-case study evaluating the effects of implementing RDI strategies with clients suffering from chronic PTSD (Korn & Leeds, 2002). Since Leeds's first introduction of RDI strategies, there have been a number of other resource development and installation variations and innovations to assist clients in preparing themselves for EMDR processing.

CAVEATS

Many clients are ready for EMDR reprocessing and do not need any resource development other than the installation of a Safe/Calm Place. However, with RDI's growing popularity, many clinicians are either unnecessarily introducing extensive RDI work prior to EMDR reprocessing or mistakenly seeing the positive state change that often occurs with RDI work as trait change and then not bothering to do EMDR processing (Shapiro, 2004). Trait change is the ultimate goal of EMDR, while state change provides coping skills clients may use until their traumatic issues have been reprocessed by EMDR. Remember, trait change is the removal of any distress related to the presenting problem, while state change is the temporary shift in emotional state as a result of some coping strategy. As an example, a client with anxiety about public speaking may use coping strategies (Safe Place, container, resources, relaxation) to change his anxious state and manage a public presentation. Trait change, on the other hand, would be the total removal of any inappropriate anxiety over public speaking. As we discuss the various RDI solutions outlined in the chapter, please note that these interventions are utilized sparingly and are directed to helping the client prepare, as quickly as possible, for EMDR target reprocessing.

IMPORTANT CONSIDERATIONS WHEN DEVELOPING RESOURCES

When developing resources, you'll have many things to consider. These include: how, how much, and when to use Dual Attention Stimulus (DAS); accessing channels of positive association; whether to use actual or imagined resources; using a focus on body sensations and posture to enhance the resource; and whether to focus on the resource itself or the process the client uses to establish that resource.

Using DAS

Regardless of the type of resource you choose to install using Dual Attention Stimulus (DAS)—whether it be eye movements, tapping, or audio—remember to start with slow short sets (4–6 passes). Be concerned that DAS may illicit negative channels and begin trauma reprocessing. Prior to beginning the resource development and installation remind clients, *If you feel uncomfortable in any way, or if distressing material arises, tell me immediately and we'll stop.* If clients begin to run into traumatic or negative affect of any kind, stop the procedure. Some clients can tolerate only one or two sets of DAS. Others thrive with installations using many sets of DAS. If clients begin to report and show positive feelings, emotions, and body sensations, consider extending the sets in order to capitalize on the positive impact. Watch your clients carefully. Always be on the alert to cut back on the DAS or stop focusing on a particular resource altogether should clients report anything negative. Just as a Safe Place may become contaminated, so may a resource. If clients are unable to tolerate the use of DAS or unable to develop a resource, all attempts to use DAS and EMDR should stop until the clients have been fully screened and treated for dissociation.

Channels of Positive Association

In EMDR processing we focus on a target or node, and the clients naturally move to associated channels (Shapiro, 2001). As we reprocess negative target nodes, the associated channels' material often moves from negative to neutral to positive. I have found that similar processing exists when working with resources except in reverse! If we pick a positive resource (let's call it a resource node), it may also have associated channels. These associated channels may be various memories or incidents that are connected with that resource node. When installing this resource node with DAS, clients will process material within those associated channels. If you use long DAS sets or stay focused on a specific channel too long, you may notice the clients' reports moving from positive to neutral to negative. If you notice any neutral, instead of positive, report, it's best to shift to another memory of that resource or stop installing that resource all together.

Developing Resources: Actual or Imagined?

Ideally, when helping clients identify and develop their resources, try to help them remember actual times when they have successfully accessed and used that resource. Using actual past events when the clients have used that skill is the most effective resource. If the clients are unable to recall or have never experienced that skill, then helping them identify someone or some thing (real or imaged) who has that skill may be necessary. When accessing an external resource, it may take far more work for the clients to be able to access and utilize that resource in session and in their daily life.

Body Sensations

Use body posture and movement to help strengthen a resource. Once the clients have gotten in touch with their resources, and the image, emotions, and sensations have been accessed and enhanced, ask them to assume the posture or create the body movement that would best represent the resource. As they experience that body posture, enhance it with short sets of DAS.

Process versus Image

What do you choose to emphasize in the resource development process? Are you going to focus mainly on the image of the resource and the positive emotions and sensations that accompany that image, or are your going to focus on the process the clients used to establish that resource? Are you going to focus on strengthening the positive sensations the clients have when thinking about a friendship, or are you going to focus on the process they followed in developing that friendship, such as taking risks, setting boundaries, being assertive, and resolving conflict? In many cases, it will be beneficial for the clients to understand the skills they used in establishing the friendship rather than the positive feelings they experienced when thinking of their friend.

USING RESOURCES DURING EMDR'S
CLIENT PREPARATION PHASE

Most resource development strategies follow the basic framework outlined by Francine Shapiro's "Creating a Safe Place" protocols (Shapiro, 1995). These include, but are not limited to, developing an image of the desired resource, expanding the vividness of the images, accessing and expanding the positive feelings, emotions, body sensations, and positive beliefs about oneself associated with the resource, then enhancing and deepening the client's positive experiences with DAS. Modify or add to this basic framework depending upon what type of resource you seek to develop and install and the outcomes you desire that resource to accomplish.

Some clients lack the ego strengths, the ability to manage and control affect, or the sense of safety and internal control to begin EMDR target reprocessing. For these clients, the solution is to front-load them with internal skills, strengths, or resources in preparation *before* doing the EMDR reprocessing. This front-loading occurs during the Preparation Phase and often results in that phase being extended for a number of sessions before beginning the EMDR reprocessing.

It's useful for these clients to be able to access and utilize their resources effectively between treatment sessions. Once they are able to master the ability to effectively access and utilize their resources in between sessions, they often gain the confidence to proceed with EMDR target reprocessing. The solution to this Preparation Phase challenge is to utilize what I call the Extending Resources Protocol.

The Extending Resource Protocol

Problem: The client has difficulty managing his anger and often yells at peers, his spouse, and his children. Although he is willing to address this issue with EMDR target reprocessing (trait change), while he is working on desensitizing traumatic memories, he needs immediate help in managing his anger at home and work (state change).

Solution: The Extending Resource is designed to help this client begin to cope with his anger by identifying anger management skills he needs and then integrating them into his daily life. This is accomplished by

1. Helping him identify, enhance, and install with DAS skills he has successfully used to manage his anger.
2. Helping him imagine how these skills help him manage his anger.
3. Helping him integrate those skills into his life by reevaluating the between-session situations where he needed or used those anger management skills.

PROTOCOL STEPS
1. Identify image of desired resource
2. Elicit positive feelings and emotions related to the resource
3. Enhance the feelings, emotions, and body sensations
4. Use DAS to install the feelings, emotions, and body sensations
5. Develop a cue word
6. Self-cuing
7. Cuing with disturbance

8. Self-cuing with disturbance
9. Rescripting a recent past experience
10. Rescripting an anticipated future disturbance
11. Closure
12. Reevaluation

This protocol differs from the Creating a Safe Place exercise by its use of rescripting recent past and anticipated near future events. I picked up the idea of using rescripting from Landry Wildwind (1998) who uses rescripting to help clients create and install essential childhood experiences. Having clients practice using their newly developed resource in recent past and near future situations seems to help them regain some level of control in their lives and prepare more quickly for EMDR reprocessing.

CASE EXAMPLE

Presenting problem: The client has difficulty managing his anger.

The Extending Resource Protocol

This example contains most of the 12 steps of the Extending Resource Protocol.

1. Identifying the Desired Skill (Image)

Therapist: *I'd like you to think about what skills you will need to successfully manage your anger.*
Client: Well, I'd like to remain calm under pressure and not take things personally.
Therapist: *When in the past have you been able to remain calm under pressure and not take things personally? Certainly there have been some times when you did this—perhaps earlier in your life—maybe during high school or college.*
Client: Well, now that you mention it, when I played basketball in high school, that was one of my strengths.
Therapist: *Bring up a memory of a time when you were playing basketball and remained calm.*

Client: I remember a game in the city finals when the guy guarding me kept fouling me. He kept doing underhanded things behind the ref's back, hoping I would retaliate and get called for a foul.

2. Feelings and Emotions

Therapist: *Focus on that experience and notice what positive feelings and emotions you are experiencing right now as you remember that situation.*
Client: I really feel calm, confident, and actually playfully in control. No matter what he did, I knew I could handle it even though I didn't think it was fair. I wasn't going to let him get the best of me. In fact, I got the best of him because eventually he got caught often enough that he actually fouled out!

3. Enhancement

Therapist: *As you think of that situation, where in your body do you notice those positive feelings and emotions. And, as you notice those body sensations, how would you position yourself in a way that would show me how confident you feel?*
Client: I feel it in my chest. I'd be more upright, my chest out, shoulders back, head up, and I'd feel some positive tension in my arms.

4. Installation (DAS)

Therapist: *Okay, assume that posture. Notice how it feels in your chest and arms, and follow my fingers.* (DAS: six passes.) *What do you notice now?*
Client: I feel really calm and confident. I actually beat him at his own game, and I was really in control.
Therapist: *Go with that.* (DAS: eight passes.) *What do you get now?*
Client: Still really comfortable.

5. Cue Word (Positive Cognition)

Therapist: *As you think about this situation, notice the positive sensations you are experiencing. What positive statement would best describe what you believe about yourself?*

Client: I can be in control of myself.

Therapist: *Okay, hold that thought, You can be in control of yourself, along with the positive feelings, emotions, and body sensations you are experiencing. Follow my fingers.* (DAS: 10 passes.) *What do you notice now?*

Client: I really did control myself well, often under a lot of stress, not only on the basketball court, but also in other situations. I remember one professor who used to try to get my goat, and I handled that situation really well, too.

Therapist: *Go with that.* (DAS: 10 passes.) *What do you notice now?*

Client: During high school and college, I really was rather laid back and didn't let things get to me very much.

Therapist: *So if you could give this skill of being able to remain in control a name or an image, what would it be?*

Client: I see myself as a basketball player.

Therapist: *So thinking or imagining a basketball player connects you with all those positive feelings and emotions.*

Client: Yes.

Therapist: *Focus on that.* (DAS: 12 passes.) *What do you notice now?*

Client: Those positive feelings come to mind and my posture feels confident.

6, 7, 8. Self-cuing, Cuing with Disturbance, and Self-cuing with Disturbance

Comment: These Safe Place Protocol steps could have been implemented at this time; however, the client seemed to be reporting a lot of positive affect, so they did not seem necessary. Therefore we moved directly to the next step.

9. Rescripting a Resent Disturbance

Therapist: *Can you think of a recent situation, perhaps in the last week or so, when you lost control of your temper?*

Client: Yes, last Thursday I yelled at my son when he kept playing his video game while I was talking to him.

Therapist: *Okay, now I'd like you to rescript that incident, except this time, I want your basketball player to handle the situation. Just notice how he would do things differently. And, that doesn't mean your son would do anything differently.* (DAS: 14 passes.) *What happened?*

Client: Well, I was able to remain in control. I could see that he was just into his game, really focused. I waited until he finished that part of his game, then talked with him.

Therapist: *Okay, focus on the positive feelings and body sensations you have right now after seeing how your basketball player handled that situation.* (DAS: 10 passes.) *What do you notice now?*

Client: I feel really pretty calm. I handled that situation really well.

10. Rescripting a Future Anticipated Disturbance

Therapist: *Now I would like you to imagine a situation that may come up between now and when we meet again where you might lose your temper.*

Client: That's easy. We have a staffing meeting next week, which almost always results in me losing my temper.

Therapist: *Okay, I'd like you to imagine that meeting, except this time, see yourself going into the meeting as the basketball player. How would you handle things differently?* (DAS: 14 passes.) *What did you notice?*

Client: Well, I see myself recognizing how each member of the meeting plays—each has his strengths and weaknesses. One guy in particular actually reminds me of that high school player. He likes to get my goat. This time, I stayed in control and didn't respond to his behind-the-back fouls.

Therapist: *As you focus on being in control, notice what feelings, emotions, and body sensations you are experiencing.* (DAS: 10 passes.) *What do you notice now?*

Client: I feel that calm, confident feeling in my chest. I see myself sitting up confidently at the meeting table, breathing calmly, shoulders back, and I'm smiling inside. I know what game he's playing!

Therapist: *Go with that.* (DAS: six passes.) *What do you notice now?*

Client: I feel really good, confident, chest and body strong.

11. Closure

Therapist: *I'd like you to take this index card on which I have written "basketball player." Try to look at it at least once a day, especially in situations where you might lose your temper. In fact, take a moment and imagine yourself, just before your staffing meeting, looking at the index card and getting in touch with your "basketball player." (DAS: six passes.) What do you notice now?*

Client: I see myself looking at the card and feeling confidence, standing confidently.

Therapist: *Okay. So between now and next week when we meet again, try to use your "basketball player" as often as possible. Try to keep a log of the situations that come up during the week. Next week we'll review the situations in which you successfully managed your anger and also look at situations when you either forgot to use your "basketball player" or he wasn't enough. We'll either rescript those, or see whether you needed another "team member" to help you out. See you next week.*

12. Reevaluation

Reevaluation should occur every week to check on how the client has been accessing and utilizing his resource(s). In some situations, the original resource is all the client needs. In others, additional resources may be necessary. In those cases, utilize the Extending Resource Protocols to develop and install each needed resource. The reevaluation phase of the Extending Resource Protocols may be used before, during, and after EMDR targeting. Often, taking 5 minutes of each session to review the previous week is all that is necessary to maintain the client's momentum for using his resource(s). The remainder of the treatment session, once the client has demonstrated the ability to access and utilize his resource, may be devoted to EMDR reprocessing.

As you can see, the clients have the opportunity to access and utilize new skills in their lives. To give them an out, I tell them that I do not expect them to come back the following week having always used these new skills. However, to help them remember and do what they have learned, I will often write down their cue word or ask them if there is some object they can carry with them as a reminder. When we reevaluate how the week went in between sessions, we will first review the positive experiences, use DAS to solidify those experiences, and then focus on the times when they were unable to utilize their resource. Then we will rescript those unsuccessful events, using either the already developed resource or a new resource that can be added to the client's "toolbox" of coping skills. This strengthening, reviewing, and rescripting provides clients with the "constant mind awareness" that they have resources and skills that will assist them in managing their lives. It is important that the clients not only develop a resource, but that they be able to access and utilize it during reprocessing and between sessions. With repeated reevaluation, rescripting, and use of the resource, clients gain the confidence and skill necessary to address their traumatic issues with EMDR.

THE RESOURCE FOCUSED PROGRESSION

Clients come to our office presenting a continuum of readiness for the EMDR Standard Protocol. For many clients, at the higher functioning end of the continuum, EMDR targeting and treatment may begin shortly after their initial appointment. Other clients need more "front loading" before they are prepared to begin EMDR target reprocessing. Dissociative clients, those who easily flood as they tell their story, who have difficulty maintaining some level of consistency in their lives, or who generally present themselves as being internally or externally chaotic or unstable, would be good candidates for RDI "front loading." My assessment of the clients' appropriateness and preparedness begins with my first face-to-face meeting. Seeing the clients through the lens of EMDR's Adaptive Information Processing Model not only helps me begin to formulate my treatment plans, but also helps me formulate what type of RDI interventions the clients may need to help them prepare, as soon as possible, for EMDR processing.

Any of the protocols mentioned under the Resource Focused Progression (Kiessling, 2001) may be implemented during the Preparation Phase of the Standard 8-Phase EMDR Protocol (see Table 2.1). These protocols are designed to help stabilize and prepare a client for the traditional EMDR targeting protocol. Beginning with the least stable to the most stable client, the RDI interventions I plan to discuss are Identifying, Accessing, Focusing, and Reminding. These stages fit within my overall conceptualization of a continuum of client presentations.

Identifying Positives

This is my interpretation of intervention strategies Kay Werk (EMDR Institute Senior Trainer) and I have informally talked about over the

TABLE 2.1
THE PREPARATION PHASE RESOURCE FOCUSED CONTINUUM

STABILITY CONTINUUM

| Unstable for EMDR | Stable Enough for |
| Target Reprocessing | EMDR Reprocessing |

→

| Identifying | Accessing | Focusing | Reminding |

RESOURCE INTERVENTIONS

years at various trainings and conferences. This Identifying protocol works well with individuals who may be more practical and concrete, preferring strategies that require less imagination.

Goal

You want to help clients reestablish the ability to access images, thoughts, emotions, and body feelings that have a positive valence. As is demonstrated by the "yes-no" exercise in the EMDR Institute's training, thoughts and words have a resonance in the emotions and the body. This method of RDI works with words and thoughts to activate desirable emotions, body feelings, self-esteem, and even worldviews. It allows a bridging of positive affect, enabling clients to access more positive states of mind in a way that is logical and straightforward from their point of view.

Clients who are preoccupied with any unpleasant states of mind have often been giving too much attention to thoughts and experiences that support that frame of mind (i.e., material in the same or similar information package). Refocusing on images, thoughts, emotions, or body feelings that bridge to positive affect may offer stabilization, perspective, considerable relief, and access to a different information package that provides positive networks both in preparation for EMDR and for learning when desensitization and reprocessing occur at a later time. Once EMDR is experienced in this way, clients can often identify when the time is right to begin desensitization and reprocessing.

Protocol

- Explain to clients how focus on any chain of association usually leads to thoughts connected with similar emotional valence. For example, worry about any topic leads to other worrisome aspects of that or similar topics. Identify that the same dynamic applies to positive things: as they think of one positive thing, clients often associate and spontaneously come up with another positive perception.
- Ask the clients if the two of you can identify *any* positive aspects in the situation being targeted. (There are almost always positive aspects once the question is asked.) If *no* positive aspects relative to the presenting situation can be identified, ask the clients to identify anything in their life that creates some sense of uplifting as they focus on it. (This usually indicates that a functional network has been accessed.)
- Record each of the aspects generated and ask the clients to consider them to see if a similar positive statement might also be true. Recording these in some metaphor that suggests movement may be helpful: a circle (like spokes in a wheel), a drawing of a stream. A list certainly works also, especially with arrows from one point to another to suggest movement or momentum from beginning to end. A summary statement may be placed in the center or highlighted in whatever way works for the clients. Later this summary may become a preliminary positive cognition, but only if it arises naturally for the clients.
- If the clients cannot honestly identify any positive perspective on their situation or can generate no valid positive emotion around the aspects identified, it may be necessary to access positive images, thoughts, emotions, and body feelings on a subject that is less directly related to the current issue. Some clients cannot identify positive aspects of the presenting issue but can access positive feelings about their children or their pets or other aspects of their lives. As they focus on these, they often begin to realize that some aspects of their world are positive. In later sessions, these clients may be able to relate more directly to the presenting issue or they may become strong enough to do reprocessing and desensitization according to the usual protocol.

- Once the items are recorded, review to determine if each does provide some lift of improved perspective as it is considered. If it does, the more functional emotions and sensations provide confirmation that the item is useful as a resource. If not, note the item for later EMDR processing, but do not attempt DAS on the item at this time.
- Once the clients have been able to successfully identify the positive aspects of the situation (or, failing that, the positive aspects of their life), and if a check of each item reveals that it is still experienced as positive, ask the clients to notice emotions or sensations as they think about each positive point.
- Link each with very slow short sets of DAS (2–4). Stop if anything negative arises and redirect attention if possible.
- Usually new positives arise as the clients focus on the identified material. Install any newly associated positive points with more DAS.
- If possible, have clients develop a summary statement based on the material that has been generated.
- Copy the positives that have been generated and the summary statement and send them home with the clients.

Examples of Therapist Input

The tendency of channels of association to generate new thoughts of a similar resonance has been discussed and is understood by the client.

Therapist: *So, let's try to come up with anything at all positive about this situation* [presenting issue—loss of job and income] *if we can. It does have to be believable to you. The mind won't allow you to lie to it. In other words, when you think about it, it has to feel a little bit better—or at least you need to feel like, well, yes, that's an okay (or truthful) thought. It feels a little better. We're looking for things that your mind recognizes as at least a little improvement. We will deal with disturbing aspects a little later—we've identified many of those but for today, let's see if we can identify any positive aspects in the situation at all.* [This client's main barrier is the loss of self-esteem related to the job loss. However that cannot be addressed until the client is

feeling more hopeful about the process of therapy and the effectiveness of EMDR.]

Client: Well, I do have savings.

Therapist: (Record the statement.) *How does that feel when you think
about it?*

Client: It's good. (This indicates the thought has some validity for
the client.)

Therapist: *Can we record that? Can you notice a little sensation of relief?*

Client: Yes.

Therapist: *Do any other positives come to mind? Something about
which you can feel a little relief and acknowledge yes, that's true.*

Client: Silence (Give the client a little time, but not enough to set
up feelings of failure to accomplish the exercise.)

Therapist: *Would it be fair to say the savings are an advantage?*
[Strengthening the point the client already made.]

Client: Yes, of course. (Record that savings are an advantage.)

Therapist: If nothing else comes to the client's mind after a short
pause, *This may sound a bit silly, but let's itemize how the savings are
really an advantage.*

Client: Well, it allows me time to consider my options.

Therapist: *Let's record that if it is a truthful and helpful thought.*

Client: It is.

Therapist: *Anything else?*

The client is then able to identify additional positive points related
to her situation: that the family can eat; that she can cook less expen-
sively now that she has more free time; that she now has more time for
other things, like being with her son whom she seldom saw when she
was working long hours; that her house is nearly paid for; that she has
a secure place to live; that her savings give her time to consider alterna-
tives. The final sections of this indicate how the channels of association
can strengthen from the exercise.

Therapist: *So, let's write that. I did make a good choice to keep some
money available.* (If client generates no more points) *Would it also
be believable if I wrote, "I did make some good choices"?*

Client: Yes, my friends tried to get me to buy more stock (they all
have more stocks than I do) but I resisted for some reason.

Therapist: (Record it as the client said it.) Usually the client will now initiate some more positives. However, if not, the clinician can ask, *Would it be truthful to say, "I was able to listen to my own judgment"?*

Client: Yes, and it worked!

Therapist: *OK, I'm writing that down: "I did listen to my judgment." Then another statement: "And it worked!"*

This continues as long as it flows easily—usually about 4–12 statements. Sometimes quite surprising positive aspects occur when the positive information networks are accessed. When the exercise becomes difficult, stop. If the client can generate positives without coaching, fine; however, the therapist may have to be active to get the process started. Therapists should never push for something the clients don't believe. Once initial thoughts have been recorded, review each statement to see if it still has a positive resonance for the clients. Now the therapist offers fewer comments, focusing on the clients' reactions to each statement. If some are negative, mark them out and assure the clients that they will be dealt with when you are doing desensitization and reprocessing. If they are positive, the therapist can be encouraging. Thinking of truthful positive aspects to the situation is often somewhat new to clients, and they may feel foolish without honest encouragement.

For each statement ask how it feels now, and, if positive, leave the item on the worksheet. Review all the items and see if others emerge and if the clients can identify a kind of summary statement that can be recorded and highlighted. It may become a positive cognition for later processing (only if that occurs spontaneously), or it may be useful as a cognitive interweave.

On a third review of the items identified, if the client continues to feel positive, ask *What positive feeling or body sensations are you experiencing as you think about this?* Install with 4–6 slow DAS. If the client identifies additional positives (often they do), record and install them as long as they are experienced as positive. Alternatively, if the clients are unable to identify any positive perspectives on the current situation, attention may be directed to anything in their life that allows them to link to and strengthen the connection to a positive information package. If this occurs, usually more strengthening is needed before going to desensitization and reprocessing.

ACCESSING

Accessing is a strategy designed to help clients get in touch with resources and coping skills that will strengthen their internal system, help them manage their current life, and strengthen them to the point where they are ready to begin EMDR reprocessing. Often, once these resources are identified, developed, and installed in your office, it is extremely helpful for the clients to apply these skills in their lives.

In the Accessing phase, resources may be real or imagined. Ideally, try to help clients identify times in their lives when they have previously used the desired resource. If there are none, help them identify a real or imagined person or archetype that represents how they would like to be. Once identified, use the Extending Resource Protocols to develop, install, and strengthen the client's ability to access and utilize it in their daily life.

Client Population

Most clients are not so overwhelmed by their traumatic experiences that they need the basic Identifying Protocols. They may still perceive their lives, however, as being out of control and chaotic. They may also need immediate coping skills to manage their lives. Until they have been able to find some level of control or the ability to cope, they are not yet ready to do EMDR reprocessing.

Accessing Case Example

A client came into my office, having just discovered his spouse was having an affair. As a result, he had not been able to sleep, eat, or keep his mind off obsessing about his wife and the affair. He was unable to parent or work and needed help to survive the weekend, knowing that she would be with the other man. He saw things as being chaotic and out of control. I used the Accessing strategy to explore when in his life he had handled chaos and being out of control. I asked him "when" rather than "if" since this implies he most likely has handled these things in the past. It may be necessary to help the client remember incidents, by probing, questioning, or reminding him of things he has already mentioned. In this case, he was able to remember leaving home at eighteen, living alone, working two jobs, and dating. Though it was chaotic, he was having the time of his life. I introduced the RDI Protocol to help develop, enhance, and install those experiences. In this case it was helpful to have him posture or move in a way that showed confidence and the ability to handle chaos. I strengthened his memories and the associated body posturing and movements with DAS. I then used the Extending Protocol to solidify his coping skills, especially in handling the upcoming weekend when his wife would not be home. During our next meeting the client indicated that this intervention had helped him realize that he could handle things. Over the weekend, he slept a little better, was able to eat, and managed through the weekend knowing his wife was with the other man. While this intervention did not solve everything, it did stop the out-of-control feelings he had and gave him hope that he could work through this issue.

Focusing

Focusing is a term I use for target-specific resources. When clients have the internal skills and strengths to address their target memory and still express fear or apprehension about "doing the work," it's necessary to help them access coping skills that would aid reprocessing traumatic memories. Target-specific resources are those resources that are directly related to the identified EMDR target. These resources often parallel or enhance clients' desired positive cognitions. The Extending Protocols may be helpful in solidifying their coping skills and in preparing them for EMDR target reprocessing. If they can find no current skills, then identify a person or image that would represent how they would like to be. Repeated use of the Extended Protocol may be necessary to help clients integrate those resources into their own systems and is essential before we are ready for EMDR target reprocessing.

Focusing Case Example

A client of mine wanted to focus on a specific issue for EMDR target reprocessing. As we began the Assessment Phase, she stopped me, indicating that she was getting in touch with some intense rage and that she did not know if she could handle it. She feared she might lose control during or after the session. She was afraid she might hurt herself, others, or me. Certainly cause for concern! Using the focusing strategy,

I asked her whether she had ever managed intense rage. She replied, "Well yes, I handled a terrible divorce and often felt enraged." As she remembered more and more of the ways she handled her rage, her affect and body posture became more positive. As a result, we installed her positive memories with a couple of short sets of DAS. Focusing on her skills and coping abilities helped her gain a greater perspective of the situation. In this case, discussing how she had handled rage in the past helped her realize that the issue we were planning to address did not come close to what she had handled in the past. As a result, she said, "Let's work on that issue now. Compared to what I have lived through, this issue will be easy." We were then able to set up the target and process it without significant difficulty.

Reminding

As with the Safe Place, once we have developed the resources and before we begin the Assessment Phase, we want to remind the clients of their skills.

RK: *Now I would like you to imagine that these skills/strengths are sitting with you on the train or on the sofa as you prepare to watch the traumatic material on your TV. Remember, you can ask for their help anytime the material becomes too stressful.*

Added Benefit! You also now have a ready-made, client-constructed, adult perspective to use as a cognitive interweave to assist in the client's processing of looping or stuck material when the standard mechanical strategies (changing DAS, stimuli, processing modality, etc.) fail.

DEVELOPING AND USING A CONFERENCE ROOM OF RESOURCES FOR CLIENT STABILIZATION

Some clients' negative belief systems are taking up all their energy and attention. In situations such as this, EMDR target reprocessing is premature. The clients first need to regain some level of control over their lives before they will be able to have the time and energy to work on their traumatic issues. One effective preparation strategy is to help them develop a "conference room" of resources and then to extend those resources into their daily lives (Kiessling, 2000).

Discussion

This strategy, while a complex process, often is helpful when the clients' negative belief systems are strongly impacting their daily lives. First, help the clients identify "target specific" resources that would help change how they cope with present triggers that are activating the original traumatic memories (target nodes). Once the target-specific resources are developed, begin to link them with the negative belief system so the clients begin to learn alternative coping skills (state change) when being triggered. To accomplish this, first we invite the negative belief into the room as a child ego state. We acknowledge its efforts and ask whether it is willing to let the team of adult parts assume responsibility for handling current issues. This way, we are introducing an adult perspective and helping the clients, when triggered, to look at the present trigger from that adult perspective. The extending protocols incorporated into the rescripting and future scripting process help solidify that adult part's role in handling the present trigger.

Example

A client's presenting problem is his anxiety when giving presentations. He is driven by perfectionism and an inappropriate level of responsibility for his students.

1. Conference Room Setup

Therapist: *I'd like you to imagine you are the head of a business, and you are sitting in an empty conference room. You are sitting at the head of the table, and you can invite into the room, one at a time, members you want to join your team.*

2. Developing Resources and Their Images

Therapist: *As you think about being relaxed, comfortable, and confident when giving presentations, I'd like you to invite into the room, one at a time, the skills and strengths you think will help you. What skill would walk in first?*

Client: I see courage walking in.

Therapist: *What form or image represents courage?*

Client: I see a lion.

Therapist: *Okay, what other skill would you want to join you and the lion. What form does it have?*

Client: Acceptance, the willingness to make mistakes and learn from them. That looks like a clown. Clowns don't mind making mistakes and can laugh at themselves when others are laughing at them. And sometimes they use humor to teach. They don't always just fool around.

Therapist: *Anything else you want on your team?*

Client: Yes, I need to have a better balance of responsibility, knowing what I am responsible for and what my participants are responsible for.

Therapist: *What represents being able to set boundaries and know what you are responsible for and what others are responsible for?*

Client: I see a professor. He has a strong boundary. While he is committed to others, he knows his job is to teach to the best of his ability and provide an environment for learning. How much his class learns is also their responsibility.

Therapist: *Anything else you would like to invite in?*

Client: No, that team feels complete.

3. Enhancements and Installation

Therapist: *Now I'd like you to focus on your team and the skills they have. What feelings and emotions are you beginning to experience as you look at your team?*

Client: It feels really good. I'm calm, confident in their ability, and a little excited to see them work.

Therapist: *Where do you feel that calmness and excitement in your body? What posture would you have sitting in your director's chair right now as you look at your team?*

Client: I feel confident. I'd be sitting upright, leaning forward a little. (Client assumes that posture in his chair.)

4. Installation

Therapist: *I'd like you to look at your team, notice your confident body posture, and follow my fingers.* (DAS: six passes.) *What do you notice now?*

Client: It feels really good.

5. Gaining Team Consensus

Therapist: *Now I'd like you to ask each member of your team if they are willing to work together and with you to accomplish your goals.*

Client: Yes, everyone seems eager to be part of the team and want to work with me.

6. Rescripting Recent Disturbance

Therapist: *Now I'd like you to recall the last time you were making a presentation that was difficult for you. This time, however, I want you to rescript it and notice how it would have gone differently if your team had helped you.* (DAS: 10 passes.) *What do you notice now?*

Client: Well, I see myself going into class with confidence. My lion walked in ahead of me. My professor assured me we were prepared. I handled questions pretty well; in fact, I messed up on one answer, and my clown stepped forward and laughed, and then turned that into his advantage and used humor as a teaching tool to help the class learn. They laughed, too. I think it ended up giving them permission to ask more questions. Seems as though they had been a little shy about asking foolish questions.

Therapist: *Go with that, and especially notice how you feel that in your body.* (DAS 14 passes.) *What do you notice now?*

Client: I feel much calmer, more relaxed.

7. Inviting in the Negative Belief

Therapist: *Now I'd like you to invite the part that feels he has to be perfect into the room. Since we often develop these feelings about ourselves in childhood, it wouldn't surprise me if a child walked into the room. And I'd like you to realize that at the time, he felt being perfect was a way to make things work, so be supportive since he was doing the best he could under whatever circumstances existed at the time he learned it was his responsibility to be perfect.*

Client: I see him coming into the room. He's about eight years old. He seems a little intimidated, although he seems to like the clown.

Therapist: *I'd like you to thank him for coming in and for doing all the hard work he's done to be responsible and perfect. And, I'd like you to ask him if he would be willing to let your team take over handling things now, so he doesn't have to be as responsible.*

Client: Well, he's a little reluctant, but he may consider it.

8. Reviewing Previous Rescripting Event

Therapist: *Okay, what I'd like you to do is review that classroom experience we just did with your team, except this time, let your childlike part observe how the team handled things and see whether he feels comfortable letting them take over things.* (DAS: 14 passes.) *What was the child's reaction?*

Client: He seems more relaxed, a little relieved in fact.

Therapist: *Okay, assure him that he can step in anytime if he really feels the need, although your team of adults is more than willing to assume responsibility for taking care of things. He may want to consider just being an eight-year-old now that he knows adults are willing to take care of the adult problems you have.* (DAS: six passes.)

Client: Okay, he'll think about it.

9. Scripting a Future Anticipated Disturbance

Therapist: *Now I'd like you to think about the next presentation you are going to give. I'd like you to imagine your team helping you handle things. Your child may or may not decide to go to the class with you. Often eight-year-old boys aren't particularly interested in teaching classes or going to things adults have to do. He may want to stay outside and play. It will be up to him. Now imagine yourself teaching your class with the help of your team.* (DAS: 16 passes.) *What do you notice?*

Client: Actually things went okay, and in fact, the boy came with us and sat in class for a little while, then got bored and went into the hall to play. The class went well. I did an okay job, not perfect, but I was okay with that.

Therapist: *And how does it feel to not be so responsible or having to be perfect?*

Client: It feels pretty good.

Therapist: *Notice how you are feeling that in your body.* (DAS: eight passes.)

10. Closure

Therapist: *I'd like you to take this note card with you and look at it every day to remind yourself of your team. Try to look at it whenever you anticipate your feelings of having to be perfect or responsible may come up.* (Note card has LION/COURAGE, CLOWN/LEARNS FROM MISTAKES, AND PROFESSOR/BOUNDARIES written on it.) *And next week we will review how things went: when you remembered and things went well; when you remembered and things didn't go as well as you had hoped; and times when you may have forgotten about your team altogether. I look at this a little like preseason or a shakedown cruise. You and your team will need to practice some, so I don't expect you to utilize it effectively every time. And we may discover that you need more team members. If so, we'll invite them to join you.*

Client: Okay, I'll do the best I can.

Therapist: *That's fine, and I don't expect you to be perfect!*

11. Reevaluation

Discussion: Spend the next session reviewing how the week went. Target each successful event and enhance with DAS. Review any events that didn't go as well as hoped to see whether additional skills need to be added to the team, whether he forgot to use the team, or if there was a saboteur on the team (another blocking belief). On some occasions, team members have to be kicked off the team and other skills added.

Once the client in the example gained confidence and control of his current situation, we explored where he learned his "I am responsible and have to be perfect" script. While accessing and utilizing his team of resources may have changed his behaviors when giving presentations, these are state changes. Remember that our goal with EMDR is

to achieve "trait" change. Therefore, once we have developed a comprehensive targeting sequence through our history taking, we follow
the 3-Pronged Targeting Approach (past targets, present triggers, and
future templates) and the Standard EMDR Protocols and Procedures to
achieve reprocessing and trait change.

USING RESOURCES AS COGNITIVE
INTERWEAVES DURING REPROCESSING

Until now we have been discussing interventions that "front load" the
client and are being implemented in the Preparation Phase (Phase 3) of
the Standard 8-Phase EMDR Protocol. When properly utilized, resources may also be effective as cognitive interweaves.

Before going into detail about using resources as cognitive interweaves, it is important that we understand some key concepts regarding EMDR. Recall that one of the key goals of EMDR is that it strives
for trait change, not state change (Shapiro, 2003). During the Preparation Phase, resources normally are effective in providing state
change. They help our clients cope with and manage a stressful state.
We have them access their Safe Place to feel calmer. We are, in effect,
helping them change their current anxious state. However, the goal of
EMDR is to change the client's trait, which means that our goal is to
eliminate their tendency (trait) to become anxious, not just to manage it.

The second key concept concerns our use of the cognitive interweaves.
Recall that our goal is to allow the Adaptive Information Processing System to work in a natural, uninhibited way. That's why, when a client begins looping, we intervene as unintrusively as possible. We first change
the external: change the direction of eye movements or switch to tapping
or auditory DAS. If those don't work, then we change the processing
modality, changing the image to a sensation, the sensation to an image or
thought. Only after those interventions fail do we cautiously consider
putting something into the system, a cognitive interweave.

The Cognitive Interweave

For our purposes, recall that cognitive interweaves (Shapiro, 2001) are
designed to link up the frozen or dysfunctional neural network with
the more adaptive network. Interweaves include

1. providing new information
2. stimulating held information
3. the adult perspective
4. "I'm confused"
5. "What if it were your child"
6. metaphors/analogies
7. "Let's pretend"
8. the Socratic method

Resources may be structured within any of these approaches to form effective cognitive interweaves.

One of the values of developing "focused resources" is that they are specific skills, strengths, or resources that will help clients address their target issues. Therefore, by their very nature, they are often valuable as cognitive interweaves. If clients become stuck, what better interweave than to help them link up a developed resource with the frozen memory network.

Be careful that you do not misuse the resource. Improperly applied, accessing a resource may take the client out of processing. When clients give us the "stop" sign and ask to go to their Safe Places, we are temporarily taking the clients out of processing (state change, *not* trait change). Once they are stabilized, we help them get back into processing. This is the proper use of a resource to change clients' states. When properly used as cognitive interweaves, however, resources may help the clients move processing toward total desensitization and installation, that is, trait change.

Case Examples

Here are some case examples. The first example shows the use of a resource as a cognitive interweave. The second shows how not to use a resource.

Proper Use of a Resource as a
Cognitive Interweave

If you recall the example I used earlier in the chapter of a focused resource, it involved a client who was fearful of her rage. She stopped the Assessment Phase because she anticipated experiencing intense rage. We accessed, developed, and installed her previous experiences in successfully handling rage. Then we resumed desensitization of her select target. Let's suppose that as we were in the process of desensitizing that target, she began to loop. She became fearful of the rage that came up and repeatedly stated, "I can't handle it, I can't handle it." Useful Cognitive Interweave strategies are: (a) Adult perspective: *What would that part of you who had handled intense rage during your divorce say to you now?* or (b) I'm confused: *We talked about how you have handled much more intense rage before. I'm confused as to why this situation seems so overwhelming.* Or, (c) Calling on past resources: *Let's suppose you had the skills available that you used when dealing with your divorce. How would you handle this situation?* Each of these interventions would help connect up existing memory network systems with the frozen system and allow processing to continue.

Improper Use of a Resource

Suppose a client had caused an auto accident. During your intake interview, he discloses that he had been a pilot in the Marine Corps and that that time in his life was very positive. You install the attributes of his being a Marine Corps pilot. You target the accident, and the process becomes stuck with his repeatedly saying; "It's my fault, it's my fault." So you try this as your cognitive interweave: *Let's get in touch with your Marine pilot. Imagine flying around in the sky, feeling fully in control.* And then you enhance his flying his aircraft. What have you done? You have taken him out of processing. Although he may report being in a more relaxed state, that intervention has not assisted him in changing his trait or unblocking his loop of "It's my fault."

An effective cognitive interweave might have been either the "I'm confused": *I'm a little confused. You had mentioned you were a Marine pilot. Certainly you would have made some mistakes and, because of the situation, had to learn from those mistakes and continue on your mission?"* or the Adult Perspective: *What would your Marine pilot have said to someone who had made a mistake?* These strategies would have helped link up the adaptive adult perspectives with the stuck materials and allowed processing to continue.

These illustrations point out how resources you have developed during the Preparation Phase of treatment may be valuable in assisting clients to process traumatic material. So, as you develop clients' resources, write them down and store them in the back of your mind for future reference. If clients become stuck, these resources may be very effective in helping clients to resume processing. Since they are interventions that you and the clients have already developed, they are already part of the clients' systems and readily accepted.

Therapists' versus Clients' Issues

Developing and integrating resources can be very helpful, and at times essential in helping clients prepare for EMDR target reprocessing. Many clients do not need much, if any, resource work before being prepared for EMDR targeting. If you find yourself using a lot of resource work and, therefore, delaying EMDR targeting work, is it because your clients need that much preparation, or are you doing all this "front loading" as a means of managing your own anxiety? Remember that clients are tremendously resilient. The processing work they are willing to do validates their internal strengths and resilience. If you are reluctant to start EMDR processing even though they are eager and willing to "go into the valley" of processing and can contain their affect, perhaps you need to work on your own issues, of having to be perfect, competent, and in control! You may need to develop a few of your own resources or see an EMDR clinician yourself.

SUMMARY

There are many ways to integrate resource installation strategies into your EMDR practice. Focusing on resources can help stabilize clients in their present lives and prepare them for EMDR processing. Regardless of the intervention(s) we choose to utilize, they are providing state change and helping strengthen the clients' internal coping systems. We have looked at how these resources may be utilized in stabilizing our clients, strengthening their ability to manage life and preparing them for the EMDR work that will help them change the traits that are causing current difficulties and will cause future problems. Unnecessary use of resources can interfere with clients doing the EMDR target reprocessing work. Having clients *identify* themselves with concrete, positive external resources can slow down their sense of being overwhelmed. *Accessing* resources is helpful in drawing the clients' attention to the internal resources they already may have or in helping them identify and practice new resources that will help them manage their lives. By *focusing* on target-specific resources, we are preparing clients for target reprocessing and helping them address some of the present triggers that are causing anxiety. At the same time, we are developing potential cognitive interweaves. Whenever we get ready to start the Assessment Phase of EMDR reprocessing, it is beneficial to *remind* clients of their resources, Safe Place, container skills, or internal strengths that may be beneficial during desensitization and, especially, during abreactions or stuck processing.

The basic RDI protocol follows Francine Shapiro's Safe Place Protocol. The Extending Resources Protocol takes the basic resource development and installation process and integrates it into the clients' present life situation. We may choose to expand and combine those protocols to create a Conference Rooms of Resources to help clients manage *their* daily stress or a particular problem.

While most of the focus of this chapter has been in "front loading" the client during the Preparation Phase (Phase 3 of the Standard 8 Phases), we have also looked at how to appropriately use resources as cognitive interweaves. Resources as cognitive interweaves often provide the necessary adult perspective to break through looping experiences.

I hope the resource development and installation protocols in this chapter will help you get your clients ready and able to work through their traumatic experiences, accomplishing the goal of EMDR: "To achieve the most profound and comprehensive treatment effects possible in the shortest period of time, while maintaining client stability within a balanced system" (Shapiro, 2001).

REFERENCES

Kiessling, R. (2000, September). *Using a conference room of resources to process past, present, and future issues*. EMDRIA International Conference audio production, Toronto.

Kiessling, R. (2001, December). Resource focused progression. *The EMDRIA Newsletter, 6* (4, pp. 35–36).

Korn, D. L., & Leeds, A. M. (2002). Preliminary evidence of efficacy for EMDR resource development and installation in the stabilization phase of treatment of complex posttraumatic stress disorder. *Journal of Clinical Psychology, 58*(12), 1465–1487.

Leeds, A. (1997, June). *Shame, dissociation, and transference—PTSD and attachment disorders* [audio tape]. EMDRIA International Conference. Denver, CO: Audio Productions.

Shapiro, F. (1995). *Eye movement desensitization and reprocessing: Basic principles, protocols and procedures.* New York: Guilford Press.

Shapiro, F. (2001). *Eye movement desensitization and reprocessing: Basic principles, protocols and procedures* (2nd ed.). New York: Guilford Press.

Shapiro, F. (2003, September). *Plenary lecture.* Paper presented at the EMDRIA Conference, Denver, CO.

Wildwind, L. (1998, June). *Using EMDR to create and install essential experiences.* Paper presented at EMDRIA International Conference audio production. Baltimore, MD.

Chapter 3

EMDR for Clients with Dissociative Identity Disorder, DDNOS, and Ego States

Joanne H. Twombly

Using EMDR with clients with dissociative identity disorder (DID) and other dissociative disorders (DDs) requires careful adaptation (Shapiro, 2001) to allow the unique benefits of EMDR to be used productively, without risking unleashing a flood of traumatic material and destabilizing the client. In this chapter I will discuss adaptations for each stage of treatment for dissociative clients. While I'll focus on work with DID (formerly multiple personality disorder) and dissociative disorder not otherwise specified (DDNOS), the EMDR adaptations and protocols taught in this chapter can be used with people with other DDs and complex posttraumatic stress disorder (PTSD), and in ego-state work.

Many clinicians come to working with people with DID after beginning to use EMDR and suddenly uncovering DID in one of their clients. Others have already been working with DID and then learn EMDR. Therapists who want to use EMDR to facilitate the treatment of DID should have thorough training in both. This recommendation is echoed in the EMDR Dissociative Disorders Task Force recommended guidelines (Shapiro, 2001). This ideal combination of expertise is often not possible or practical. Newly diagnosed clients with DID, for example, may wish to continue in treatment with their therapist if there has been a long-standing established treatment relationship. Other clients may lack the resources to pay for the services of a specialist, or there may not be a specialist within driving range.

Although many of the techniques and EMDR adaptations described in this chapter can be used by any therapist, it is strongly recommended that therapists who do not have training augment this chapter with trainings, other readings, and consultation. My own clients, many of whom have come to me after years of treatment with other therapists, ask me to tell therapists that it is the clients who pay for the wrong kind of treatment, with years of additional pain, diminished quality of life, and high financial cost. Therapists without training should, at the very minimum, read a summary article on working with DDs (e.g., Kluft, 2003) before applying any of the material in this chapter.

ABOUT DID

The most recent research indicates that dissociative symptoms develop in people who as infants experienced neglect, had primary caretakers who were emotionally unavailable during the first 2 years of the children's lives, and who exhibited disorganized attachment (Lyons-Ruth, 2003). Research also shows that infants who exhibit disorganized attachment develop it in relation to mothering that is either "frightened or frightening" (Liotti, 1999). Abuse frequently occurs in the kinds of families that neglect or abandon their infants. Maltreatment or abuse then causes further dissociation. It is important to realize that a foundation of neglect underlies the reported traumatic material. This foundation must be treated along with the attachment disorder.

Chu described the internal world and external presentation of clients with an overt DID presentation as follows: "switching of personalities, the dissociative and amnestic barriers, and the complexity of internal psychic structures and identity . . . periodic intrusions of re-experiencing phenomena, including flashbacks, nightmares, overwhelming affect, and even somatic sensations lend a sense of chronic instability . . . comorbid characterologic difficulties including patients' intense interpersonal disturbances, affective instability, and impulsive and self-destructive behavior add to the sense of ongoing crisis and chaos" (1998, p. 147).

On the other hand, many presentations of DID may not be as dramatic or overt. One man following referral to an EMDR clinician was described by his former therapist as a very nice, very competent professional who "just needed a little EMDR" to take care of a couple of stuck areas that his "very helpful" twenty-five-year therapy couldn't resolve. He was later diagnosed with DID. It is important to become familiar with different presentations and symptoms that would indicate the possible presence of a DD.

Remember that DID and DDNOS clients live with what Kluft terms a "multiple reality disorder." They live in "several parallel but incompletely overlapping constructions of the world and of life experience" (1993b, p.147). In practice, therapists must remember:

- The part of the DID person who shows up for treatment, and seems like a whole person, is not.
- Parts not addressed directly frequently are not listening, and they probably won't be learning whatever you're teaching.
- Many parts may be stuck in the past, that is, believing they are still children, living where they grew up, with their parents, and during years long past.

The following points, though directed at therapists by Courtois (1999), are also important for clients to understand:

- The therapist strives to practice from a neutral perspective regarding memory.
- The therapist understands the malleability of human memory and the differences between historical and narrative truth.
- The therapist's goal in attending to traumatic memories is to facilitate mastery and resolution.

This chapter is divided into three sections, summarizing the treatment of DDs within the three stages of standard phase-oriented trauma treatment. These three phases have been variously titled beginning with Janet (1898). However there is consensus as to their content (Brown, Scheflin, & Hammond, 1998). EMDR adaptations and uses will be detailed within each stage.

For clarity and consistency, the following terms will be used: *part* or *part of the mind* will be used, rather than the more common terms *alter* and *personality* as a gentle reminder to clients that any perceived separateness is more illusion than reality. The parts of the clients who have primary responsibility for their daily life and usually are the ones who bring everyone to treatment are referred to as the *host*. The word *system* is used to describe all the parts of one person. For patients with complex systems, a *daily life team* is identified or developed. This daily life team is made up of parts that already function in that capacity, and at times other parts who add in something useful. A final note: Janet's (1898) descriptions of the three phases of the treatment of trauma will be used as headings to each section.

PHASE 1: SYMPTOM REDUCTION
AND STABILIZATION

The initial task of this first phase of treatment is to establish the frame. This provides a foundation for the therapeutic relationship and allows the treatment to unfold. As Kluft noted, DID "is a condition created by broken boundaries. . . . Therefore, a successful treatment will have a secure treatment frame and consistent boundaries" (1993a, p. 26).

DID- and DDNOS-specific tasks in this phase include identifying and connecting with the more accessible parts of the mind (either separately or through the host) and developing internal communication and cooperation (Kluft, 1999) among parts. These tasks can be enhanced by EMDR adaptations.

During this phase of treatment, clients are encouraged to continue dissociating any and all traumatic material related to the past. Although some clients will initially be disappointed, they need to appreciate that processing trauma requires the development of new skills that would have been acquired during a healthier childhood. These skills include affect tolerance, self-soothing, and the ability to identify needs and feelings. This treatment phase begins to repair and develop what was neglected and interfered with during childhood.

Although formal trance work is often unnecessary, hypnotic techniques are invaluable in working with DDs and are often easily taught through imagery facilitated by hypnotic language. As Kluft stated, "With such highly hypnotizable patients, who spontaneously demonstrate dissociative and hypnotic phenomena and use defenses that incorporate these phenomena, it is impossible to treat DID without the treatment's being suffused with hypnosis" (1994, p. 207). Clients often find it reassuring that dissociative defenses, such as losing time, amnesia, and parts switching, that is, symptoms that often necessitated treatment, can be developed into coping skills proactively used to facilitate the treatment process.

SAFE SPACE IMAGERY

Safe Space Imagery (SSI) is a relatively easy hypnotically informed exercise (Twombly, 2001) taught to facilitate stabilization, and it tends to be one of the first coping skills taught. With regular practice, SSI lowers clients' biological reactivity level, provides self soothing and respite, and facilitates trauma processing. It is an excellent coping skill that, aside from beginning to give the client a sense of self-efficacy and control, helps to develop positive attachment between therapist and client by providing a positive experience early in the treatment process. I present it in depth because of its usefulness.

There are many scripts available for teaching SSI. Given the natural trance ability of dissociative clients, however, the use of hypnotic language will enhance its impact Brown, (1990) and Kluft, (1992) inform my explanations of SSI language and benefits. The benefits of SSI include:

- It is an exercise that will help clients learn to reach a state of relaxation and block out intrusive thoughts and feelings.
- The process of learning SSI will help clients begin to learn to use their dissociative symptoms (like amnesia or numbness) proactively. To raise their expectation of positive results, evidence that suggests their future success is helpful. For instance, to a client who had amnesia for much of her life prior to the age of 11, I might say: *You've already been able to unconsciously block out lots of things that happened before you were 11. Now we're going to work on you learning to consciously block things out.* These kinds of comments begin to reframe some of the clients' troublesome symptoms as abilities they will learn to use to help with the healing process.
- SSI is a helpful coping skill to have during trauma processing, both to provide respite from excessive negative affect and to

help ground the client following the trauma-processing part of the session (Shapiro, 2001).

- In practice, use of SSI daily over time helps lower clients' biological reactivity level, resulting in clients feeling calmer over all.
- Mind-body savvy professionals state that everyone should be doing some kind of meditation, SSI, or progressive muscle relaxation every day. They say it makes us physically healthy by strengthening our immune systems. This normalizes the practice of SSI by giving clients a non-trauma-based reason to do this exercise. Even therapists should be doing it!
- Since intrusions often occur, predicting their possibility and normalizing intrusions as part of the learning process decreases distress over what might otherwise be perceived as failure. Useful wording that states this while not inadvertently giving the negative suggestion that intrusions will happen is: *This process works differently for different people. Some find a safe space that feels safe and comfortable right away while others may get intrusions and need to work on learning to block them out. Either way is just fine.*
- Although many scripts for SSI ask clients to close their eyes, in this one clients are given the free choice of closing their eyes, keeping them open, or experimenting during the process. This gives clients permission to do what's right for them and guards against the reflexive compliance some were forced into as children.
- Clients are told there will be talking throughout the exercise so the therapist can help with the learning process. Some clients will require that their Safe Space be secret. When this is necessary, the clients are reminded about the importance of the Safe Space being somewhere where no one has ever been hurt, and a place that is not from their childhood. They are asked to let the therapist know right away if something isn't working for any part or if there are questions. It's also important for the therapist to check in with the clients regularly during the process.

Once the explanations are out of the way, I begin the following process, which is specifically designed for DD clients. It's concrete, it channels them into positive imagery, and it offers choices. The availability of choices is especially helpful to those clients whose ability to generate imagery or to imagine possibilities has become impaired in the struggle to avoid intrusions.

A common error of therapists is to assume that if you work on SSI with a DD client (or even in some ego-state work) that all parts will automatically be included. This rarely, if ever, happens. Parts need to be referred to, or they won't think a communication applies to them. Often a client who has done well developing a Safe Space in session can't access it following the session. It turns out that an unidentified ego state or child part has interfered, believing that any relaxation would bring doom.

Creative use of SSI can assist with the treatment process. Examples include:

- Orienting to the present can be facilitated by adding concrete information about the present (e.g., a current calendar, picture of current home) and with the post-hypnotic suggestion comment: *As* (the part) *is in her/his Safe Space she/he will be learning more and more about how things are different* (in the present vs. the past).
- Attachment to the therapist and object permanence can be facilitated by noting appointment dates on the imaged calendar, by an imaged picture of the therapist, and simply because SSI itself is a transitional object of sorts as it's developed in session with the therapist and used between sessions.
- Growth and learning are facilitated by incorporating whatever is needed into the Safe Space. For instance, the Safe Space developed for a part who head-banged incorporated walls that perfectly cushioned the head, so each time the part head-banged he was reminded that "things are different now, he's no longer allowed to hurt himself, and no one is allowed to hurt him."
- The host can develop Safe Spaces for other parts who are too young or too distressed to be able to develop their own Safe Spaces. These Safe Spaces can be used to soothe parts who are having flashbacks, or to contain parts who might pop out at inappropriate times, such as at work.

SAFE SPACE IMAGERY PROCESS

As previously stated, DD clients are highly hypnotizable and unconsciously have developed dissociative defenses that make use of hypnotic phenomena. Because of this, the protocol for SSI incorporates hypnotic language to facilitate access to the benefits of trance, including increased imagery and increased problem solving (Brown & Fromm, 1986).

There are two approaches to beginning SSI work with clients. The first is to have all parts work simultaneously on developing Safe Spaces. This approach works well when the relationship with the therapist feels safe enough to permit all to engage in the task at same time. The second is to have one part volunteer to go first while the others watch. This approach works well when there are protective or suspicious parts that need to stay hypervigilant. Parts are told: *Watch carefully so you can help other parts learn how to do SSI too.* Their need to be hypervigilant is used in the service of healing. Internal communication and cooperation are supported. In addition this approach models one of the ways of using SSI to cope with daily life, such as having one or more triggered parts use their Safe Space while others handle the daily life situation (parenting, work, or driving).

Approach #1: *We're going to work on SSI together. I'd like all of you who are willing to work on this to follow along with me. While we're doing the exercise I'd like everyone to ask me any questions you have and if you need help, just let me know. Okay, now I'd like all of you to find a space or a place together or apart where you've felt safe before, or where you'd like to feel safe.* Continue on adapting the wording to fit the group. Wording that's important to take note of is "all of you" because this phrase includes every part that's known, while also covering the possibility that unknown parts are listening. I also ask for "willing" parts, which decreases the likelihood of arguments and is more respectful to "unwilling" parts. Parts who are unwilling, or aren't ready to do the exercise, don't have to.

Some clients easily come up with an image of a Safe Space, and when they don't, it often helps to provide a few suggestions. I often suggest that they imagine a condominium complex where each part can have his or her own space and there are common rooms where groups of parts can come together. This is an example of a Safe Space that allows for current and future communication and takes care of individual needs at the same time. Sometimes more separateness is needed; for instance, one client's parts made Safe Spaces on different planets. Although this person's parts could not tolerate any closeness, the exercise was done together with some internal cooperation and respected the parts' need for space. This facilitated the development of internal relationships.

Approach #2: *Is there anyone who's willing to try this Safe Space exercise out? Okay, great, I'm going to talk directly to Mary now and everyone else can listen and watch how it's done so later you can help each other learn how to do it.*

Standard wording for developing SSI follows. Pauses should be made to give the client a chance to come up with imagery, and the therapist should periodically ask the client to describe what's happening.

- *Pick a space or a place not from your childhood* . . . Many people had places they felt safe in as a child, but inevitably they had to go home where they were possibly abused. In practice, these safe spaces get contaminated quickly.
- . . . *where nothing bad has ever happened* . . . For some, the safest times were after being abused, and they could count on it not happening again for the rest of the night. These also get contaminated rapidly.
- . . . *where you've felt safe before or would like to be able to feel safe, or a place or space that's completely or partially made up* . . . The goal is a positive, calm, relaxed physical state, not factual accuracy. One client's Safe Space was "nowhere," as no one could hurt her if she was nowhere. At times the Safe Space may seem negative to the therapist although it may make sense to the client; one client's Safe Space was in a coffin because if the perpetrator thought she was dead, he wouldn't look for her. Since the goal is the felt body sensation of safety and relaxation, these Safe Spaces are fine, although it's often helpful for the therapist to make suggestions that add comfort. The coffin, for example, was made large, had a soft blanket in it, a pillow, snacks, and a fresh air supply.

It's best if the images and process come from the clients themselves. At times it needs to be a joint process, with me using whatever information I have about the clients, to make suggestions: a beach, a mountaintop, an island, another planet, surrounded by music or soft blankets. Suggestions often appear to help clients come up with their own imagery and ideas.

- *Imagine or put yourself in your Safe Space*... Use wording the client has come up with wherever possible, for example, *So, imagine now that you're at that beach in Maine, or put yourself in that space where you're surrounded by blackness feeling soft blankets around you*... *and look around with all your senses*... Use of as many senses as possible enhances the imagery and deepens the experience, which has a positive effect on the exercise's impact.

- *... and notice everything about it that makes it safe to be there*... Using positive suggestion is helpful and enhances the possibility that the client will come up with positive imagery. To deepen the imagery and the experience, it's helpful to underline what the client is experiencing. For instance, the client might have noticed she is alone on a beach; she can feel the sun and hear seagulls. The therapist can underline this by saying: *So, you're on a beach, you can feel the sun and hear seagulls*... It also lets the clients know you are there with them, in a shared experience, which facilitates the development of the treatment relationship (Brown & Fromm, 1986). The next step anticipates intrusions and begins the process of teaching the client to handle them.

- *Look around your Safe Space with all your senses and notice if there's anything you see (hear, smell, taste, touch) that doesn't feel quite right and if there is, just look around and as you look around you'll either see (hear, smell, taste, touch) something that will help, or some thoughts will occur to you that will help*... This wording provides further positive suggestion while making use of the trance dynamic of increased access to imagery and problem solving (Brown & Fromm, 1986). Often even in a very light trance, this will result in the client being able to look around and see (hear, smell, feel, or touch) something helpful, or a helpful thought will pop into the client's mind. Ask: *What are you noticing? Focus on it and notice what changes. What ideas come to mind? Focus on them and notice what changes*... Sometimes what's noticed doesn't make sense, and the hypnotic trait of trance logic may be in effect (Brown & Fromm, 1986).

Don't have clients focus on overtly traumatic images; one client visualized being on a beach, and as she looked around the ocean turned to blood. There are times when I will offer a client a choice and say: *Would you like to continue to work with this Safe Space or would you like to move on to a new one that's even safer?* There are also times when it appears that the Safe Space is too contaminated, where I say: *You'll find yourself moving away from this Safe Space, and as it's getting further and further away, you're getting closer and closer to a new even safer Safe place.*

When there has been an intrusion, most often the clients who look around with all their senses will notice something that helps. The therapist can say: *Focus on _____ and notice what happens . . .* Often the intrusion will go away or lessen. If some of the intrusion remains, the clients are reinforced for the progress with an ego-strengthening comment: *You're just learning this technique and already you have been able to get rid of some of that intrusion . . .* The clients are then instructed to keep looking around. Clients who have totally gotten rid of an intrusion can be given more comprehensive ego-strengthening statements.

Carefully watch and listen for clients who aren't able to get rid of intrusions. When this happens, I work with them by making suggestions to add or subtract something that makes it safer. This teaches the clients a problem-solving process to deal with intrusions as they work on SSI at home:

1. *First look around and you will see something . . .*
2. *Or a thought will occur to you . . .*
3. *Or you can try adding or subtracting something . . .*
4. *If that doesn't work then move to a new even safer Safe Space . . .*
5. *Sometimes it helps to draw a picture of it, and then draw in improvements . . .*
6. *If that doesn't work or if at any step along the way it gets too scary, stop, write down what happened, and we'll work on it next session. This will give us information about how your intrusions work.* The subtext of this is that even something that looks like a failure can be helpful.

Once clients have dealt with whatever intrusions there are and has reached a state of peaceful, calm relaxation, continue by saying:

You can just settle in to being there, breathing in all the feelings of (whatever the clients have identified) *and feeling those feelings settle deep inside every cell of your body* . . . Use words the clients have used to describe their experience. For example, if the client has described being surrounded by music and she feels peaceful and calm, the therapist would say: *Just settle there surrounded by music, feeling peaceful and calm* . . .

Research has shown that trauma has an impact on a cellular level (van der Kolk, 1994). This suggestion is made to suggest the possibility of cellular repair and is a message that the body is learning to relax on a deeper level than it ever could before.

Before ending the exercise, make a post-hypnotic ego strengthening comment, such as *You've just started learning this, and already you're learning to create an environment in which you can really relax. As time passes you will find more and more ways to use SSI in your daily life* . . . Or *As you continue to practice SSI, you will notice that every time you block out intrusions you get better and better at it* . . . These positive comments may have a greater impact due to the likelihood of the client being in a trance.

To end the exercise: *In a way that's right for you, you'll find you can bring yourself back from your Safe Space to this office* . . . This gives the clients control over being in the Safe Space or taking themselves out of it and is very important not to forget. The therapist then asks the clients for questions and feedback about the exercise. And finally, clients are instructed to practice SSI everyday, whether or not they feel stressed.

INSTALLATION OF COPING SKILLS

Install SSI and other coping skills using short sets of Dual Attention Stimuli (DAS). The client's task is to hold on to the positive feeling and knowledge of the skill during the installation. Use short sets because longer ones run the risk of activating traumatic material. I start with three to five pairs of alternating stimuli and will lengthen the next set if the client is successful or shorten it if the client isn't successful in holding the positive feelings. With practice, clients tend to make progress and get better at holding on to positives. This installation process appears to solidify knowledge, making it more readily accessible in the future (Shapiro, 2001). Use DAS to facilitate communication of coping skills to other ego states or parts (providing parts are willing to receive the information). Installing and communicating coping skills offer an easy, nonthreatening introduction to EMDR.

Standard Resource Development and Installation (RDI) is also helpful. "RDI refers to a set of EMDR related protocols which focus exclusively on strengthening connections to resources in functional (positive) memory networks while deliberately not stimulating dysfunctional (traumatic) memory networks" (Korn & Leeds, 2002, p. 1469). Again, developed resources can be communicated with DAS to any parts willing to receive the information.

The three EMDR adaptations (Twombly, 2000) that will be presented here in detail are Installation of Current Time and Life Orientation, Height Orientation, and Installation of the Therapist and the Therapist's Office. They each make use of DAS-facilitated communication and were developed through my work with DD clients. These techniques work to facilitate internal communication and cooperation, decrease anxiety, increase grounding in the present, and decrease negative transferences. They are presented along with a protocol for clients with no oriented parts (Fisher, 2000).

It is important to attend to the timing and use of these techniques. Although these techniques do not interfere with the dissociation of traumatic material, they do increase a system's overall knowledge and awareness of the present. For some, this can cause distress. As Loewenstein pointed out, "The selectively focused attention of the MPD patient often helps to maintain dissociation so intensely that any movement toward greater awareness may be experienced as dysphoric" (1993, p. 63). When such a dynamic is present, the use of these techniques must be postponed.

TECHNIQUE #1: INSTALLATION AND TRANSMISSION OF CURRENT TIME AND LIFE ORIENTATION

It is difficult to appreciate the tenacity of multiple reality disorder, even in clients who have been in extended treatment. My appreciation of this was heightened by a largely integrated child part in a complex system that had had much successful trauma work. Although this part knew the correct year and that the office and her apartment were in Massachusetts, she believed that once she left the office, she walked into both her past and her original home state. This belief caused her to feel considerably at risk of dangers from the past and led her to block present efforts to process traumatic material. Following this experience, I began looking closely for similar discrepancies and have used this intervention with the goal of reducing anxiety and increasing clients' ability to differentiate the past from the present:

A. Beginning with the host or other oriented parts, discuss all or some of the following:

   1. How they know what year it is
   2. How many years it has been since they were last abused
   3. How they organize life so they are safe, for example
      a. Where they live
      b. How they know their husband (wife, roommate, etc.) does not abuse them
      c. Place of work, that they drive

   Identifying concrete differences between the past and the present helps the client differentiate past from present. In addition to a verbal list of the differences, have the host visualize the information in pictures and videos. Thus the host might visualize their current home with a visually detailed picture and a fast-forward visualized video of their history in the house from when they moved until the present. Visual information helps with communication to nonverbal parts and adds a time-span dimension increasing the credibility of the communication. At times, gathered information needs to be adjusted to the targeted parts. For instance, child parts may respond more fully to childlike observations. Symbolic of how their wishes and needs were heard and responded to now versus in the past, one client installed child parts having cocoa whenever they wanted.

B. After information between past and present is detailed and listed, the therapist installs it with DAS. This process may be done silently, or the host can verbalize the information. The advantages of doing the installation process verbally are that the therapist can add any missed information, make sure there are no intrusions, and immediately install additional spontaneous information.

C. Request that the part or parts to whom the information is directed be open to receiving it, without the expectation that they believe it. For example, say: *Could Susie and Bud be open to listening and watching the information Sarah is going to give you? You don't have to believe her, just take it in. Once you've received it, you can ask any questions you have. When you leave here, please check out the information for yourselves. Next week it will be interesting to hear what you agree or disagree with. Do you have any questions before we start?* Arguments about veracity are minimized by not expecting belief.

An alternative, with the advantage of extending the potential impact of the exercise, is to make the statement more inclusive: *Could Susie and Bud and anyone else who needs this information . . .*

At times, it is not clear what part of the dissociated system will be receiving the information. In this case, the instruction is more general. For example, say: *Would parts please be open to listening, watching, and taking in this information? You don't need to believe it. You can check it out later.*

D. Ask the host and/or other oriented parts to broadcast the information to the parts that are to receive it. DAS is used in this step during the broadcasting because it appears to facilitate communication among parts. Use DAS continuously or to broadcast each item separately.

E. Ask the host and/or other oriented parts how the process went and ask parts who received the information if they have any questions. It is common for parts to verbalize disbelief or to feel "tricked." Alternately, they might feel some cautious relief.

F. Homework consists of parts checking out the information with the host and/or other oriented parts supporting that process by pointing out concrete detailed evidence, for example, *Here is our white house with the green shutters (not the brick one we grew up in).*

G. Follow up in the next session.

Example: A female client entered treatment for a long-term anxiety disorder that had not been helped by her long-term treatment. Once diagnosed with DID, it was clear that most parts thought they were still living in the 1970s, in the home where they grew up, being abused and terrorized. As parts became oriented to the present, although initially suspicious, their anxiety decreased significantly.

Example: A 41-year-old male in the process of taking his first college class in 20 years noted that he was having trouble completing a take-home exam. Asking inside yielded the information that a part was preventing him from doing the work to protect him from negative reactions his mother had when he was a child. The host identified concrete evidence of how his mother had changed, including her now showing interest in his class work and praising his good grades. This information and visualization of these interactions were installed and then communicated with DAS to the part. The host reported that the part argued but then agreed to let him complete the take-home exam once as a trial experience. The part, age 12, then came out, agreed to check out the mother's reactions for himself, and began yawning and feeling waves of fatigue. He explained that for the first time ever, he felt he could relax.

Example: A woman with a childhood history of many traumatic surgeries began to install and communicate details regarding the location and interior of her current home. During this DAS-facilitated communication process, she experienced intrusive imagery suggesting some child parts believed they still lived in the hospital. After reminding parts that there was no expectation of belief and requesting that they simply take in the information, she was able to communicate and install the current-day visualization. In between sessions she called to report that she had awakened the next morning smelling ether, and reinstalled "the present" by asking parts inside to watch during a tour of the apartment, using walking as the DAS (Grand, 1998). By the next session, she reported noticing she could now see her apartment more completely, realized she had always viewed her home in sections as if she had been wearing blinders, and noted her general anxiety level had decreased.

Example: An adult client, abused on a beach during childhood, became suddenly anxious and nauseous during a walk on a beach. As no one responded when she asked inside herself about the cause, she made an educated guess that there was at least one part of her who was confusing the past with the present. After stating that any concerned parts did not have to believe her and requesting that they just listen and watch, she installed and then broadcast the following

statements and pictures: how this beach looked different from the one
in the past, that her abusive uncle had been dead for 25 years, a picture
of their last sight of him alive when he was very old, and a view of his
grave site. She immediately felt relief and was able to continue her
walk.

As in the above example, clients are encouraged to try using this
technique on their own when they are triggered by reminders of their
past. Clients have used bilateral tapping, walking, and bilateral movement, standing and shifting their weight from one foot to the other
(Withers, 1999) as the DAS to facilitate communication when using this
process out of session. Obviously, this technique requires at least one
part that is grounded in present reality. Persons for whom this technique has not worked have been poorly grounded overall and lacked
parts who could reasonably identify facts about the present.

PROTOCOL FOR CLIENTS WITH NO
ORIENTED PARTS

This protocol is very useful for clients who seem to have no oriented
parts or whose rapid switching makes continuity difficult (Fisher, 2000).
Fisher recommends standing up with the client using bilateral movement (stepping from side to side) as the DAS. The bilateral movement
is mirrored by the therapist who speaks continuously, orienting the
client with some repetitive combination of *I want all of you to be present
in my office, and all of you to look around and notice what it's like. You can
tell you're in my office because there's the* (mention some concrete details),
*and we're both here together, and in this moment in time nothing bad is hap-
pening. I want all of you to feel the feeling of your feet on the ground, your ankles, your legs, the feel of your clothes, and want all of you to look around and
see you're right here in my office, it's* (state the year), *and in this moment in
time everything's okay, just look around and everyone just keep looking
around and get to know what it's like to be here in my office, see that nothing
bad is happening right now. Notice if you feel any tension, you can put your
attention on it and let it come up and go by, just notice it* (increasing mindfulness) . . .

I recommend doing this exercise for 5–10 minutes every session
(usually depending on what the client can tolerate) until enough parts
are oriented to begin to learn other coping strategies.

This protocol helps disoriented clients' systems begin to become oriented and grounded and to develop a systemwide awareness of the present. After a few sessions, one client who had very little connection with her system and had argued that no place was safe, began to feel more settled in my office, noticed more of herself was present, and began to have communication with more of her system.

TECHNIQUE #2: HEIGHT ORIENTATION

Orientation, usually thought of in terms of time (past vs. present), can be applied to personal physical size. Child parts often experience themselves as child-sized. Orientation to height lessens anxiety and gives child parts concrete proof of another way the present is very different from the past.

A child part is asked to volunteer to try an experiment or to be co-conscious with an adult part and with that support try to see if they can reach something, for instance, on the top shelf of the book-case. Child parts tend to be extremely surprised when they can easily reach much higher than expected. This effect appears to be heightened by DAS and the adult height awareness is then installed. Responses to height orientation can be idiosyncratic. One part wondered if the book-shelf had been shrunk by magic. Note that the part's perceived age does not appear to change with their change in perceived body height.

Obviously, this technique is not appropriate for parts who believe that growing up or being large is in some way dangerous; therefore the timing of its use has to be evaluated. In addition, some child parts appear to be unable to reach higher than the dictates of their perceived height.

Example: A child part, despite appearing fully oriented to the present, believed that she was trapped in the office and that she was too small to unlock the door. With some encouragement, she managed to tolerate her terror enough to be able to test out how high she could reach. She was astonished to find out she could reach all the way to the top of the door and open it easily. The awareness of her ability was installed, and she was asked to check out all the doors in her home and learn, assisted by older parts, how to lock and unlock them. This was particularly important for this client who as a child had been too short to unlock a door to escape the room in which she was being abused.

Example: In preparation for trauma work, it was decided to try to orient a group of anxious young ego parts to their current height. With much trepidation, a child part volunteered to try first and was surprised to see he could easily reach higher than the top of a door. He then exclaimed that the therapist looked short to him for the very first time. This knowledge of height was installed and communicated systemwide. The host/daily life team and several parts reported that their overall anxiety was reduced significantly.

Note: I found it necessary to ask the host or daily life team to renew some limits with these parts, since some felt being tall meant they could drive and emerge at work.

TECHNIQUE #3: INSTALLING THERAPIST AND THERAPIST'S OFFICE, MAINTAINING DUALITY

This technique is useful for increasing cooperation between the therapist and dissociative system. Although a comprehensive discussion of transference is beyond the scope of this chapter, it is clear that DID clients' transference reactions are complicated and that they vary among ego states. Lowenstein described that there are (often covert) "negative transference concerns about the therapist's trustworthiness, inherent dangerousness and potential abusiveness" (1993, p. 66). This technique can help to at least minimize some negative transferences by using DAS-facilitated communication to share information among parts and to invite protective parts to continue checking out the therapist.

In addition, this technique is a concrete way to enhance and maintain the client's dual awareness during the processing of traumatic material. Maintaining duality is part of standard EMDR practice, which keeps the client grounded in the present and connected to the therapist (Shapiro, 2001). Van der Hart and Steele stated (in reference to DD clients) that "a modulated and controlled process (re trauma processing) should take place, in which the patient is helped to remain oriented in the present, i.e. to be certain that the current experience is a representation of a prior event" (2000, p. 4). The section on targeting traumatic material will incorporate this technique into a structured format for processing traumatic material.

Specifically, when the client has had enough experience with the therapist and therapist's office, it is helpful to list, install, and communicate concrete knowledge and observations to any parts willing to accept the information. Parts are then asked to keep watching, keep gathering information, and keep testing the therapist's trustworthiness. This process seems to enable parts previously living in the past to begin to gather information about the present.

Helpful information to install includes:

A. Factual information about the appearance of the office, including orientation information such as a current year calendar or modern computer.

B. Safety-oriented information

   1. That the client sits on a chair across from where the therapist sits
   2. Circumstances of any physical contact between the therapist and client (e.g., a handshake)
   3. That abuse is not allowed in the office and has never happened
   4. Any information a particular client might need (e.g., that no one is hiding in the closet)

C. Significant interactions between the client and therapist

   1. When a client got angry and the therapist responded non-punitively
   2. When the therapist went on vacation and returned
   3. When disagreements were worked out
   4. Occasions when the therapist was empathic.

D. A fast-forward video spanning the treatment from beginning to end helps to decrease some parts' needs to evaluate the therapist as if each session were the first one.

Example: The information to be installed and communicated can be quite tentative. A client of 3 years could identify only that the therapist had never yelled at, laughed at, hurt, or used anything she had said against her. This was installed and communicated. Parts who received the information then argued that the therapist was still dangerous because some of the people who had hurt them had "acted nice" at first. The host and therapist managed to identify one important difference. The people who had hurt her had "acted nice" for only short amounts of time, while the therapist had been "acting nice" for 3 years. This difference was installed and communicated verbally and with a fast-forward video of the 3-year treatment process, along with encouragement to keep watching and checking the therapist out.

Example: A client with little internal communication suddenly said she had a "weird sense of not being sure" she was in the therapist's office or somewhere else. After installing and communicating a quick review of weekly sessions for the past two years, plus how this therapist differed from the previous therapist (the client is not expected to know all the answers, the current therapist's voice is more confident, and she is taller), this client felt grounded.

THE MIDDLE PHASE: TREATMENT OF TRAUMATIC MEMORY

This format (Twombly, 2000) was developed to provide a safe, controlled way to begin using EMDR to process traumatic material with DID clients. Its goal is to teach clients to have control during processing and to enhance the ability of parts to work together. Clients are told: *You did not have control of what went on in your childhood, but you need to have control of your healing.*

This format combines adaptations of EMDR with standard techniques used in the hypnotic processing of traumatic material. The hypnotic techniques create the safety and control necessary to be able to use EMDR with this fragile population and are similarly used in Fine and Berkowitz's Wreathing Protocol (2000). It was developed from Fine's earlier work with Lazrove (1996) on the use of EMDR with DID clients, with additional structure added to limit the number of parts involved in processing, and to enable the client to start and stop the process. This process is a useful way to initiate trauma work wherever there is concern for the client's stability and ability to maintain duality.

Because maintaining stability in daily life is crucial, the host or daily life team is protected from the impact of trauma work for as long as possible. "Thus, the affect initially gets contained, retained, and processed within clusters and among like-personalities. Consequently, by the time the affect seeps to other personalities outside the original cluster or to the host, it will be more diluted and less 'raw'" (Fine, 1991, p. 672).

Processing with clients who are unable or unwilling to work in this way must be handled more carefully to protect their stability. For example, although a DDNOS client could not dissociate the host during the processing, it was possible to limit parts that needed to be present, as some child parts were willing to stay in their Safe Space. The trauma work was done very slowly, and sessions were held at the end of the day so the host would not have to go from session to work.

Once a target is chosen, the target and work on it are fractionated. This method was developed by Kluft and expanded upon by Fine: "The therapist-patient dyad deconstruct(s) the traumatic memory into constituent components with manageable amounts of affect and sensation. Individual fragments then serve as discrete targets for separate sessions during which the fragments are re-engaged and re-experienced" (1991, p. 672). This process "guard(s) against uncontrolled affect bridging, i.e., the EMDR activating and linking into other traumatic material and overwhelming the process" (Lazrove & Fine, 1996, p. 290). The following strategies further limit the possibility of affect bridging and limit the presence of parts during processing to those parts targeting traumatic material and parts helping.

COPING SKILLS TO HELP MANAGE AND
TITRATE THE TRAUMA WORK

The following is a list of key coping skills used in the trauma processing protocol.

A. SSI or "provision of sanctuary" (Kluft, 1988) provides a place for all parts not involved to go during the processing. Variations on SSI that I regularly use include: (a) adding sound-proofing and affect-proofing to the walls of the Safe Space to insulate parts from the processing, (b) secure Safe Spaces to protect parts who may not understand the need to stay separate from the EMDR (e.g., nonverbal parts), or who may sabotage it, and (c) protective walls to block unknown parts from joining in.

B. During trauma processing, it is very easy for parts to lose duality, that is, lose awareness of the present during the trauma processing. To prevent this, I frequently use an updated version of
the Television Technique (Brown & Fromm, 1986), which uses
Picture in a Picture (PIP) TV technology designed to "watch"
two programs at once, one on a tiny box in a corner of the large
screen. This imagery allows the client many options, for example, the boundaries of the PIP can be very strong (to contain the
traumatic piece), it can be turned on or off, the volume can
be turned down, or the client can focus on the large screen and
see the PIP only in peripheral vision. I think of this also as an
unexpressed metaphor for a goal of treatment, to put the past in
its proper place, as a small part of a person's life that does not
need to be her sole focus.

C. Therapeutic sleep (Kluft, 1988) is a technique where tired or
overwhelmed parts can go to their safe space and go into deep
trance, into a deep dreamless sleep until rested. This is useful
because trauma work is tiring.

D. Container imagery (Kluft, 1988) is used to teach parts to volun-
tarily dissociate incompletely processed feelings and memories
until the next session and to contain aspects of trauma not directly targeted by storing the material and affects in the container. Variations of containers often used include bank vaults,
computer files, boxes of every style and material, which are
sometimes further contained in larger boxes, buried, placed on
another planet or in the therapist's closet. Whatever the container, inherent in its development is the message that there is a
commitment to working on the stored material and affect. Without this message, parts will sometimes refuse to store material,
thinking if it's stored it will be "forgotten about," as clients often
have the understandable desire to banish traumatic material
forever. Another version suggested by Omaha (2004) is a sign
stating: "To be opened only when it serves my healing."

E. Affect dial (Brown & Fromm, 1986) or dimmer-switch imagery
to teach parts to reduce affects or body sensations to a manageable level or to turn them off. On a practical note, I put a Subjective Units of Distress Scale (SUDS) on the dimmer switch to
facilitate both teaching affect regulation and reporting affect

level. With clients who have trouble keeping affects at manageable levels, I put a block, similar to that of a telephone block preventing long distance calls, on the dimmer switch at a SUDS level of 3, 4, or 5 (depending on what the client can manage). I tell the client: *The harder you try to turn up the dimmer switch, the stronger the block becomes.* This hypnotic language helps reinforce the block. Note that the specific imagery is not important and can be adapted to work for different clients.

INITIAL TARGETING OF TRAUMATIC MATERIAL: STEPS

The process of preparation for memory work may take a number of sessions. Often other concerns and resistances will need attention first, for example, some parts will need a Safe Space, or some will worry something bad will happen if traumatic material is addressed. These parts must be attended to before trauma processing is begun.

A. The client and therapist identify a piece of traumatic material that appears to be less difficult and is held by a cluster of parts that are not part of the work or daily life team. Therapist and client identify parts that need to be involved in the processing and ask one to three additional parts to volunteer to help. Ideally, these "helper parts" should not be part of the work or daily life team and should not have been involved in this particular piece of material. Thus, they can remain grounded, remind other parts about coping skills, and warn the therapist if there is a problem.
B. Request that all other parts go to their Safe Spaces and isolate themselves from sound and feelings by raising autohypnotic walls around themselves. The therapist needs to ascertain if the host and daily life team can be dissociated. If not, the processing must be done very carefully so that current life functioning is not disrupted.
C. The client and therapist decide together how to fractionate the trauma work. Options include, but are not limited to, parts

participating one at a time or processing one BASK (Behavior, Affect, Sensation, Knowledge) dimension (Braun, 1988) or one aspect of the trauma at a time.

Example: A memory was broken down into three components: physical pain, emotional pain, and screaming. It was decided to begin with the screaming, which was further broken down into the following four categories: father screaming at her, her screaming in pain, screams of other children being hurt, and silent internal screaming. The silent screaming was targeted first. All traumatic material not directly targeted was stored or dissociated away in an imaged vault to ensure the patient was not flooded by it.

D. Identify a negative and positive cognition (per the EMDR Standard Protocol), unless doing so disrupts this controlled process. Alternatively, identify a general goal for the work, for example, *Traumatic material causes symptoms 1, 2, and 3, and we want to process the trauma to eliminate the symptoms.* Or: *We're going to process this past traumatic event so it goes from feeling like it's occurring in the present to realizing it really happened in the past.*

E. Develop and install any additional necessary resources and coping skills. Reinstall the presence of the helpers, therapist, and therapist's office. Ask the patient if there is anything that would be helpful for the therapist to say during the processing and install those remarks, for example, *It's old stuff. Remember, you are here in my office. You can feel the chair's arm. You can stop anytime you want.* I operate from the principle that it is better to be safe than sorry, so I would rather install too many resources than too few.

F. Practice with TV and Picture in a Picture (PIP) imagery, having the clients "turn on and off" the PIP initially for very short amounts of time to teach them control and to provide safety checks on the process. This process concretely helps the client maintain duality. Instruct parts to put an image of the office with the client and therapist present on the whole screen, turn on the PIP to a benign or mildly annoying scene, then after 2 seconds switch the PIP off and return to the whole screen showing the office. Initiate DAS when the whole screen is imaged: parts are asked to say when the PIP is turned on; therapist counts 2 seconds then reminds the client to switch it off. Continue this practice with 2-second sets until the client has confidence in controlling the PIP. Increase the length of sets gradually as the client's confidence and control increase.

Other coping skills may need to be developed, incorporated, and practiced in this step, for example, use of an affect dial to modulate painful affect.

After necessary skills are in place, participating parts allow the PIP to be on for 2 seconds of the targeted material. Clients are instructed to allow the processing to go for 2 seconds unless they want to stop it sooner. The emphasis is on control being exercised by parts that are processing and by helper parts, with the therapist functioning as an emergency brake. Once the client can turn on and off the traumatic material, processing continues for longer periods of time and looks more similar to standard EMDR processing, with the exception of the PIP being turned off in between sets. Note that some of the trauma work has already been occurring along with the skill building. Parts now have control over material and choices they previously lacked.

G. At the end of the memory-work portion of the session, if the target has been fully processed, install the positive cognition or whatever else is relevant. For example, some clients feel enormous somatic relief. Install it! Often, work on a target will take more than one session. As in any incomplete EMDR session, ask helpers and processing parts what was the most important thing they learned and install that with DAS (Shapiro, 2001). Then put remaining traumatic material away, using the established container imagery reinforced by DAS.

Parts are then asked what would be helpful, the main options being resource installation, going to their Safe Space and resting, or doing deep-trance dreamless sleep. An advantage of working with parts that are not part of the daily life team is that they are not needed for the rest of the day and can rest. Before the end of the session, ask other parts to return from their walled-off Safe Spaces (when appropriate) and provide information about the trauma work as necessary. Answer questions, check on the system's stability, and set up the plan for the next session.

H. After one fragment of traumatic material is processed, the next
    one is selected and processed.
I. As traumatic material is successfully processed, groups of parts
    often integrate. When this occurs, there is a need to acknowl-
    edge and discuss this to facilitate the system's adjustment to the
    change. Parts who have completed trauma work often become
    very effective helpers when it's time for other parts to work on
    their trauma experiences.

Example: A 36-year-old woman's system consisted of three parts, a
host/adult, a teen, and a child. Initial preparation for memory work
covered several sessions and included all parts. In these sessions
coping skills were reinforced, practiced, and installed with DAS, including an affect dial, SSI, and deep-trance, deep dreamless sleep. Before preparation for work on the specific target was initiated, the host
went to her Safe Space and put sound/feeling proofing up. She placed
nontargeted traumatic material in a "bank vault," and the teenage part
agreed to help the child part who held most of the traumatic memories. Resources the child had identified were installed (with DAS), including feeling the teen's arm around her shoulders, feeling an imaged
blanket wrapped around her, and an antenna to watch out for danger. I
suggested that the antenna could also be noticing current-orientation
reminders. These reminders are included whenever possible to maintain focus on current reality. Once these resources were installed the
patient decided to hold a Teddy bear, which was then included in the
installation of being in the office with me. At this point, TV and PIP imagery were initiated and practiced with DAS while the teen part
helped the child notice that she could turn off the PIP or shift her attention to the rest of the screen and see the PIP only peripherally. This was
practiced first with mildly annoying scenes and then with 2-second
blips of the targeted traumatic material, the fear that she would die
during the abuse. In this first session of targeting the traumatic material directly, the child part only wanted to bring it up in 2-second
blips on the PIP and shut it off over and over. At one point, the
helper/teen part suggested to the child part that the affect dial be
turned down and fixed so it would be blocked from going above a
SUDS of 3 and that block was installed with DAS. At the end of the
trauma-work part of the session, processing was shut down by having the child and teen parts put all traumatic material away in the

bank vault. The vault was equipped with a night deposit slot in case any subsequent material arose that needed to be put away in between sessions. With DAS, we installed the lock on the vault and the commitment to continue working on the contained traumatic material when the time was right.

During this session, what was most important for this client was that the memory work process felt very different from what she had gone through in a previous treatment: "This time I did not get lost in it, and I could start and stop it!" We installed this awareness. Then the child and teen decided to go to their Safe Space and do deep-trance deep-dreamless sleep until rested, and the host returned.

Example: This client had already done much EMDR-facilitated processing. After integrating a large portion of her dissociated ego system, a 38-year-old woman found several deeply dissociated parts who had been responsible for episodic violent acting out and homicidal feelings. Because of concern for potential violence, this client took a dose of Ativan (a prescription medication often used as for needed calming) prior to beginning processing. Ativan increased her sense of control and she described a sense of "everything slowing down." These effects were installed with DAS and then broadcast in the direction of parts that were not in contact with the host. In spite of the host's lack of direct connection with these parts, she had a sense of useful pre-established resources. They included allowing her body to become so heavy that she could only move slowly—the faster she tried to move, the slower she would go (note the hypnotic language)—and an image of a cool mountain stream to reduce physical pain. These were reinstalled with DAS and then broadcast along with the information that she was in my office where she had never been hurt even when she was vulnerable. During sets, the client asked me to remind her that she was in my office, to open her eyes and see that she was not alone and that she could switch to the stream or turn the PIP off at any time. This was also installed with DAS and broadcast along with the sound of my voice (useful because during the traumatic work, she would at times see me as the perpetrator but could ground herself with my voice). She then practiced using the TV with PIP imagery focusing on a work issue. What worked best for her was first to visualize the big-screen picture of my office. Then I turned the DAS on, and she practiced allowing the PIP to come into focus, pushing it back out of focus to a dot and turning it off. Once she was back to the big-screen picture, the DAS was turned off, and, per standard protocol, she took a deep breath in and let it out. We then practiced beginning with 2 seconds of allowing the PIP with the targeted issue to come into focus, my counting 2 seconds off and saying, *Okay, you can send the PIP back now.* After the second 2-second trial, she reported that what came up was "too dark and overwhelming." A "healing light" resource was installed with DAS. With that, the client felt ready for a 5-second trial. After two 10-second trials, she felt ready to do up to a 45-second set. More standard processing followed with the exception that the sets ended with the client de-focusing the PIP and returning to awareness of being in my office.

As the processing proceeded, the client became aware that the parts holding the traumatic material were a 4-year-old who was terrified that the 2-year-old part she was holding was dead. Once the traumatic material was cleared out, the two parts were given Safe Spaces with images of sunshine and the host's current pets (orientation information). The host observed that the baby had been "smart to shut down and not give life energy to being hurt," noting, "If they can't reach you, you can't die." We installed this validation of inner resourcefulness with DAS.

At this point, the host became aware of intense, potentially uncontrolled rage that the baby had been in this position, coupled with intense protective feelings. We tried to put the rage away in a vault; however, since the host was not connected to the parts holding it, not all of the rage could be put away. The host solved this by placing an imaged heavily reinforced wall between the host parts known to her and all other parts. Along with the wall, we installed (with DAS) the message that the host was committed to working with parts behind the wall and would in the next session. If that session was canceled or missed, another plan would be made. Specificity and commitment in messages appears to decrease the necessity for parts to act out for attention. As the wall was installed, the host felt calmer, and the sensation of calmness was also installed. The host agreed during the week to reinforce the wall, reinforce the commitment, and work gently on orienting the child parts to their current life.

Using this format, over the next 3 weeks, traumatic material contained by the parts behind the imaged wall was fractionated and systematically processed by the host. Once that was done, a body scan revealed some residual traumatic material. After processing that, the involved parts integrated with the host.

THE LATE PHASE: PERSONALITY INTEGRATION

As traumatic material is processed, the need for dissociative boundaries becomes unnecessary and integration either occurs spontaneously or can be assisted by the therapist. Usually the process is gradual, with groups of parts integrating over time rather than all at once.

Once clients appear to have worked through all traumatic material and are in the first stage of final integration, it is useful to have them review their life from their earliest memory or bit of information (e.g., how their parents felt about the pregnancy) to the present. DAS is used during the review and the client is instructed to stop if any affectively charged material is discovered. Negative material is processed; positive is installed. This review also appears to facilitate access to any remaining parts.

Life as an integrated being requires considerable adjustment on the client's part. Clients must master "how to live in the world without the use of pathological dissociative defenses and structures." (Kluft, 2003, p. 82) EMDR facilitates this process with Resource Installation, through processing fears about the future and through installing future templates (Shapiro, 2001). This allows the client to practice future situations, bringing new coping skills and resources into EMDR facilitated visualizations.

CONCLUSIONS

EMDR and adaptations of EMDR have much to offer to the treatment of people with DID and DDNOS throughout the entire treatment process. In the first stage of treatment, DAS can be used to facilitate communication across dissociative boundaries, productively orienting dissociated parts of the mind to the present with respect to time, place, height, and relationships. It thereby decreases anxiety and negative transferences caused by parts who had been living as if the past were the present. In addition, DAS can be used to strengthen, install, and communicate resources and coping skills. In the second stage of treatment, the Standard Protocol must be altered to protect DID clients from decompensation. With additions to the protocol, EMDR facilitates the processing of traumatic material. In the post-integration phase of treatment, EMDR can be used to process fears about the future and help clients with their adjustment to life without dissociative defenses.

The process of healing from a DD, even under optimal circumstances, requires commitment from the client, special training for the therapist, and then several years of often painful and difficult treatment. EMDR adaptations and the addition of coping skills and control to the Standard Protocol allows these clients, otherwise too fragile, to benefit from its accelerated information-processing effect, helping them maintain their highest level of functioning while providing protection from the risk of decompensation. The addition of EMDR to the treatment process, where appropriate, facilitates the stabilization process, streamlines the processing of traumatic material, and is a gift to the healing process.

RESOURCE

International Society for the Study of Dissociation (ISSD): www.issd.org

REFERENCES

Braun, B. G. (1988). The BASK model of dissociation. *Dissociation, 1*, 4–24.

Brown, D. P. (1990, April). *Hypnotherapy and posttraumatic stress disorder.* Workshop presented at Harvard Medical School CE Division, Cambridge, MA.

Brown, D. P. and Fromm, E. (1986). *Hypnotherapy and hypnoanalysis.* Hillsdale, NJ: Erlbaum.

Brown, D., Scheflin, A. W., and Hammond, D. C. (1998). *Memory, trauma, treatment and the law.* New York: Norton.

Chu, J. (1998). *Rebuilding shattered lives: The responsible treatment of complex post-traumatic and dissociative disorders.* New York: Wiley.

Courtois, C. A. (1999). *Recollections of sexual abuse: Treatment principles and guidelines.* New York: Norton.

Fine, C. G. (1991). Treatment stabilization and crisis prevention: Pacing the therapy of the multiple personality disorder patient. *Psychiatric Clinics of North America, 14*, 661–676.

Fine, C. G. (1996, July). *EMDR-facilitated trauma work in patients with dissociative identity disorders.* Paper presented at the EMDRIA Conference, Denver, CO.

Fine, C. G., and Berkowitz, S. A. (2001). The wreathing protocol: The imbrication of hypnosis and EMDR in the treatment of dissociative identity disorder and other dissociative responses. *American Journal of Clinical Hypnosis, 43* (3, 4), 275–290.

Fisher, J. (2000, November). *In the service of stabilizing dissociative symptoms.* Paper presented at the International Society for the Study of Dissociation Annual Meeting, San Antonio, TX.

Grand, D. (1998, July). *Innovation and integration in EMDR-based diagnosis, technique, teaching, performance enhancement, and creativity.* Paper presented at the EMDRIA Conference, Baltimore, MD.

Janet, P. (1898). Traitement psychologique de l'hystérie [Psychologic treatment of hysteria] In A. Robin (Ed.), *Traité de thérapeutique appliquée* (pp. 3–4). Paris: Rueff.

Kluft, R. P. (1988). Playing for time: temporizing techniques in the treatment of multiple personality disorder. *American Journal of Clinical Hypnosis, 32,* 90–98.

Kluft, R. P. (1992, February). *Hypnosis and multiple personality.* Workshop presented at Daniel Brown and Assoc., Cambridge, MA.

Kluft, R. P. (1993a). Basic principles on conducting the psychotherapy of multiple personality disorder. In R. P. Kluft and C. G. Fine (eds.), *Clinical perspectives on multiple Personality Disorder* (pp. 19–50). Washington D. C.: American Psychiatric Press.

Kluft, R. P. (1993b). The initial stages of psychotherapy in the treatment of multiple personality disorder patients. *Dissociation, 6,* 145–161.

Kluft, R. P. (2003). Current issues in dissociative identity disorder. *Bridging Eastern and Western Psychiatry, 1*(1), 71–87.

Kluft, R. P. (1999). Current issues in dissociative identity disorder. *Journal of Practical Psychiatry and Behavioral Health, 3,* 19.

Kluft, R. P. (1994). Applications of hypnotic interventions. *Hypnos, 21,* 205–223.

Korn, D. L., and Leeds, A. M. (in press). Preliminary evidence of efficacy for EMDR resource development and installation in the stabilization phase of treatment of complex posttraumatic stress disorder. *Journal of Clinical Psychology.*

Lazrove, S., and Fine, C. G. (1996). The use of EMDR in patients with dissociative identity disorder. *Dissociation, 9,* 289–299.

Liotti, G. (1999). Disorganized attachment as a model for understanding dissociative psychopathology. In J. Solomon and C. George (Eds.), *Attachment disorganization* (pp. 297–243). New York: Guilford Press.

Loewenstein, R. J. (1993). Posttraumatic and dissociative aspects of transference and countertransference in the treatment of multiple personality disorder. In R. P. Kluft and C. G. Fine (Eds.), *Clinical perspectives on multiple personality disorder* (pp. 51–85). Washington, DC: American Psychiatric Press.

Lyons-Ruth, K. and Jacobvitz, D. (1999). Attachment disorganization: Unresolved loss, relational violence, and lapses in behavioral and attentional strategies. In J. Cassidy and P. R. Shaver (Eds.), *Handbook of attachment: Theory, research, and clinical applications* (pp. 520–554). New York: Guilford Press.

Lyons-Ruth, K. (2003). Dissociation and the parent-infant dialogue: A longitudinal perspective from attachment research. *Journal of the American Psychoanalytic Association, 51,* 883–911.

Omaha, J. (2004). *Psychotherapeutic intervention for emotional regulation.* New York: Norton.

Shapiro, F. (2001). *Eye movement desensitization and reprocessing (EMDR). Basic principles, protocols, and procedures* (2nd ed.). New York: Guilford Press.

Twombly, J. H. (2000). Incorporating EMDR and EMDR adaptations into the treatment of clients with DID. *Journal of Trauma and Dissociation, 1*(2), 61–81.

Twombly, J. H. (2001, December). Safe place imagery: Handling intrusive thoughts and feelings. *The EMDRIA Newsletter, Special Edition,* 35–38

Van der Hart, O., and Steele, K. (2000). Critical issues column. *International Society for the Study of Dissociation: Newsletter, 18*(2), 4–5.

Van der Kolk, B. (1994). The body keeps the score: Memory and the evolving psychobiology of post traumatic stress. Available at http://www.traumapages .com

Withers, D. (1999, June). *EMDR bilateral movement therapy.* Paper presented at the EMDRIA Conference, Las Vegas, NV.

Chapter 4

EMDR Processing with Dissociative Clients: Adjunctive Use of Opioid Antagonists

Ulrich F. Lanius

DISSOCIATIVE SYMPTOMS ARE COMMON IN TRAUMATIC STRESS SYNDROMES (e.g., complex posttraumatic stress disorder [PTSD], disorder of extreme stress, not otherwise specified [DESNOS], borderline personality disorder, and dissociative disorders). They commonly interfere with psychotherapy including EMDR treatment. It appears that the adaptive information processing system gets overwhelmed and shuts down, thereby barring the integration and resolution of traumatic experience and thus precluding positive treatment outcomes. A series of case studies by Ferrie and Lanius (2001) found that the administration of an opioid antagonist prior to EMDR treatment significantly reduced dissociative symptoms, somatization, and numbing, as well as aiding trauma processing. The present chapter describes the relevant scientific research, as well as a theoretical rationale and a protocol, for the use of opioid antagonists in trauma processing with EMDR.

DISSOCIATION AND DISSOCIATIVE PROCESSES

The essential feature of dissociative processes is a disturbance or alteration in the normally integrative functions of identity, memory, and consciousness (American Psychiatric Association, 2000). Dissociation includes three distinct but related mental phenomena (van der Kolk, 1996). *Primary dissociation* refers to the inability to integrate what is happening into consciousness, with sensory and emotional elements of the event not being incorporated into personal memory and identity, thus remaining isolated from ordinary consciousness. *Secondary dissociation* refers to the dissociation between observing ego and experiencing ego, for example, mentally leaving one's body at the moment of the trauma and observing what happens from a distance. *Tertiary dissociation* refers to when people develop distinct ego states that contain traumatic experiences consisting of complex identities with distinct cognitive, affective, and behavioral patterns.

Dissociation and somatoform dissociation (Nijenhuis, 1999) can present in a variety of ways that include perceptual alterations in the experience of time (e.g., flashbacks), changes in self-experience (e.g., depersonalization) and in the perception of reality (e.g., derealization), amnesia, and fugue states. Attentional impairment, as well as alterations in somatic and sensorimotor phenomena that include but are not limited to sensory distortions, motor weakness, freezing, numbing, paralysis, tremors, shaking, and convulsions, are also common. Severe dissociative and somatization symptoms are common in patients with PTSD, particularly if the stressor is of an interpersonal nature and there is a history of repeated traumatization. The resulting constellation of symptoms is frequently referred to as complex PTSD (Herman, 1992) or DESNOS (van der Kolk et al., 1996).

Van der Kolk (1996) has suggested that the experiences of day-to-day, nontraumatic events are integrated into consciousness without the sensory aspects of the event being registered separately. Flashbacks, on the other hand, lack such integration of experience. Indeed, they have been described as timeless, predominantly nonverbal, imagery-based memories (Brewin, Dalgleish, & Joseph, 1996; Lanius et al., 2004; van der Kolk & Fisler, 1995), lending support to the notion that the failure to integrate traumatic memories into the present context accounts for their ongoing disturbing nature (Lanius, Bluhm, Lanius, & Pain, in press).

Essentially, dissociation results in an alteration in consciousness that disrupts the integration of information, resulting in an inability to integrate memories into the present context, as well as an inability to integrate the totality of what is happening into personal memory and identity. Thus these memories remain isolated from ordinary consciousness (e.g., van der Hart, van der Kolk, & Boon, 1996).

OPIOIDS AND OPIOID ANTAGONISTS

Exogenous opiates (e.g., codeine, opium, morphine, heroine, Demerol) are most commonly used as analgesics but are also substances of abuse. Endogenous opiates, such as endorphins and enkephalins, are produced within the organism itself. They are released in response to a variety of stressors including pain and anticipatory pain, childbirth, surgery, exercise, social conflict, and starvation. Opioids have an anxiety-relieving as well as analgesic effect and inhibit cardiovascular response to stress.

Opioid antagonists block the effects of both exogenous and endogenous opiates by binding preferentially to opiate receptors. The two commonly used opioid antagonists are naloxone (Narcan) and naltrexone (Revia). Naloxone is injectable; naltrexone is in pill form. Both are nonselective opioid antagonists, that is, they bind to all different types of opiate receptors in the brain that include μ (mu), δ (delta), and κ (kappa) receptors, resulting in powerful opiate blockade. A standard dose of 50 mg of naltrexone will block the effects of 25 mg of intravenously administered heroin.

ATTACHMENT AND ENDOGENOUS OPIATES

Human attachment is, in part, mediated by the endogenous opiate system. Brain circuits involved in the maintenance of affiliative behavior are precisely those most richly endowed with opioid receptors (Kling & Steklis, 1976). Behavioral studies show that the endogenous opioid system plays an important role in the maintenance of social attachment (van der Kolk, 1989).

In animals, the separation response can be inhibited with morphine, abolishing both the separation cry in infants and the maternal response to it (e.g., Newman, Murphy, & Harbough, 1982; Panksepp, Nelson, & Sivey, 1994; Panksepp, Sivey, & Normansell 1985). Furthermore, lack of caregiving during the first few weeks of life decreases the number of opioid receptors in the cingulate gyrus in mice (Bonnet, Hiller, & Simon, 1976).

Schore (2001) suggested that abuse or neglect over the first 2 years negatively impacts the major regulatory system in the human brain, the orbital prefrontolimbic system. He further suggests that the resulting hyperarousal and dissociation set the template for later childhood, adolescent, and adult PTSD. This raises the question of whether lack of caregiving and neglect in humans also impact the opiate system, resulting in fewer opioid receptors. This potentially reduces human capacity to experience pleasure, at the same time making their brains more vulnerable to the effects of opiates, resulting in a predisposition toward dissociation.

ENDOGENOUS OPIATES, STRESS RESPONSE, AND PARASYMPATHETIC REGULATION

Dissociation in response to early trauma that is experienced as "psychic catastrophe" has been described as "detachment from an unbearable situation," "the escape when there is no escape," and "a last resort defensive strategy" (Schore, 2001). Essentially, dissociation is a parasympathetic regulatory strategy (Kaufman & Rosenblum, 1967, 1969).

It involves much increased vagal tone, resulting in decreased blood pressure and heart rate despite increasing amounts of circulating adrenaline. In this passive state, endogenous opiates become elevated, blunting and numbing emotional pain. These opioids, especially enkephalins, instantly trigger pain-reducing analgesia and immobility (Fanselow, 1986), as well as inhibiting cries for help (Kalin, Shelton, Rickman, & Davidson, 1998). Infants lose postural control, withdraw, and self-comfort, reminiscent of the withdrawal of Harlow's isolated monkeys or of the infants in institutions observed by Spitz (cited by Bowlby, 1978).

Moreover, Perry (1999) has suggested that bradycardia (abnormally slow heartbeat), cataplexy (rigidity of the muscles caused by shock or extreme fear), and paralysis are opioid-mediated dissociative responses to childhood trauma. In an evolutionary sense, dissociation is a "profound detachment" (Barach, 1991), a disengagement "to conserve energies . . . to foster survival by the risky posture of feigning death, to allow healing of wounds and restitution of depleted resources by immobility" (Powles, 1992, p. 213).

DISSOCIATION AND LEARNED HELPLESSNESS

The above descriptions are very much reminiscent of what is commonly referred to as learned helplessness, a research paradigm that purports to be a model of depression but indeed fits better with dissociation. Hemingway and Reigle (1987) suggested that the endogenous opiate system is involved in the induction and expression of learned helplessness and stress-induced analgesia (reduced sensitivity to pain). That is, animals exposed to inescapable shock develop stress-induced analgesia when reexposed to stress shortly afterward.

In addition, animal research suggests that naltrexone and naloxone reverse conditioned and unconditioned freezing. For instance, naltrexone blocked immobility in a forced swimming test, an animal model of depression (Makino, Kitano, Komiyama, Hirohashi, & Takasuna, 2000). Furthermore, naloxone readily reverses the stress-induced analgesic response (Kelly, 1982). Finally, opioid antagonists reversed anhedonia (lack of pleasure) and enhanced emotional reactions to novel stressors secondary to early exposure to chronic variable stress (Zurita, Martijena, Cuadra, Brandao, & Molina, 2000).

TRAUMATIC STRESS AND
ENDOGENOUS OPIOIDS

Abnormalities in the endogenous opioid system have been identified in PTSD clients. For instance, PTSD clients, as compared to controls, show significantly higher levels of analgesia in response to specific (trauma-related stimuli) and nonspecific (exercise) stress (Hamner & Hitri, 1992; Pitman, van der Kolk, Orr, & Greenberg, 1990).

Furthermore, Gold, Pottash, Sweeney, Martin, and Extein (1982) found that when people who were traumatized as adults were reexposed to situations reminiscent of the trauma, this evoked an endogenous opioid response. This is analogous to the response of animals that are exposed to mild shock after having previously been subjected to inescapable shock. Moreover, Pitman and colleagues (1990) and van der Kolk, Greenberg, Orr, and Pitman (1989) reported that Vietnam veterans with PTSD experienced a 30% reduction in perception of pain when viewing a movie depicting combat in Vietnam. The analgesia produced was equivalent to the injection of 8 mg of morphine. Naloxone, however, reversed this response. Thus, it appears that repeated exposure to uncontrollable stress results in changes in the endogenous opioid system that can manifest as dissociative symptoms and stress-induced analgesia.

THERAPEUTIC USE OF OPIOID
ANTAGONISTS IN TRAUMATIC STRESS
SYNDROMES

Schmahl, Stiglmayr, Böhme, and Bohus (1999) administered naltrexone (50mg qid, p.o.) to female patients with borderline personality disorder (BPD) over a period of several weeks and reported a decrease in dissociative symptoms. Similarly, Bohus, Landwehrmeyer, Stiglmayr, Limberger, Bohme, and Schmahl (1999) reported a reduction in tonic immobility, analgesia, and flashbacks in trauma patients who were administered naltrexone (25–100 mg qid) for a 2-week period.

Glover (1993) administered the opioid antagonist nalmefene to PTSD veterans and found a decrease in intrusive symptoms, rage, vulnerability, startle response, and emotional numbing. Similarly, veterans given naltrexone showed decreased hypervigilance, anxiety, panic, flashbacks, and intrusive thoughts. Rage reactions decreased whereas appropriate assertiveness increased. Traumatic memories began to surface spontaneously and resolved if the patient could tolerate the accompanying affect. Frequency of disturbing dreams increased, often with bizarre or changed content (Maurer & Teitelbaum, 1998). Nuller, Morozova, Kushnir, and Hamper (2001) administered naloxone to 14 patients with depersonalization disorder. Eleven patients received single doses (1.6 mg or 4 mg i.v.) and 3 others received multiple infusions, with the maximal dosage being 10 mg. In 3 of 14 patients, depersonalization symptoms disappeared entirely and 7 patients showed a marked improvement.

On the other hand, Lubin, Weizman, Shmushkevitz, and Valevski (2002) administered naltrexone (100–200 mg per day) to 6 males and 2 females with chronic PTSD. While they obtained a decrease in intrusive and hyperarousal symptoms, they judged them as not clinically significant. Furthermore, they found that significant side effects limited dosage. It should be noted that no mention is made whether there was an ongoing therapeutic relationship with patients in any of the studies, with the exception of the Bohus and colleagues (1999) study, where patients were in an ongoing dialectical behavior therapy (DBT) program.

Opioid antagonists, above and beyond affecting opioid binding to receptors, will also influence hypothalamic pituitary axis (HPA) activity. While HPA activity is increased secondary to acute stress, in chronic stress and PTSD, HPA activity is commonly inhibited with a concurrent reduction in cortisol levels (Yehuda, 2001). Administration of naltrexone will increase HPA axis activity, as well as cortisol plasma levels and ACTH plasma levels in both humans (King, et al., 2002) and primates (Williams, Ko, Rice, & Woods, 2003). That is, opioid antagonists appear to counteract a chronic stress or PTSD response.

DISSOCIATION, PSYCHOTHERAPY, AND EMDR

Dissociative and somatoform symptoms can often be severe and interfere with psychotherapy in general and trauma processing in particular. Peritraumatic dissociation occurring at the time of the trauma is adaptive to the extent that the associated narrowing of consciousness will reduce the impact of overwhelming duress at that point in time. On the other hand, dissociation during psychotherapy generally interferes with overcoming the effects of traumatic events. Dissociative symptoms such as depersonalization, freezing, numbing, unpredictable ego-state shifts, and excessive somatization commonly block effective treatment. These symptoms essentially interfere with the mindfulness, dual awareness/focus, and awareness of one's own body, necessary for successful psychotherapy in general and EMDR treatment in particular.

In EMDR treatment, dissociation often presents as a blocked response where either nothing comes up or the client is unable to connect to any emotion or body sensation. Alternatively, it may result in either severe somatization (e.g., headache activity, pain sensations) or ongoing severe abreaction without any decrease in Subjective Units of Distress Scale (SUDS) level. The latter scenario is usually highly aversive and retraumatizing for the client. It potentially results in treatment avoidance and reinforcement of such negative beliefs and cognitions as "I can't get over it," "I am powerless," "I cannot succeed," "I am permanently damaged," and "I am a failure."

EMDR can also break through dissociative barriers (Paulsen, 1995; Shapiro, 2001), and it appears to directly affect dissociative processes. Insufficient affect management skills and inadequate client preparation may result in uncontrolled affect bridging and lead to a significant deterioration in a client's functioning. Consequently, EMDR training emphasizes extensive preparation and precautions with regard to the use of EMDR in individuals with significant dissociative symptoms.

At the same time, EMDR may work exactly because it breaks through dissociation. Stimulating the Adaptive Information Processing System by means of Dual Attention Stimulation (DAS) may affect the underlying neurological mechanism of dissociation and thus aid the integration of information (Lanius, 2002, 2004b). If there is limited traumatic material, information processing usually occurs rapidly without overwhelming the system. However, when the magnitude of traumatic material is too extensive to be integrated, hyperarousal or dissociative processes may be triggered, resulting in impaired information processing.

For clients with significant dissociative symptoms, stabilization is always indicated prior to trauma processing. This has prompted the incorporation of stabilization techniques into the EMDR protocol (Shapiro, 1995/2001), such as DBT (Linehan, 1993), Resource Development and Installation (Korn & Leeds, 2002), ego-state (Forgash, 2002), and body-oriented approaches. Specialized protocols developed for EMDR processing with dissociative clients include fractionated abreaction (Lazrove & Fine, 1996), ego-state approaches (e.g., Paulson, 1995; Twombly, 2000, and this volume, Chapter 3), body-focused psychotherapy (e.g., Fischer, 2003; Ogden, 2004; Ogden & Minton, 2000), as well as an eclectic comprehensive approach that integrates body and ego-state approaches with recent developments in neuroscience research (Lanius, 2000). Nevertheless, the effective resolution of traumatic material in clients with significant dissociative symptoms often remains difficult at best.

USING OPIOID ANTAGONISTS
FOR THE FIRST TIME

I started seeing Sarah in early 1999. Sarah had developed PTSD after being assaulted and raped at gunpoint. Subsequently, her assailant had stalked her in the community. In addition to PTSD, Sarah had a preexisting severe dissociative identity disorder (DID) that was exacerbated by the recent assault, resulting in much increased fragmentation of the self. Sarah's dissociative disorder (DD) was attributable to a childhood history of profound physical, sexual, emotional, and psychological abuse by multiple perpetrators, her parents among them. Whereas prior to the assault, Sarah had been able to function relatively well in her daily life, she was now completely overwhelmed not only by the most recent assault but also by intrusive symptoms relating to her childhood experiences.

After spending some time on stabilization, we had progressed to EMDR. To facilitate processing, we used fractionated abreactions, ego-state work, and body-oriented work, as well as a wide array of other techniques. Treatment was difficult. There was a lot of blocking, and Sarah frequently went blank during processing, experiencing significant depersonalization. Despite that, Sarah felt that she was making good progress. She stated that EMDR was the only thing that had ever helped her, despite the fact that her SUDS level in most of those sessions never went anywhere near 0 or 1.

At the same time I was seeing another client, Zoltan, who had survived a severe head-on collision that left him crippled, with chronic pain and severe PTSD. Zoltan was making good progress with EMDR, when one day he came in and EMDR processing suddenly came to a halt. In fact, his processing that day very much resembled that of Sarah (whom I had just seen in the session prior to Zoltan) when she was having a bad day. When I checked for the body sensation, Zoltan responded with "nothing." Responses after sets included "nothing," "just blank," and "I don't get anything." It became clear that Zoltan was experiencing significant depersonalization. Zoltan eventually volunteered that he had just been prescribed a large dose of Tylenol 3 (an analgesic that contains the opiate codeine) for pain control, as he had reinjured his leg in a fall. Zoltan's response to EMDR during that session when he was on Tylenol 3 was strikingly similar to that of Sarah on occasions when she was experiencing dissociative and depersonalization symptoms after overshooting the therapeutic window. In both cases, information processing had essentially ceased.

During that same week I attended the International Society of Traumatic Stress Studies (ISTSS) conference in Miami, Florida. Dr. Rachel Yehuda held a keynote address on HPA axis functioning. During her presentation she skipped over a slide showing a correlation between Dissociative Experiences Scale (DES) scores and opioid levels. Although the slide was projected onto the screen for only a few seconds, it had been permanently etched into my memory.

Upon my return home to Vancouver, I conducted a Medline search and came across a recently published article noted above by Bohus and colleagues (1999). They found that administration of the opioid antagonist naltrexone significantly reduced dissociative symptoms in many of their borderline clients with PTSD. I showed the article to Sarah, and we both decided that it was worth giving naltrexone a try. I had been seeing Sarah for close to a year when her general practitioner prescribed continuous-dose naltrexone, as described in the studying Bohus and colleagues at 50 mg qid (a total of 200 mg per day). Sarah responded extremely well to the medication. EMDR processing suddenly improved and she was able to process multiple traumatic events for the first time, achieving a SUDS of 1 or 0. Interestingly enough, with Sarah on the naltrexone, we were able to use the Standard Protocol without needing to resort to alternative protocols to deal with dissociative symptoms. Also the level of visible abreaction had been strikingly reduced.

Unfortunately, Sarah developed endometriosis-related pneumothorax, requiring emergency medical care. Since she was now at ongoing risk of needing emergency surgery and opioid blockers would interfere with anesthesia, Sarah chose to discontinue the naltrexone. However, when we did EMDR processing, it almost appeared as if Sarah was still on naltrexone—there was no longer any undue dissociation, as if the blockage had been removed. Apparently, after the trauma processing with naltrexone, the reduction in dissociative symptoms remained, even after discontinuation of the medication.

Only when we proceeded to target the traumatic memories of sexual abuse by her father that had occurred during her childhood over a period of many years did dissociative symptoms emerge again. It was at this point that Sarah wondered about going back on naltrexone. Given the ongoing risk of possible emergency surgery, she was curious whether naltrexone would work if taken just prior to the session. After consulting with her physician, we went ahead and Sarah took 50 mg of naltrexone 45 minutes prior to the session. We worked through the traumatic memory again with very little visible abreaction and ended up with a SUDS of 1. Once again, EMDR proceeded well, so that Sarah decided to take naltrexone prior to additional EMDR sessions concerned with severe abuse by her primary caretakers. Using naltrexone, Sarah continued to process these traumatic memories, some of which she could speak about for the first time. The EMDR processing of these traumatic events resulted in a profound improvement in Sarah's overall psychological functioning. Sarah was able to extricate herself from an abusive relationship. She returned to work at a new job and eventually enrolled in a number of courses and continued her education.

When I talked about Sarah's case in a presentation on dissociative processes and EMDR at the EMDR Association of Canada (EMDRAC) meeting in Vancouver in 2000, it caught the attention of Dr. Robert Ferrie. This led to a collaboration in the series of case studies described below involving the use of opioid antagonists We presented those data for the first time at the EMDR International Association (EMDRIA) conference in Austin, Texas, in 2001, and then again at the EMDRIA conference in San Diego, California, in 2002.

OPIOID ANTAGONISTS AND EMDR:
A SERIES OF CASE STUDIES

Since it appeared that opiate blockade enhanced the effectiveness of EMDR processing with dissociative clients, both Dr. Robert Ferrie and I were curious to see whether these initial impressions would hold true with other clients who had difficulties with EMDR processing. In this way, we embarked on a series of case studies, finding additional support for this initial impression.

Our series of case studies included 16 clients that met criteria for a variety of diagnoses that included PTSD and partial PTSD, DID, dissociate disorder not otherwise specified (DDNOS), obsessive-compulsive disorder (OCD), and BPD. They all had gone through a stabilization phase and we had an ongoing therapeutic relationship with all of them. Each had some experience with EMDR, but the application of standard and modified EMDR protocols had been unsuccessful. EMDR had been discontinued because of depersonalization or derealization, severe somatization or lack of change on SUDS ratings of the target memory. In other words, in each case a therapeutic impasse had been reached.

Clients were administered either naltrexone (modal dosage 50 mg; dosage range 25–125 mg) 30–60 minutes prior to the EMDR session or 1 mg of naloxone injected subcutaneously immediately prior to EMDR. That is, rather than continuous dosing, opioid antagonists were only administered prior to EMDR sessions.

The results can be summarized as follows: Thirteen clients were able to process the traumatic memory down to SUD rating of 0 or 1, with a markedly improved body scan. Twelve reported elimination of somatization and depersonalization. Seven went on to successfully process other memories without naltrexone. On average, clients underwent five sessions using either naltrexone or naloxone. In four cases, ongoing improvement with regard to dissociative symptoms occurred after only one session, whereas other cases needed more frequent sessions—up to a maximum of 15 sessions. Eleven clients showed long-term improvement in presenting complaints after opioid antagonist pretreatment. Two showed no therapeutic effect. Gastric distress is a common side effect of both naltrexone and naloxone. However, in our sample, naloxone was better tolerated than naltrexone: six clients had adverse gastrointestinal reactions to naltrexone that included abdominal pains, nausea, vomiting; those who were prescribed naloxone did not report any adverse effects.

None of our clients exhibited increased anxiety, even though this is a commonly noted side effect with opioid antagonists. At the same time, we observed that opiate blockade resulted in higher initial heart rate but not to an extent where it became distressing to our clients. Increased heart rate has been shown to correlate with treatment outcome in exposure therapy for PTSD (Jaycox, Foa, & Morral, 1998), whereas lowered or unchanged heart rate has previously been associated with dissociative symptoms (e.g., Lanius, et al., 2002). The lack of self-reported anxiety may be attributable to the fact that none of our subjects were undergoing substance withdrawal and were generally very much aware of their anxiety-related symptoms prior to the use of opioid antagonists. Furthermore, the ongoing psychotherapeutic relationship and the experience of increased mastery over symptoms after EMDR with opioid antagonists may have reduced rather than exacerbated anxiety symptoms.

Depression has also been reported secondary to the use of opioid antagonists in the treatment of substance use disorders. Again, this was not evident among our clients. However, a slightly lowered mood appropriate to the issues being targeted with EMDR was evident. When previously there had been an air of "la belle indifference" or inappropriately positive or ebullient affect, there now appeared to be a more somber countenance. In general, mood stability appeared to be enhanced rather than compromised by the use of opioid antagonists.

Furthermore, we noted a rapid reduction of flashbacks and intrusive symptoms, as well as decreased hypervigilance. Fearfulness, anxiety, and panic symptoms were significantly diminished. In particular, we noted that in our client sample, mindfulness and dual attention were greatly improved. Moreover, body awareness was heightened with a concomitant decrease in alexithymia—our clients now knew what they were feeling.

Rather than EMDR breaking through dissociative barriers, clients seemed to be able to effectively synthesize and integrate the dysfunctionally stored information, as well as make choices about what material they wanted to work on. Clients who had previously looped at a high level of disturbance with significant abreaction were now able to utilize the Standard Protocol effectively without any additional interventions by the therapist. Instead, clients seemed to spontaneously integrate previous ego-state techniques, inner-child work, as well as to access resources into their processing using the Standard Protocol, without the need on the part of the therapist to facilitate such a process.

Overall, there appeared to be much decreased primary and secondary dissociation. Tertiary dissociation was reduced with concomitant increase in co-consciousness between ego states. In one case, there was a decrease in "dissociative voices" that previously had not responded to neuroleptic medications. Somatization was greatly reduced. In one case where a client reported the onset of migraine headache activity prior to EMDR processing, the pain stopped almost immediately after naloxone injection. In some clients with more complex dissociative disorders, there appeared to be spontaneous recovery of previously dissociated traumatic memories. This did not seem to pose a problem to individuals who were processing these events in treatment but could be disturbing to those who receive opiate blockade without the benefit of an established therapeutic relationship.

Finally, the severity of visible abreaction was minimized and processing appeared to occur more rapidly. There appeared to be much-increased self-regulation and affect tolerance during EMDR processing that coincided with greater ego strength and ability to tolerate the traumatic material. This suggests that dissociation associated with reaccessing traumatic material interferes with affective regulation. This is illustrated by the following quotes from clients:

CLIENT RESPONSES AFTER OPIOID
ANTAGONIST MEDIATED EMDR SESSIONS

Clients' subjective experiences reflect the reduction of dissociative symptoms after using opioid antagonists in EMDR processing.

Robbie:	"Wow it's nice to feel the ground. I've never felt my feet on the ground before."
Chris:	"I couldn't have faced that without the naloxone."
Winona:	"A wave of numbness went through my legs and out."
Lois:	"I can't seem to back away from it the way I usually do, and yet it wasn't so bad."
Becky:	"The voices have stopped, my groin doesn't hurt anymore, the headaches are gone for the first time in 10 years."
Felicia:	"I like it; it makes me not sad, sort of dozy. It stops my worry thoughts."

CAVEATS AND CONTRAINDICATIONS FOR
THE USE OF OPIOID ANTAGONISTS

Opioid antagonists should be used only within an established psychotherapeutic relationship, as their use can be experienced as aversive if an attachment figure or transitional object such as the therapist is not available. Therefore, the use of an opioid antagonist should never be initiated prior to the primary therapist going away on vacation.

Furthermore, opioid antagonists will result in profound avoidance reactions to aversive or threatening stimuli. For instance, they may result in some circumstances in a client leaving an abusive relationship. However, this is only possible if there is a potential escape route or place for the client. If such is not available, being in an abusive relationship while on opioid antagonists is at least very aversive and potentially traumatizing if adequate resources, either internal or external, are not available.

Furthermore, because of increased behavioral avoidance, homework assignments that include exposure should be avoided until traumatic material is completely processed. The therapist needs to ensure that such behavioral avoidance is not ecologically appropriate (e.g., the return into an abusive relationship or to a workplace where harassment is likely to occur).

In general, do not use the described protocol with clients who continue to exhibit severe affect dysregulation and significant amnesia for significant parts of their lives. That is, the reduction in primary and secondary dissociation can result in clients spontaneously recovering previously dissociated material. Such memories may be overwhelming. Even relatively large dosages of opioid antagonists may be insufficient to keep the client from dissociating all over again, making such an experience retraumatizing. Thus, in the face of a lack of sufficient affect dysregulation or insufficient ego strength to manage this material, a resurfacing of traumatic memories may result in a sudden deterioration in functioning. While this does not preclude the use of opioid antagonists, focus needs to remain on stabilization rather than trauma processing and different dosage regimes may be more appropriate in this kind of population (e.g., Lanius, 2003, 2004a).

The following adverse effects of naloxone have been reported to occur in a significant percentage of patients: nausea, vomiting, sweating, tachychardia, increased blood pressure, and reversal of analgesia. With naltrexone, these symptoms can also hold true and, in our experience, the likelihood of gastric distress (abdominal pains, nausea, vomiting) is much more likely to occur.

With regard to blood pressure and heart rate, in our client sample we found generally slightly increased heart rate and blood pressure. Clients who exhibited extremes in both directions generally exhibited less lability. However, it should be noted that Ibarra and associates (1994) described a case of a 32-year-old male with PTSD, from a sample of 24 patients who exhibited an unusual behavioral and cardiovascular reaction during opioid blockade with naltrexone. He experienced significantly increased ambulatory blood pressures during the 24-hour period following naltrexone, as well as feelings of rage, explosive behavior, and other unpleasant symptoms.

Naltrexone has clear hepatotoxic (liver toxicity) potential, particularly at higher doses. While this is less of an issue with single dosing prior to the session as compared to continuous dosing, a liver function test should be obtained at the discretion of the prescribing clinician prior to prescribing opioid antagonists. The use of naltrexone is contraindicated in acute hepatitis or liver failure.

Clients should be opiate free (street drugs, painkillers) for 7–10 days prior to using naltrexone or naloxone with EMDR, as opioid antagonists can precipitate an acute withdrawal reaction. In particular, ongoing opioid use is of concern. As naltrexone preferentially binds to opioid receptors, opioid users will sometimes turn to huge amounts of opioids to override the blocking action of naltrexone, thereby potentially negatively affecting liver functioning. This can be fatal. Thus, clients need to be cautioned never to attempt to override the antinarcotic effects with large doses of opiates. If there is any doubt about ongoing opioid use, a so-called Narcan (naloxone) washout prior to commencing naltrexone is recommended.

Clients need to be advised that naltrexone in the described dosages results in a significant reversal of analgesia. Clients on these medications need to know that while the drug is active they will have an impaired ability to respond to opioids for pain relief and may require the use of nonopioid analgesics, benzodiazepines, spinal block, and general anesthesia in cases of emergency. While this is a much-reduced problem with single doses prior to sessions, it is nevertheless important that clients are aware of potential complications in case of medical emergencies or injuries (e.g., motor vehicle accidents). The use of a Medicalert bracelet is recommended.

Opioid antagonists can affect appetite and food intake. With repeated administration in previously overweight clients, some weight reduction commonly occurs with eventual stabilization. With regard to bulimia, some positive effect with regard to reduction of bingeing has been noted. On the other hand, some caution is indicated in clients with a diagnosis of anorexia. Reduced appetite in two clients with both dissociative disorders and anorexia was noted. Another client with anorexia who did not exhibit severe ego-state fragmentation showed improved appetite.

Some clients report feeling intoxicated or high upon the initial administration of an opioid antagonist. This commonly diminishes with prolonged or repeated usage and it may be attributable to a partial reversal of opioid tolerance. Therefore, it is recommended that clients be advised not to operate a motor vehicle until their response to opioid antagonists has been established.

Some clients with complex dissociative disorders will occasionally report visual disturbance (e.g., seeing multiple images in their visual field). This may represent an epiphenomenon of partial co-consciousness. If clients are advised about this prior to experiencing it, it usually does not present a problem and they don't experience much anxiety.

As noted earlier, one client, while on a continuous dose of naltrexone (50 mg qid) developed endometriosis-related pneumothorax. However, whether there is any causal connection to the use of naltrexone remains to be established.

Apart from opioids, the use of other medications while undergoing opioid antagonist–mediated EMDR sessions has not posed a problem— some of the clients in our case studies were on antidepressant medications (selective seretonin reuptake inhibitors [SSRIs]), as well as atypical neuroleptics. Nevertheless, there is some suggestion that opioid antagonists may influence the absorption rates of other medications (Nuller and colleagues, 2001). We observed changes in international normalized ratio (INR) levels in one client who was on warfarin (Coumadin), a blood thinner and anticoagulant. If there is any doubt, the prescribing physician or a pharmacologist should be consulted regarding possible drug interaction effects.

Finally, caution with regard to administration to mothers of newborns is indicated because of the endogenous opioid system's involvement in attachment. For instance, even though animal research suggests that opioid antagonists increase care-taking behavior, they may decrease the quality of such behavior.

PROTOCOL FOR THE ADJUNCTIVE USE OF OPIOID ANTAGONISTS FOR EMDR PROCESSING

Therapist Considerations: Therapists who consider using opioid antagonists should have experience with treating dissociative symptoms and disorders. They should be able to draw on the standard repertoire of techniques used with this population and should be comfortable treating clients with those symptoms. If in any doubt, clinicians should obtain supervision prior to proceeding with treatment. As attachment is at least in part mediated by opioids, blocking the opioid system can be aversive during times when the therapist is on vacation or unavailable. Therefore, therapist availability is essential.

Preparation Phase: Opioid antagonists should only be initiated when a therapeutic relationship with good rapport has been established. I refer the reader to the relevant section in *Eye Movement Desensitization and Reprocessing.* Client readiness and client safety factors are paramount (Shapiro, 2001). Ensure that the client's current living situation is sufficiently stable.

Adequate client preparation is essential. This should include an adequate amount of time spent on stabilization prior to embarking on metabolization of traumatic events. In my experience clients will often utilize previously learned self-soothing skills and stabilization techniques on their own once an opiate antagonist is administered, even though they may previously have had some difficulty applying these strategies without therapist assistance.

Client Factors/Informed Consent: Clients who exhibit a lack of response to EMDR due to excessive dissociative symptoms or somatization may be good candidates. Specifically, the adjunctive use of an opioid antagonist may be considered if there is evidence for significant dissociation or somatization, including depersonalization, derealization, cognitive looping, or a lack of body awareness during EMDR processing that precludes successful treatment.

Clients should be familiar and comfortable with the EMDR process. They need to be informed about the rationale of using an opioid antagonist. Potential caveats, contraindications, and side effects need to be discussed by the therapist, including the experimental nature of this approach.

Prescription: If the client feels comfortable to proceed, the therapist, unless also the prescribing clinician, needs to contact the prescribing clinician. As this is an off-label prescription, the prescribing clinician will usually require some background information regarding the use of opioid antagonists in populations with dissociative symptoms and traumatic stress syndromes.

This can usually be accomplished by providing an abstract of one of the cited articles. I commonly use the Bohus and colleagues (1999) article.

Opioid Antagonist Choices and Dosages: With regard to possible opioid antagonists, there is either naltrexone (Revia, oral) or naloxone (Narcan, injectable).

Naltrexone was administered 30–60 minutes prior to the session, with an initial dosage of either 25 mg or 50 mg. The standard dosage for naltrexone is 50 mg. The range of dosages in our series of case studies was 25–125 mg, with the doses above 50 mg being slowly titrated upward if there was ongoing depersonalization. Naltrexone is appropriate for longer sessions but is more likely to produce gastrointestinal side effects. If there is ongoing blocking on 50 mg of naltrexone, usually more time needs to be spent on client preparation, but in some cases increasing dosage may also assist the client to work through the traumatic memory.

Naloxone needs to be injected subcutaneously at 1 mg subcutaneously at the beginning of the session, which usually limits its use to a clinician who has prescription privileges. Due to the short half-life of naloxone, it is important that EMDR processing begin immediately after injection without delay, as the effects of naloxone essentially wanes after 60 minutes. Naloxone appears to be the preferred choice if there are significant adverse gastrointestinal symptoms.

Choice of Protocol: Opioid antagonists may be used with any protocol suitable for the population being treated. As noted above, in many cases the Standard Protocol appears to be sufficient, but in more complex cases, specialized protocols may be necessary to optimize treatment effects.

DISCUSSION

Administration of an opioid antagonist to clients with severe traumatic stress syndromes prior to EMDR processing suggested that managing these symptoms with opiate antagonists may facilitate

EMDR processing, especially in cases where there is evidence of severe dissociation or somatoform dissociation. When an opioid antagonist was administered prior to treatment, clients who had previously been unable to benefit from EMDR, even when special protocols for Dissociative Disorders were utilized, were now able to undergo EMDR and process traumatic material to resolution or to a level of decreased disturbance. Clients appeared to be able to stay with the process much better without undue dissociative symptoms when having been administered an opioid antagonist.

These findings are consistent with a phasic activation of the endogenous opioid system during reaccessing of traumatic memories in dissociative clients, and they support the notion that increased activity of the opioid system contributes to dissociative symptoms. Moreover, rather than continuous dosing being necessary, use of an opioid antagonist just prior to the EMDR session seems sufficient to facilitate and maintain this treatment effect, thus much reducing the risk of untoward side effects and potential complications.

Interestingly enough, the administration of naltrexone prior to an EMDR session greatly reduces visible abreaction in clients, lending credence to notion that the concept of abreaction be replaced with one of synthesis (van der Hart, Steele, Boon, & Brown, 1993). That is, opioid blockade appeared to result in much less distress during the accessing of the traumatic material, by potentially allowing for improved self-regulation, contributing to more effective information processing.

Opioid antagonists may not only facilitate EMDR processing using the Standard Protocol but also greatly enhance client response to other interventions, such as RDI, Safe Place, ego-state therapy including inner-child work, and other hypnotically based stabilization techniques (Ferrie & Lanius, 2002). In addition, opioid antagonists appear to have beneficial effects on DBT (Bohus et al., 1999) and sensorimotor psychotherapy (Lanius, 2003). Therefore, the use of opioid antagonists may allow for a shortened period of stabilization and preparation. At the same time, opioid antagonists clearly do not obviate the use of appropriate stabilization and preparation prior to venturing into trauma focused work. It should be noted, however, that when using opiate antagonists for stabilization, different dosages may be appropriate (Lanius, 2003, 2004a), particularly in cases where there is significant amnesia and a lack of co-consciousness between ego states.

Furthermore, initial observations suggest that the timing of the use of opioid antagonists is crucial to maximizing their effectiveness.

Based on my familiarity with several cases, the potential aversiveness of using opioid antagonists appears to be minimized when used within an established therapeutic relationship, when compared to the effects when used outside such an established relationship. This may be attributable to the fact that the opioid system is significantly involved in attachment.

In summary, the use of opioid antagonists in conjunction with EMDR treatment is an innovative method that conjoins pharmacological interventions and psychotherapeutic interventions. Particularly, this approach shows potential with regard to the treatment of traumatic memories in clients who exhibit significant dissociative symptoms or are experiencing excessive somatization, as it appears to reduce dissociative symptoms, thereby enhancing EMDR information processing. Nevertheless, even though the above-described therapeutic effects are promising, the use of opioid antagonists in conjunction with EMDR treatment should be considered an experimental treatment until these findings can be replicated in a placebo-controlled, double-blind study.

REFERENCES

American Psychiatric Association (2000). *Diagnostic and statistical manual of mental disorders,* (4th ed., text revision). Washington, DC: author.

Barach, P. M. M. (1991). Multiple personality disorder as an attachment disorder. *Dissociation, 4,* 117–123.

Bohus, M. J., Landwehrmeyer, G. B., Stiglmayr, C. E., Limberger, M. F., Bohme, R., & Schmahl, C. G. (1999). Naltrexone in the treatment of dissociative symptoms in patients with borderline personality disorder: An open-label trial. *Journal of Clinical Psychiatry, 60,* 598–603.

Bonnet, K. A., Hiller, J. S., & Simon, E. J. (1976). The effects of chronic opiate treatment and social isolation on opiate receptors in the rodent brain. In H. W. Kosterlitz (Ed.), *Opiate and endogenous opioid peptides* (pp. 335–343). Amsterdam: Elsevier.

Bowlby, J. (1978). Attachment theory and its therapeutic implications. In S. C. Feinstein & P. L. Giovacchini (Eds.), *Adolescent psychiatry: Developmental and clinical studies* (pp. 5–33). Chicago: University of Chicago Press.

Bowlby, J. (1997). *Attachment.* London: Pimlico.

Brewin, C. R., Dalgleish, T., & Joseph, S. (1996). A dual representation theory of posttraumatic stress disorder. *Psychological Review, 103,* 670–686.

Fanselow, M. S. (1986). Conditioned fear-induced opiate analgesia: A compelling motivational state theory of stress analgesia. *New York Academy of Sciences, 467,* 40–54.

Ferrie, R. K., & Lanius, U. F. (2001, June). *Opioid antagonists and EMDR*. Paper presented at the EMDRIA Conference, Austin, TX.

Ferrie, R. K., & Lanius, U. F. (2002, June). *The neurobiology of opiates: Opioid antagonists and EMDR*. Paper presented at the EMDRIA Conference, San Diego, CA.

Fisher, J. (2003, September). *Minding the Body: Integrating EMDR and Somatic Psychotherapy*. Paper presented at the EMDRIA Conference, Denver, CO.

Forgash, C. (2002). *Deepening EMDR treatment effects across the diagnostic spectrum: Integrating EMDR and ego state work* [Video]. http://www.emdrandego statevideo.com. Self-published.

Glover, H. (1993). A preliminary trial of nalmefene for the treatment of emotional numbing in combat veterans with post-traumatic stress disorder. *Israel Journal of Psychiatry and Related Sciences, 30*, 255–263.

Gold, M. S., Pottash, A. C., Sweeney, D., Martin, D., & Extein, I. (1982). Antimanic, antidepressant and antipanic effects of opiates: Clinical neuroanatomical and biochemical evidence. *Annals of the New York Academy of Sciences, 398*, 140–150.

Hamner, M. B., & Hitri, A. (1992). Plasma beta-endorphin levels in post-traumatic stress disorder: A preliminary report on response to exercise-induced stress. *Journal of Neuropsychiatry and Clinical Neurosciences, 4*, 59–63.

Hemingway, R. B., & Reigle, T. G. (1987). The involvement of endogenous opiate systems in learned helplessness and stress-induced analgesia. *Psychopharmacology, 93*, 3353–3357.

Herman, J. L. (1992). *Trauma and recovery*. New York: Basic Books.

Ibarra, P., Bruehl S. P., McCubbin, J. A., Carlson, C. R., Wilson, J. F., Norton, J. A., & Montgomery, T. B. (1994). An unusual reaction to opioid blockade with naltrexone in a case of post-traumatic stress disorder. *Journal of Trauma Stress, 7*, 303–309.

Jaycox, L. H., Foa, E. B., & Morral, A. R. (1998). Influence of emotional engagement and habituation on exposure therapy for PTSD. *Journal of Consulting and Clinical Psychology, 66*, 185–192.

Kalin, N. H., Shelton, S. E., Rickman, M., & Davidson, R. J. (1998). Individual differences in freezing and cortisol in infant and mother rhesus monkeys. *Behavioral Neuroscience, 112*, 251–254.

Kaufman, I. C., & Rosenblum, L. A. (1967). The reaction to separation in infant monkeys: Anaclitic depression and conservation-withdrawal. *Psychosomatic Medicine, 40*, 649–675.

Kaufman, I. C., & Rosenblum, L. A. (1969). Effects of separation from mother on the emotional behavior of infant monkeys. *Annals of the New York Academy of Sciences, 159*, 681–695.

Kelly, D. D. (1982). The role of endorphins in stress-related analgesia. *Annals of New York Academy of Sciences, 398*, 260–271.

King, A. C., Schluger, J., Gunduz, M., Borg, L., Perret, G., Ho, A., & Kreek, M. J. (2002). Hypothalamic-pituitary-adrenocortical (HPA) axis response and biotransformation of oral naltrexone: Preliminary examination of relationship to family history of alcoholism. *Neuropsychopharmacology, 26*, 778–788.

Kling, A., and Steklis, H. D. (1976). A neural substrate for affiliative behavior in non-human primates. *Brain Behavior Evolution, 13*, 216–238.

Korn, D. L., & Leeds, A. M. (2002). Preliminary evidence of efficacy for EMDR resource development and installation in the stabilization phase of treatment of complex posttraumatic stress disorder. *Journal of Clinical Psychology, 58*, 1465–1487.

Lanius, U. F. (2000, April). *Dissociative processes and EMDR—staying connected*. Paper presented at the North West Regional EMDR Conference, Vancouver, British Columbia.

Lanius, U. F. (2002, November). *Trauma, neuroscience and EMDR*. Paper presented at the EMDRAC AGM. Vancouver, BC.

Lanius, U. F. (2003, October). *The neurobiology of attachment and dissociation: Clinical implications*. Paper presented, Complex Trauma Treatment Approaches, Loch Lomond Shores, Balloch, Glasgow, Scotland.

Lanius, U. F. (2004a, September). *Attachment and dissociation: The role of endogenous opioids*. Paper presented at the EMDRIA Conference, Montreal, Quebec.

Lanius, U. F. (2004b, September). *PTSD, information processing and thalamocortical dialogue*. Paper presented at the EMDRIA Conference, Montreal, Quebec.

Lanius, R. A., Bluhm, R., Lanius, U. F., & Pain, C. (in press). Neuroimaging of hyperarousal and dissociation in PTSD: Heterogeneity of response to symptom provocation. *Journal of Psychiatric Research*.

Lanius, R. A., Williamson, P. C., Boksman, K., Densmore, M., Gupta, M., Neufeld, R.W., Gati, J. S., & Menon, R. S. (2002). Brain activation during script-driven imagery induced dissociative responses in PTSD: A functional magnetic resonance imaging investigation. *Biological Psychiatry, 52*, 305–311.

Lanius, R. A., Williamson, P. C., Densmore, M., Boksman, K., Neufeld, R.W., Gati, J. S., & Menon, R. S. (2004). The nature of traumatic memories: A 4-T FMRI functional connectivity analysis. *American Journal of Psychiatry, 161*, 36–44.

Lazrove, S., & Fine, C. G. (1996). The use of EMDR in patients with dissociative identity disorder. *Dissociation, 9*, 289–299.

Linehan, M. M. (1993). *Cognitive-behavioral treatment of borderline personality disorder*. New York: Guilford Press.

Lubin, G., Weizman, A., Shmushkevitz, M., & Valevski, A. (2002). Short-term treatment of post-traumatic stress disorder with naltrexone: An open-label preliminary study. *Human Psychopharmacology, 17*, 181–185.

Makino, M., Kitano, Y., Komiyama, C., Hirohashi, M., & Takasuna, K. (2000). Involvement of central opioid systems in human interferon-alpha induced immobility in the mouse forced swimming test. *British Journal of Pharmacology, 130*, 1269–1274.

Maurer, R. G., & Teitelbaum, P. (1998, November). *PTSD, opioids, and antipredator behavior: A pilot treatment study with naltrexone*. Paper presented at the annual meeting of the International Society for Traumatic Stress Studies, Washington, DC.

Newman, J. D., Murphy, M. R., & Harbough, C. R. (1982). Naloxone-reversible suppression of isolation call production after morphine injections in squirrel monkeys. *Society for Neuroscience Abstract, 8*, 940.

Nijenhuis, E. R. J. (1999). *Somatoform dissociation*. Assen, Netherlands: van Gorcum and Comp. B.V.

Nuller, Y. L., Morozova, M. G., Kushnir, O. N., & Hamper, N. (2001). Effect of naloxone therapy on depersonalization: A pilot study. *Journal of Psychopharmacology, 15*, 93–95.

Ogden, P. (2004, September). *Empowering the body: Somatic awareness and physical action in the treatment of trauma and dissociation.* Paper presented at the EMDRIA Conference, Montreal, Quebec.

Ogden, P., & Minton, K. (2000). Sensorimotor sequencing: One method for processing trauma. *Traumatology, 6.* Available at http://www.fsu.edu/~trauma/v6i3/v6i3a3.html

Panksepp, J., Nelson, E., & Sivey, S. (1994). Brain opioids and mother-infant social motivation. *Acta Paediatrica, 397* (Suppl.), 40–46.

Panksepp, J., Siviy, S. M., & Normansell, L. A. (1985). Brain opioids and social emotions. In M. Reite & T. Fields (Eds.), *The psychobiology of attachment and separation* (pp. 3–49). Orlando, FL: Academic Press.

Paulsen, S. (1995). EMDR and its cautious use in the dissociative disorders. *Dissociation, 8*, 32–44.

Perry B. (1999). *The memories of states.* In J. Goodwin & R. Attias (Eds.), *Splintered Reflections: images of the body in trauma* (pp. 9–38). New York: Basic.

Pitman, R. K., van der Kolk, B. A., Orr, S. P., & Greenberg, M. S. (1990). Naloxone-reversible analgesic response to combat-related stimuli in posttraumatic stress disorder. A pilot study. *Archives of General Psychiatry, 47*, 541–544.

Powles, W. E. (1992). *Human development and homeostasis.* Madison, CT: International Universities Press.

Schmahl, C., Stiglmayr, C., Böhme, R., & Bohus, M. (1999). Behandlung von dissoziativen Symptomen bei Borderline-Persönlichkeitsstörungen mit Naltrexon [Treatment of dissociative symptoms in borderline patients with naltrexone]. *Nervenarzt, 70*, 262–264.

Shapiro, F. (2001). *Eye movement desensitization and reprocessing: Basic principles, protocols, and procedures* (2nd ed.). New York: Guilford Press.

Twombly, J. (2000). Incorporating EMDR and EMDR adaptations into the treatment of clients with dissociative identity disorders. *Journal of Trauma and Dissociation, 1*, 61–81.

van der Hart, O., Steele, K., Boon, S., & Brown, P. (1993). The treatment of traumatic memories: Synthesis, realization, and integration. *Dissociation, 6*, 162–180.

van der Hart, O., van der Kolk, B. A., & Boon, S. (1996). The treatment of dissociative disorders. In J. D. Bremner & C. R. Marmer (Eds.), *Trauma, memory and dissociation* (pp. 253–283). Washington, DC: American Psychiatric Press.

van der Kolk, B. A. (1989). The compulsion to repeat the trauma: Reenactment, revictimization, and masochism. *Psychiatric Clinics of North America, 12*, 389–411.

van der Kolk, B. A. (1996). Trauma and memory. In B. A. van der Kolk, A. C. McFarlane, & L. Weisaeth (Eds.), *Traumatic stress: The effects of overwhelming experience on mind, body, and society* (pp. 279–302). New York: Guilford Press.

van der Kolk, B. A., & Fisler, R. (1995). Dissociation and the fragmentary nature of traumatic memories: Review and experimental confirmation. *Journal of Traumatic Stress, 8*, 505–525.

van der Kolk, B. A., Greenberg, M. S., Orr, S. P., & Pitman, R. K. (1989). Endogenous opioids, stress induced analgesia, and posttraumatic stress disorder. *Psychopharmacology Bulletin, 25*, 417–421.

van der Kolk, B. A., Pelcovitz, D., Roth, S., Mandel, F. S., McFarlane, A., & Herman, J. L. (1996). Dissociation, affect regulation and somatization: The complex nature of adaptation to trauma. *American Journal of Psychiatry, 153* (Suppl.), 83–93.

Williams, K. L., Ko, M. C., Rice, K. C., & Woods, J. H. (2003). Effect of opioid receptor antagonists on hypothalamic-pituitary-adrenal activity in rhesus monkeys. *Psychoneuroendocrinology, 28*, 513–528.

Yehuda, R. (2001). Biology of posttraumatic stress disorder. *Clinical Psychiatry, 62* (Suppl.), 41–46.

Zurita, A., Martijena, I., Cuadra, G., Brandao, M. L., & Molina, V. (2000). Early exposure to chronic variable stress facilitates the occurrence of anhedonia and enhanced emotional reactions to novel stressors: Reversal by naltrexone pretreatment. *Behavioral Brain Research, 117*, 163–171.

RECOMMENDED READINGS

Herman, J. L. (1992). *Trauma and recovery*. New York: Basic Books.

Levine, P. (1997). *Waking the tiger*. Berkeley, CA: North Atlantic Books.

Linehan, M. M. (1993). *Cognitive-behavioral treatment of borderline personality disorder*. New York: Guilford Press.

Nijenhuis, E. R. J. (1999). *Somatoform dissociation*. Assen, Netherlands: Van Gorcum and Comp. B.V.

Ogden, P., & Minton, K. (2000). Sensorimotor sequencing: One method for processing trauma. *Traumatology, 6*. Available at: http://www.fsu.edu/~trauma/v6i3/v6i3a3.html

Parnell, L. (1999). *EMDR in the treatment of adults abused as children*. New York: Norton.

Putnam, F. W. (1989). *Diagnosis and treatment of multiple personality disorder*. New York: Guilford Press.

Putnam, F. W. (1997). *Dissociation in children and adolescents: A developmental perspective*. New York: Guilford Press.

Schore, A. (2001a). The effects of a secure attachment relationship on right brain development, affect regulation, and infant mental health. *Infant Journal of Mental Health, 22*, 7–66. Available at http://www.trauma-pages.com/schore-2001a.htm

Schore, A. (2001b). The effects of early relational trauma on right brain development, affect regulation, and infant mental health. *Infant Journal of Mental Health, 22*, 201–269. Available at http://www.trauma-pages.com/schore-2001b.htm

van der Hart, O., Steele, K., Boon, S., & Brown, P. (1993). The treatment of traumatic memories: Synthesis, realization, and integration. *Dissociation, 6,* 162–180.

van der Kolk, B. A., McFarlane, A., & Weisaeth, L. (Eds.). (1996). *Traumatic stress.* New York: Guilford Press.

Watkins, J., & Watkins, H. (1997). *Ego states: Theory and therapy.* New York: Norton.

Chapter 5

The Phantom Limb Pain Protocol

Robert H. Tinker and Sandra A. Wilson

FOLLOWING AN AMPUTATION OF ALMOST ANY BODY PART, THE PATIENT can experience phantom limb *sensation*, which is the feeling that the limb is still there, or phantom limb *pain* (PLP), which is pain that exists after the amputation (Sherman, 1997). Often the pain after the amputation is the pain that existed before the amputation, somehow staying locked in the nervous system. The pain associated with phantom pain can be severe. On a scale of 0 to 10 (10 being most severe), around a 7 or 8 experience of PLP significantly interferes with a person's quality of life to the point that the person has difficulty sleeping, working, and thinking. The person often becomes addicted to drugs to kill the pain. Some people commit suicide because of the intractable pain and the lack of any hope of relief. The pain might be a cramping sensation, searing pain, tingling, itching, aching, or almost any other kind of pain that a person can experience. In any part of the body that's been amputated, a person can continue to feel PLP. For example, phantom tooth pain, phantom breast pain, and phantom gall bladder pain, among others, are recognized as phantom pains (Sherman, 1997). Between 60% (Jensen, Krebs, Nielsen, & Rasmussen, 1985) and 70% (Melzak, 1992) of amputees suffer pain in their phantom limbs, with such pain continuing to exist after 20 years (Sherman, 1997). Very often, the greater the pain before amputation, the greater the pain following amputation (Sherman, 1997).

As of 1996, there were 1.2 million amputees in the United States, with a 38% increase each year over the last 5 years (Amputee Coalition of America, 2004). Ninety-seven percent are lower limb amputations, with 82% being from vascular disorders (Amputee Coalition of America, 2004). Other than vascular disorders, cancer and traffic accidents account for the most amputations (Amputee Coalition of America, 2004). As more people become obese, diabetes becomes more prevalent, and as our population ages, there are more amputations per year. In the last few years diabetes among children has increased and consequently there are more amputations among children, as well. There's been a big switch from orthopedic surgeons to vascular surgeons doing the amputation (Sherman, 1997). Orthopedic surgeons usually amputate below the knee so that about 80% of the leg function remains, but vascular surgeons tend to amputate above the knee, causing the person to retain only 30% of leg functioning (Sherman, 1997). There is greater recovery of usable function following successful EMDR treatment of below-the-knee amputations.

PLP sufferers are dealing for example, with a leg or a foot that is not there, but one that causes pain as though it is. In their view, they have a physical problem. They're often worried about being judged to be crazy, so there's almost no likelihood of them going to a psychologist for treatment. The first 3 months after surgery, the wound is healing and the doctors are unlikely to recognize or treat PLP. After healing has occurred, doctors are likely to ignore PLP, as they are not aware of effective treatments for it. They might refer to another professional for relaxation training, biofeedback, physical therapy, prosthetic adjustment, or other forms of palliative care. The 50-plus known treatments for PLP have at most about 8% effectiveness that lasts over time (Sherman, 1997). The physician is likely to be reluctant to prescribe painkillers for limbs that are not there.

PLP patients deal with troubling pain that ostensibly shouldn't be there. After physical healing takes place but the PLP remains, patients don't get much help from the medical community. Instead, what happens is that the prosthetist, who forms the new prosthetic leg or arm, is the one who ends up dealing with emotional sequelae from the loss of a limb. Prosthetists report that 50% of the time the patients faint when they first see the stump. Most of the time there's an abreaction to this awful loss. The prosthetic often ends up becoming the focus of the PLP. The average prosthetic leg costs $9,000. A good one runs $20,000. An up-to-date, above-the-knee, computerized prosthetic (a C leg) costs upward of $70,000 (Amputee Coalition of America, 2004). Patients often say, "Okay, the PLP is because I don't have a good fit," so they keep going back to the prosthetist to get an adjustment or a new prosthesis. Often the prosthetist puts the prosthetic limb on the workbench, makes adjustments, listens sympathetically, and the patient will say, "Oh, it feels much better." But unfortunately the pain isn't relieved for long.

In 1996, in Los Angeles, Dr. Francine Shapiro had a facilitators' meeting that Dr. Robert Tinker and I attended. At that time, she told us what happened when Linda Vanderlaan went to Bogota, Columbia, to visit her sister, who was running an orphanage in which the children had cancer or AIDS. One of the children was an 8-year-old girl, Anna Marie, who had an amputated leg as a result of cancer. Linda began working with her, using EMDR to help reduce her trauma of the loss of her leg. After the session, the girl reported to Linda that her PLP had disappeared.

At that time Dr. Tinker and I decided to start a research study with amputees. In 1996 we did a pilot study, using a case series approach, with seven amputees. We wanted to see if EMDR could be effective in treating PLP. We thought that PLP might be similar to posttraumatic stress disorder (PTSD), in that the event is over but the pain (emotional or physical) is still there, somehow embedded in the nervous system. Since EMDR is very effective with PTSD, and it had already been shown to work in one PLP case, we thought that it might be an effective treatment for other forms of PLP. In our case series, EMDR was found to be an effective treatment for PLP (complete elimination) in leg amputations. In most of the cases, pain disappeared within three sessions of treatment after the initial diagnostic interview.

We started the study in June 1996, and it's ongoing; we've continued following patients in 2005. Elizabeth, 49 years old, was our first client. She had had a blood clot in her leg, and she refused a full amputation. As a result, the doctors waited to see what circulation remained in her leg, in order to determine how much of her leg had to be amputated. Some circulation remained to her heel, which developed extreme pain. Within a week they had made a decision to make a below-the-knee amputation. Following surgery, the PLP was concentrated in her heel. She had thought that the terrible heel pain would be gone after the surgery. She was rudely surprised and said with frustration, "They amputated the leg, but they forgot to amputate the pain." She came to us for the study after 1 year of constant PLP. She had stopped working full-time. She was depressed and crying every day. She was using medication and alcohol to lessen the pain and to attempt to sleep in spite of the pain. She had completely changed her routine. She could function only

2 or 3 hours a day. The initial clinical interview took 3 hours. After that, in the first EMDR session (2 hours in duration), her PLP disappeared and didn't come back. In the second session, we worked with her depression, following which she was able to taper off her antidepressant medication. The third session was primarily a closing session.

In the protocol approach that Dr. Tinker and I developed, we first worked on the most traumatic aspect of the loss. The worst for her was that she didn't know what she could do with the rest of her life, since she wasn't whole or capable anymore. So we worked on the trauma of her awakening after the amputation, her worst memory. When that resolved down to 0 SUDS, we then focused on her phantom pain. As she attended to that, the pain began to move and change, and finally disappeared. This process seems analogous to how emotion from trauma begins to change, shift, and disappear with EMDR.

I did a 1-year follow-up with Elizabeth, and the pain has never returned. She's working full-time; she's a registered nurse. She took up skiing. She still hikes in the Colorado Rockies, does a lot of fly-fishing with her son, and is able to stand in the water while fishing. Her depression didn't return. Her whole appearance changed once she got rid of the depression and the drug and alcohol usage to control the pain. She does more now than she did before. "I didn't know what I couldn't do. I still can't run, and sometimes I still try to put a sock on my foot, but I don't have any more pain."

Linda was our second client. She had been in a car accident and had her leg crushed 12 years prior to our treatment. Her injuries were so severe that she had had to remain in the hospital for a full year of inpatient treatment following her accident. Her PLP, again with the amputation below the knee, was a cramped foot that constantly felt like it was in a shoe two sizes too small (that she could never take off for 12 years!), with her toes painfully bent back over one another in agonizing positions. Perhaps she "remembered" that from what had happened to her foot in the accident. She had severe trauma and depression that had to be worked on in the first session to get down to 0 before we could concentrate on the cramped pain. That pain left in the second session. I did a 1-year follow-up with her. Again, lifestyle improved, and no pain returned. Following that, I did a 2-year follow-up with both Elizabeth and Linda. No pain had returned. Linda died 2 years ago, from congestive heart failure. In the years before she died, she counseled other amputees. A few months ago (in 2004) I talked to Elizabeth, and she confirmed that her PLP has never returned since her treatment 8 years before.

Then we worked with a young girl with a below-the-knee amputation. Her mother was more upset about the amputation than she was. The girl had a complicating issue of feeling like she had to take care of her mom. Her PLP went down from an 8 to only a 2 (the other two victims had gone to 0) and didn't really move much beyond that. She was okay with it, as it was her mother she was more worried about.

We worked with another woman, 52 years old. They accidentally cut the main vein in her leg during knee surgery and had to amputate her leg. She had thought she was just having a tendon fixed, but when she woke up from surgery, her leg was gone. She was furious because of what had happened, so her sessions were longer. It took about three sessions to get the traumatic aspects of the surgery over. Her SUDS level went down and stayed down. It took another series of sessions for the pain.

THE PROTOCOL

In general, the protocol for PLP consists of three parts: history-taking and relationship building, then targeting the trauma of the experience, and finally targeting the pain itself.

Phases 1 and 2: Client History and Preparation (2 to 3 hours)

That first session is about getting to understand what happened, what the injuries were, how they happened, how the amputees feel about it, what they can do. As a therapist, first you build up some trust so that the clients realize you don't think they're crazy. Take half an hour to make the patients understand that you're serious about treating a phenomenon like phantom pain that doesn't "exist" physically. You normalize their experience. They often have mental pictures; almost all amputees have frozen pictures of the stump or the accident, and they want you to see it through their eyes. Ask about getting the prosthesis, what it was like when they first saw the stump, and the first time a family member saw them without the limb.

You may lose all effectiveness if you show any revulsion. Become friends with the stump. Often, they want you to touch the stump or they want to take the prosthetic off and have you look at it and talk about it. They frequently want to talk about what functions they have with and without it.

In the second hour, you ask about the changes in lifestyle, the changes in self-esteem, and the amount of therapy and medication they have had. You ask about changes in social, occupational, recreational, and sexual lives, quality of life, family impacts, and activities in general. You get the story of the reorganization of their entire life. It used to take 20 or 30 minutes to get ready in the morning; now it takes an hour and a half. It takes an hour and a half to go to bed at night or to take a bath. I ask, *What do you really miss the most since you lost your leg?* They answer that they miss being able to cut the grass, shopping easily, climbing, hiking, or riding horses. Loss and grieving are symbolized in a lost activity. After the PLP and the trauma are gone, they often engage in that activity again. They take up golfing, go shopping, or add new activities, like learning to ski.

Ask about the family's responses. Most of the families have PTSD symptoms around the patients' traumas. For example, the children are traumatized that their mother has lost part of her leg. As a result, the children's behavior changes.

The clients develop self-esteem issues after the amputation. They don't feel valuable because of how people react to them because they have a missing limb. They all report about the constant staring and startle response of strangers, especially children. Kids point and stare because it's inconceivable to picture ourselves not whole. The clients tend to withdraw more and more as time goes by. You talk about that and then the issue of attractiveness. Women feel less attractive if their leg has been amputated, in contrast to their arms, less attractive if a breast has been amputated in comparison to an arm. Men have a loss of self-esteem around arm amputations, more than with leg amputations.

In the third hour, we go back to the limb, and we do a detailed analysis on every single part of that limb that hurts and how it hurts. We employ the commonly used Numeric Analog Scale (NAS; 0–10, with 10 being the worst pain imaginable) to rate the intensity of the pain. I also use the McGill Pain Scale in the interview. It has a drawing of the limb, and it has all the questions mentioned above. It rates several kinds of pain on four levels (none, mild, moderate, severe) including "throbbing, shooting, stabbing, sharp, cramping, gnawing, hot-burning, aching, heavy, tender, and splitting." It also rates the client's response to pain from none to severe, including "tiring-exhausting, sickening, fearful, and punishing-cruel."

Generally, by the time amputees get to us, they've tried about everything to get rid of their pain: physical therapy, massages, medications, and different routines. Often, a neuroma, which is a bundle of nerves, will form at the end of the stump, and they talk about that. That becomes a major issue. The fourth most common treatment for PLP is to surgically remove the neuroma, which shortens the limb. However, the more the surgeon shortens the stump, the more likely the patient is to lose function. When the surgeon blames the pain on the neuroma and amputates more of the limb, it's because he doesn't understand the cause of PLP.

Assessment and Desensitization
(Two to Five Sessions)

At the end of the third hour of the clinical interview, we set up the first EMDR target. We start with, *What is the worst traumatic aspect of this amputation experience?* We complete the EMDR assessment on that, and that's our first target. In the next session and beyond, if necessary, we clear out all traumatic targets around the amputation.

When the trauma targets are gone, we go back to the pain scale. The clients have previously completed an in-depth description of the pain. They have pointed to their toes or the wrist or the ankles that aren't there, which is a real confirmation of their experience. We have measured the amount of pain in the (nonexistent) big toe that's curled under. They have finally gotten to talk in detail and get some validation about their pain. When we're ready to do the processing, we're already familiar with this pain, we've cleared psychological trauma, and it's then easy to say, *Let's focus on the worst pain, the toe bent over backward, which is an 8, and let's start with that.* If you start with the worst pain, oftentimes the rest of the pain is released as well. If you don't get complete generalization, you go to the next pain, then the next pain.

However, the pain can be very complex. In a foot you might have cramping toes, a burning sensation, and a twisting sensation. You have to get a detailed description of the limb that's missing, where all the pain is, and exactly what kind of pain it is. So it might be that the calf is cramping, the ankle is twisting, the toes are cramped, the foot is cramped, and you focus on the exact pain, taking one at a time, taking the worst one first. Each one gets an NAS measure. You continue the EMDR with the client focusing on the pain until it changes or it leaves. Often the pain changes before it is eliminated, much as emotions change in EMDR as they diminish. At times there'll be initial report of tingling or a prickly feeling, followed by other changes, with the foot (for example) beginning to relax. Since I've been doing this work, *relax* is probably my favorite word, besides *love*, in the world. When people report that the limb relaxes, I know that the pain is leaving.

Arm and hand amputations need more EMDR sessions than leg amputations. The physiological explanation for that has to do with the size and complexity of the representation of the hand on the homunculus in the brain. The largest parts of the homunculus are devoted to the lip and the hand, a smaller part to the leg. The representation of the hand in the brain takes up a huge area. The thumb has its own large area; the finger, the hand, and wrist areas are smaller.

With one patient, we had more effect on PLP following an arm amputation by stimulating the upper lip, left-right, rather than using eye movements. In terms of the homunculus organization, the lip is right next to the hand. We stimulated the lip using the Tac/AudioScan, by taping the tappers, one on each side of the lip. We also still did some tactile tapping, touching left-right on the knees or shoulders. We've used EMDR with only bilateral lip stimulation. It's effective, but it processes faster for hand and arm amputations if it's done with more than one kind of stimulation.

To review: You do 3 hours of relationship building, intake, and target selection. You do one EMDR processing session, or however many it takes, with the trauma of the accident and the distress around it. You then directly focus on the pain until it goes away. When it is a leg amputation, or mastectomy, or a finger, it's generally one session. It can take more sessions with arm or hand amputations. If you use tactile stimulation on the upper lip with arm and hand amputations, the pain may process faster.

After you've cleared the pain, you can then work with the prescribing MD to have the patient withdraw from pain medication. After medication has been eliminated, you follow up to make sure the pain hasn't returned. I'm a researcher, so I do a 30-day and 60-day check. If the pain comes back, they're instructed to call back right away. There's a 1-year follow-up, and I've done much longer than that. The longest I've done has been 8 years with Elizabeth, the first patient.

Post Treatment

Dramatic things happen after clearing the trauma and pain. First, clients start to sleep. Before treatment, nearly all report that the pain is worse at night. As a result, a lot of these patients are very, very sleep deprived. After treatment, they get back to being able to sleep. Once they get sleep they feel better, and now there's no pain. Then they have energy, and they can live their life. They say their quality of life is greater than it was before. They go back to what is important: relationships, education, and however they want to spend their time. One lady said, "They didn't amputate my heart and soul."

When Elizabeth got over her pain and trauma, her 11-year-old son then went back to being more like a normal kid. He had been afraid to touch her. He wouldn't sit in her lap. He had been unrealistically good, doing extra work, but not being a normal, rambunctious youth. And it had been breaking her heart. After her pain had disappeared, she said, "He sat in my lap last night and we watched baseball together."

TREATMENT CONSIDERATIONS

The *meaning* of the amputation for the person can have a bearing on EMDR outcomes. Elective surgery can have a different feel in terms of psychological reorganization and acceptance. One woman in our case series had cancer, and because she had made the choice for amputation rather than have the cancer go through her body, she didn't regard it as a traumatic loss. Rather, she regarded her decision as lifesaving. In EMDR, she did a complete jump from an 8 to a 0 NAS.

Her acceptance was so complete after her pain was eliminated that she had no problem dancing and twirling around. One evening, while two-stepping, her partner twirled her and her prosthetic arm came off. He was standing there with her arm while she was lying on the floor laughing, but everyone around her was completely aghast. She explained that it was a prosthetic, put it back on in another room, returned, and continued dancing. There's a dramatic difference between this person and another who's lost an arm and hasn't left the house since. Again, the *attitude* of the person toward the amputation, or the *meaning* of the amputation for the person, can have an effect on the EMDR treatment.

Preamputation considerations can affect treatment. It's important to ask about any injuries to the limb before the amputation, even if they occurred years before. These experiences may become important targets for EMDR treatment. Without clearing them, the PLP may not move (J. Boel, personal communication, July 2004).

Family history can affect the treatment. A German man lost one third of his index finger. His reaction to the pain was so intense that he couldn't work, he wouldn't go out of the house, he couldn't cry, he couldn't have normal relationships, and he was having marital difficulties. I could not get this guy to move. In processing, he looped and looped. Finally I suggested a cognitive interweave. *I want you to picture yourself standing up on a stage. I want you to start with your father or your grandfather, people that you know in your heart really love you. I want them to come up and reject you now and not love you because you're missing part of your finger.* We got that set up, and he just about gave Nadia, the translator, and me heart attacks. He started with his grandfather, and suddenly he spoke emphatically and with astonishment, "Tradition! Tradition!"

It turned out that he had been the only "whole man" in the family. His grandfather lost the same finger in a woodworking accident, and his father lost the identical finger chopping wood. This guy did woodworking, and he lost his finger on the saw the way his grandfather lost his finger. As soon as it hit him that he had lost his sense of worth because there was no longer a whole man in the family, his pain went away. Then he started to cry and grieve the loss of his finger. He later said that he cried for 3 days. Then he went back to a full life. Again, the *meaning* of the pain was important to this person (but sometimes, unfortunately, the meaning is not conscious, as in this case). Things are not always easy, even with EMDR. This could easily have been an EMDR "failure" if the right key had not been found to unlock the unconscious connection.

The protocol works on other than PLP. Clinicians have found success using the PLP protocol to lower pain from car accidents. With motor vehicle accidents (MVAs), victims can have pain from structural damage (e.g., back injuries, nerve damage, closed head injuries, broken bones), as well as from whiplash syndromes and the primitive "freeze" response that remains locked in the body. It is difficult, if not impossible, to tell ahead of time whether the patient's pain is due to structural damage or whether it is a pain "memory," such as phantom pain, muscular tightness from the "freeze" response unreleased from the body, or whiplash (possibly the same thing as the unreleased freeze response). Once the trauma of the MVA has been dealt with, the pain remaining from the accident can be directly targeted, as in the PLP protocol. Alternatively, the pain itself can be targeted immediately when it comes up, in reprocessing the accident. Robin Shapiro had remarkable success using the PLP protocol with a young woman who had suffered a severe head injury. The woman's pain dropped from a life-shattering 9 to a manageable 3 (on a 0–10 scale) and her serious amnesia disappeared.

Research

When I was doing a research review on PLP, I found that there was a study being conducted at the University of Tübingen in Germany by Neils Birbaumer and Herta Flor, which was eventually published in 1997 (Birbaumer et al., 1997). They were working on a study with arm amputees using the magnetoencephalogram (MEG). The MEG has to be conducted in a vaultlike room, insulated from Earth's magnetic field. Inside the vault, a helmet that looks like a hair dryer, with 151 leads, is lowered onto the participant's head. This collector picks up and amplifies the minuscule magnetic emanations from the electrical activity in the brain. Think of it as being a multimillion-dollar improvement on the electroencephalogram (EEG), as it provides much better localization of brain activity. In studying PLP, the researchers stimulate the lower right lip 1,000 times a minute with air puffs; then they stimulate the left lower lip in the same fashion; and finally, they stimulate the unamputated thumb, 1,000 puffs per minute. From this, they can predict where the amputated thumb should be represented on the sensorimotor cortex. How far the observed scan deviates from the predicted one is directly related to the intensity of the phantom pain: the greater the reorganization (deviation from what was expected), the greater the PLP intensity. The researchers found that if they successfully induced a brachial-block anesthesia in a participant, eliminating the PLP, and then obtained another MEG reading, it was found to be reorganized back to normal, indicating no phantom pain. When the anesthesia wore off, the pain returned, and the MEG showed the prior reorganization again. What they learned from the scans was that the idle thumb neurons (from the missing thumb) had been recruited to respond as lip neurons when the lip was stimulated; the greater the recruitment, the greater the PLP.

And I'm thinking, simplistically, that we should be able to see the same changes in the MEG scans, when EMDR, instead of anesthesia, eliminates PLP. So I went over to Germany and worked with four patients at the University of Tübingen in the MEG lab. As predicted, we could see the pre–post changes. But I ran out of funding. It cost $2,000 for each MEG, and I was mostly paying for it myself. Arne Hofmann, an EMDR pioneer in Germany, also helped out with some of the funding, and he has continued to promote interest in this work.

Two years ago, Bernhard, a man with a traumatic arm amputation, came to Colorado Springs, and we worked with him for 2 weeks to eliminate his severe and intractable PLP. Because he had been a participant with the MEG, he hit upon the idea to stimulate his lips in EMDR when we were getting minimal changes from tapping his knees and shoulders. He said, "Well you know, Dr. San, they stimulated my lip to find out what the reorganization was, when they did the MEG. Why don't we tap my lip to see if it wouldn't take away the pain." It was the first time since 1996 that we got his pain down to a 0. We all cried; it was an incredible experience. And so then I trained him how to do it himself with the Tac/AudioScan. Once in a while the pain goes back up to a 2, but he can get it back down with the tactile pads taped to his lips.

Our work with PLP has caused us to think of EMDR in a more general sense, as a treatment that is effective in reducing or eliminating pain, whether emotional or physical, when the pain is a "memory" and not due to physical damage. PLP is the clearest example of a pain memory, as the body part is gone but the pain is not. Such work induces us to think of a mind-body *system,* with so many interconnections that it doesn't make sense to refer to them as separate entities. We all have a "bodymind," as Candace Pert has put it (Pert, 1997). Nowhere is this better illustrated than with EMDR work with PLP and other forms of pain memory. It is exciting to think how the use of EMDR will continue to change and illuminate our conceptions of the interactions of the brain, body, and nervous system. It is also exciting to think about how we can help people as never before.

REFERENCES

Birbaumer, N., Lutzenberger, W., Montoya, P., Larbig, W., Unertl, K., Topfner, S., Grodd, W., Taub, E., & Flor, H. (1997). Effects of regional anesthesia on phantom limb pain are mirrored in changes in cortical reorganization. *Journal of Neuroscience, 17,* 5503–5508.

Jensen, T. S., Krebs, B., Nielsen, J., & Rasmussen, P. (1985). Immediate and long-term phantom limb pain in amputees: Incidence, clinical characteristics and relationship to pre-amputation limb pain. *Pain, 21,* 267–278.

Melzack, R. (1992). Phantom limbs. *Scientific American, 266,* 120–126.

Pert, C. B. (1997). *Molecules of emotion: Why you feel the way you feel.* New York: Scribner.

Sherman, R. A. (1997). *Phantom pain.* New York: Plenum.

RESOURCES

Amputee Coalition of America, 900 E. Hill Ave., Ste. 285 Knoxville, TN 37915-2568, www.amputee-coalition.org.

Chapter 6

The Two-Hand Interweave

Robin Shapiro

THE CLIENT WAS 52, SMART, FUNNY, AND HIGHLY DISSOCIATIVE. SHE HAD just lost her seventh job in 5 years of treatment. The story was always the same: Due to her dissociation, she'd be late to work or make a major mistake. Her boss would express disapproval. My client would scream at her boss, usually with threats. She'd be escorted out of the building by security. Cognitive therapy, bibliotherapy, ego-state work, and a year of dialectical behavior therapy (DBT) group hadn't stopped the pattern. We had targeted each firing event with the EMDR Standard Protocol from various angles, many times. The new cognitions pertaining to current safety and efficacy never stuck. This time, on a hunch, I asked her if she thought that an angry boss was exactly the same as the "Man" who tied her down and raped her when she was a child.

Client: Of course they're the same!

RS: *So you think your boss is going to tie you down and rape you?*

Client: Well, he's mad at me, isn't he?

RS: *Okay. Put the man who raped you in one hand. Got it? Now, put your boss who has never raped you and just wants you to show up on time and do your job in the other hand. Just go with that.* (15 DAS [Dual Attention Stimuli], which could be eye movements, taps, or tones.) *What do you notice, now?*

Client: They're not the same person at all!

RS: *What does your boss want?*
Client: For me to do my job.
RS: *What did the Man want?*
Client: To rape and humiliate me and totally control me.
RS: *Go with that.* (24 DAS.)
Client: They want totally different things. My boss was not a threat, except that he could fire me. When I get scared, I get him confused with "the Man."

It stuck for good. And we began to differentiate between all events, feelings, cognitions, and ego states that belonged "back there," from events, feelings, and cognitions that belonged "here and now" with our new tool, the Two-Hand Interweave. After clearing the trauma with Standard Protocol, we used the Two-Hand Interweave to integrate ego states. Now, 5 years past integration and 4 years after the completion of treatment, I receive occasional e-mail updates, some of them mentioning occasions of using "that two-hand thing" when she is feeling emotions out of proportion to the present. After using it with others, I realized that I had developed a simple and effective protocol.

THE TWO-HAND INTERWEAVE

1. Client anchors one conflicting feeling, thought, choice, belief, or ego state in one hand.
2. Client anchors another feeling, thought, choice, belief, or ego state in the other hand.
3. The therapist commences eye movements or tapping, or the client can alternate opening and closing hands. *(Just notice.)*
4. If there is distress in one or both of the choices, it is cleared with the Standard Protocol. After the clearing is complete, both hands are rechecked.

Some people have suggested to me that the most positive or current situation or belief be placed in the right hand and the negatively charged or past situation be placed in the left. I allow the client to choose which hand holds which situation. *Which hand holds wanting to stay?*

I give minimal direction to the clients about what to think, after the two choices, beyond *What difference do you notice?* The answers range from, "The right hand is very light" to existential breakthroughs: "I realize that I've been held back by my old belief for my entire life and that I have a choice now."

The Two-Hand Interweave can be used as preliminary or as adjunctive to the standard EMDR protocol. The Interweave may bring up formerly unknown traumatic material that is best retargeted and cleared with the Standard Protocol.

Client: *When I focus on that choice it reminds me of when "X" happens, and I feel scared.*
Therapist: *Let's do EMDR with that. What words go with X? Where do you feel it in your body? What thought about yourself goes with that?*

In the case of looping, or at the end of a session, when a two-choice dilemma arises, it may be used as any other interweave. Often, the Two-Hand Interweave, without use of the Standard Protocol, is sufficient to provide a clear differentiation, choice, or integration of two disparate choices, ego states, or situations. It can be dropped into any discussion involving a choice or differentiation whether or not you are setting up for EMDR processing. The distress, if any, accruing to one or both of the choices may fade completely without the need for the Standard Protocol.

For example, during the check-in at the beginning of a session a client is wondering if she made the right choice in taking a new job.

Therapist: *Put the job you took in one hand and the job you didn't take in the other.* (15 DAS.)
Client: *The "new job" hand is getting lighter. The other hand is feeling like dead weight.*
Therapist: *Go with that.* (15 DAS.)
Client: I think I just had some anxiety about my choice. It's gone now. I know I took the best job.

TARGETS FOR THE TWO-HAND INTERWEAVE

The following are a few of the many ways to use this interweave. Feel free to create new uses of your own.

- To discriminate between decisions or choices: *Hold your future if you take the job in one hand and your life without this job in the other.*
- For helping people locate the source of decision-making inside of them: *Hold wanting to go in one hand, wanting to stay in the other. Where else in your body do you feel wanting to go? Where do you feel wanting to stay?*
- For alexithymic clients who may not be able to know what they feel, I ask a list of questions: *Put chocolate in one hand, vanilla in the other. Which do you want the most? Where else in your body do you feel that preference? Put romantic comedies in one hand and slasher flicks in the other. What is your body telling you now?*
- As a "float-back" or "affect-bridge" technique to find a target: *Put your current pretty good situation in one hand, and your feelings in the other.* (DAS.) *What situation or time in your past goes with the old feelings?* (DAS.) *Let's do EMDR with that past event.*
- Holding more than one emotion, especially useful with borderline or other primitive clients: *What hand is the anger in? What hand is the fear in?* (DAS.) *Is there room for both of those feelings in you?* (DAS.)
- Similar, or as an addendum to A. J. Popky's Level of Urge to Use (LOUU see Chapter 7) or Jim Knipes's Level of Urge to Avoid (LOUA see Chapter 8): *When you're home after a stressful day at work, feeling bored and lonely, how good do you feel when you think of having a drink? Put that in one hand. In the other hand, put the consequences of having that drink?* (DAS.) or *How good would it feel to continue to avoid doing your paper work? Put that in one hand. In the other hand put how it would feel to get that paperwork done?* (DAS.) *What stands in the way of you doing the paperwork?* (DAS.)
- Holding more than one feeling toward an abuser. *Hold the love you have toward your father in one hand and the disgust you feel at what he did to you in the other hand.* or *Hold the love you have for your [battering] husband when he's nice to you, in one hand and the hatred and fear you have for him when he's raging in the other hand.* Clients who have been feeling great shame for their attachment to abusers begin to understand and accept the totality of the relationship. People who are living with abusers stop flip-flopping between "I hate him. He's bad. I'm leaving" and "I love him so I

must stay." Only when they can hold both sides can they begin to make decisions such as "I love him and he's bad for me. I'm leaving" or "Sometimes he's bad for me, but I think I have the leverage to get him to treatment."

- Projections: *Hold your [abusive] father in one hand and your [pretty nice] husband in the other. Just notice.* (DAS.) *What comes up?* "My father beating me." *What thought comes up about yourself?* Proceed with the Standard Protocol around the father's abuse. When the old target is cleared with straight EMDR processing, come back to the original two-hand targets: *Now hold your father in one hand and your husband in the other. What do you get now?* (DAS.) "I get how different they are. My husband would never beat me, and anyway, I'm grown up now, and I wouldn't let him!"
- Feeling versus being (hopelessness, shame, incompetency, anxiety): *Which hand is hopelessness in? What age does it correspond to? Put your actual situation, right now, in the other hand. Just notice.* or *Which hand holds your anxiety about the situation? In the other hand put the facts, with the real probability of a bad outcome.*
- Transference: *So you're thinking I'm mad at you right now. Put me in one hand and you in the other. Which hand is holding the anger?* or else *Who might you be confusing me with? Which hand are they in? Which hand am I in?*
- Delineating ego states: There are many good ways to do ego-state work. The Two-Hand Interweave is one way to differentiate or set up interactions between different ego states.

   1. Place a different ego state in each hand.
   2. Delineate the differences, with physical, emotional, and other state-specific traits.
   3. Facilitate an interaction between the two, while applying bilateral stimulation. Keep the client accessing internally by asking feeling, sensing, wondering, or thinking questions.

- Distinguishing past situations and capabilities from present capabilities: *Hold that old feeling of compensation in one hand. Hold what you know about your current competency in the other. Remember that you were incompetent only because you were little. Notice how*

much older and wiser you are now in the other hand. What can the here-and-now part of you do that the incompetent younger self couldn't?
- Future possibilities: *Put you as you are now and your current situation in one hand and what your older, wiser self will be able to do later in the other.*

AN INTERNALIZED-ADULT/CHILD-EGO-STATE INTEGRATION

Which hand is that terrified little girl in? Can you feel how small she is? (DAS.) *Can you get a sense of her thoughts and her real vulnerability?* (DAS.) *Now find your oldest, wisest, strongest self. Hold her in your other hand. Feel how much bigger she is than that little girl* (DAS.) *Can you feel her strength?* (DAS.) *Her wisdom?* (DAS.) *Feel her competency?* (DAS.) *Notice the resources that she has.* (DAS.) *Notice what she would do, as a competent adult if she were in that situation.* (Start continual DAS.) *Bring the adult hand over to that little girl. Hold that little girl. Let her know that you are there. Let her feel surrounded with your strength, your competence, and your resources. Tell her that she lives with you now. Take her on a tour of your adult life: your job, your house, and your children. Let her see all the people who love you in your adult life. Let her see what a good parent you are and how well you take care of little girls. Let her know that you are going to handle this situation. It's your job, not hers.* (Halt DAS.) *How's that little girl now?* (DAS.) *Where's that little girl now?* (DAS.) *Is she still in your hand?* (DAS.) Client often reports that she's "inside" now. If not: *Where is that little girl going to live so that you can take care of her from here on in, and she can know that she's always got you to take care of her?* (DAS.)

Don't force integration. Rigidly dissociated fragments of traumatic experience will often integrate naturally with this method. It is useful with dissociative identity disorder (DID) after much of the clearing work is done. I've seen pieces integrate after I suggested, *Put the 4-year-old that saw the abuse in one hand and the 4-year-old that felt the feelings in the other. Are they ready to come to together now? Great. Bring them together while I tap on you.* Of course, if integration occurs naturally after clearing trauma with the Standard EMDR Protocol, you don't need this or any other interweave.

CONCLUSION

The Two-Hand Interweave can be used to "front load" EMDR processing, as an interweave during processing or on its own. In my experience, and the experience of my consultees and trainees, it helps about
95% of clients differentiate between murky feelings and choices.
Clients like it. They often come in saying that they need to "two-hand"
a decision. They report using the technique at home to make differenti-
ations and choices. Borderline clients report "holding two feelings so
that I could see that gray you're always talking about."

Chapter 7

DeTUR, an Urge Reduction Protocol for Addictions and Dysfunctional Behaviors

A. J. Popky

THE DESENSITIZATION OF TRIGGERS AND URGE REPROCESSING (DETUR) model and the theories involved are based on experience from personal client observation and anecdotal reports received from other therapists using this same protocol. It is an eclectic model and combines many methodologies, including but not limited to, cognitive-behavioral, solution-focused, Ericksonian hypnosis, narrative, object relations, and emotional freedom techniques (EFT; Craig & Fowlie, 1995), to name a few. The bilateral stimulation (BLS)* in the accelerated information-processing model of eye movement desensitization and reprocessing (EMDR; Shapiro, 1995) seems to form the catalyst for rapid processing and change, the turbocharger that speeds the healing process.

This protocol represents only a small part of a complete treatment model. The therapist's role is that of a case manager, orchestrating any resources necessary to aid the patient through recovery and relapse to a successful and healthy state of functioning and coping. The therapist has to assess the severity of the addiction and also determine any other diagnosis associated with the case. This overall treatment model includes outside help, such as referrals for medication, testing for physical

---

*Popky uses bilateral stimulation (BLS) in place of dual attention stimulus (DAS).

or neurological problems, and, depending on the situation, inpatient treatment, outpatient treatment, or detox. Other outside resources include support systems, such as 12-step groups, educational programs, skills training; couples, group, or family therapy; or acupuncture. Comorbidity issues, day-to-day stressors, and survival issues are addressed. An extremely high percentage of these populations are dually diagnosed and can therefore run the full dimensional spectrum of disorders and behaviors as described in the *DSM-IV*.

ADDICTION TREATMENT MODEL

Successful results have been reported using the DeTUR protocol across the wide spectrum of addictions and dysfunctional behaviors: chemical substances (nicotine, marijuana, alcohol, methamphetamine, cocaine, crack, heroin/methadone); eating disorders such as compulsive overeating, anorexia, and bulimia; along with other behaviors such as sex, gambling, shoplifting, anger outbursts, obsessive-compulsive disorder (OCD), and trichotillomania. Since this is an urge-reduction protocol, the scope of applications can include a wide variety of applications, for example, anxiety, panic, and phobias.

The DeTUR model is flexible and is to be tailored to the client's needs, goals, and values (see Figure 7.1). Use this therapeutic process to address core trauma events and issues underlying psychological addiction. The therapeutic interweave and interventions are determined by each therapist's training, style, and client feedback in order to assist clients in breaking blocks and reprocessing causal issues. The BLS of EMDR is the catalyst and accelerator for processing in this treatment model and the key element for accessing core events and issues for lasting change.

THE DeTUR TREATMENT APPROACH

1. As an urge protocol it treats all addictions as similar, whether chemical or behavioral.
2. Client's attention is directed toward a positive, attractive, achievable compelling goal, *not* away from a negative behavior.
3. Abstinence is not required as a treatment goal; coping and functioning in a positive manner as described by the client are.

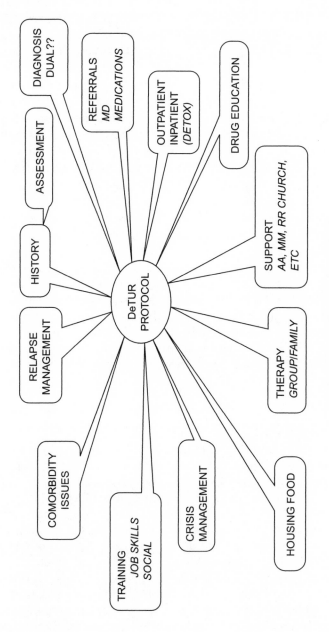

Figure 7.1 Addiction Treatment Model

4. Employs ego strength and empowerment to build coping skills.
5. Relapse is reframed as new emerging opportunities to address.
6. Abstinence is preferred but not mandatory.
7. Includes individualized therapy to address core issues causing the addiction.
8. Therapeutic interventions accommodate clinician's style and training.
9. Chemical withdrawal and anxiety appear to be addressed since the process seems to take place out of the client's level of awareness, not requiring constant attention on the part of the client. Clients often report surprise that at the end of the day they had not engaged in the negative behavior, had engaged—but not as often—or had noticed urges to engage and could put them aside.
10. Targeting triggers for systematic desensitization allow this model to be used with clients early in recovery.

Initially, it was not deemed advisable to do EMDR early in recovery since it was thought that the individual would not be able to handle the affect and would relapse. By targeting triggers instead of trauma, ego strength seems to grow as triggers are desensitized. While clearing the triggers, the client seems to be able to process trauma and core issues that arise. Targeting the triggers instead of the trauma seems a gentler method of uncovering and reprocessing traumas (see Figure 7.2).

1. Accessing Internal Resources (RA)

Usually therapy sessions start with the therapist asking the client, "What's your problem?" Beginning each session by asking clients about their problems seems to focus their energy on the problems and places them into the physiology of powerlessness. I learned from Robbie Dunton in 1990 that she had her young clients focus on their positive strengths while she did BLS. They seemed down and unhappy when they walked in. By getting them to talk about good things they had done, their physiology and demeanor changed to a more positive state. With DeTUR I begin each therapy session by asking the client *Recall a time when you felt resourceful, powerful, and in control. Focus on this experience and all the feelings involved.* I then do BLS to enhance these feelings. This appears to empower clients and allows the process to move faster. Their entire physiology shifts and they appear more energized.

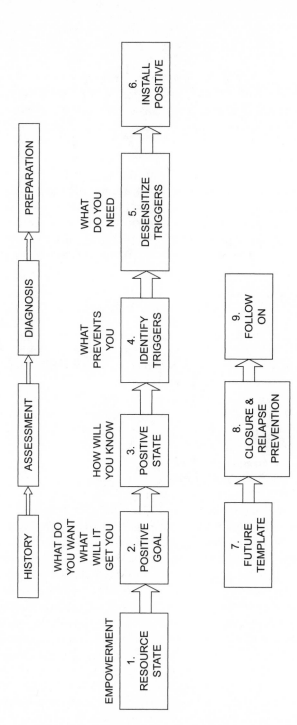

Figure 7.2 DeTur Flow Chart

Clients might only be able to momentarily bring up something positive and then immediately the scene shifts to a negative component. I have them freeze the experience and focus only on the positive element before doing BLS. *Notice what you are seeing and how it feels, breathe into it, and move around in your body. Notice how it feels and smells and take it all in.*

Some therapists report that their clients are not able to think of anything positive in their lives. Some examples you might try with them could be: participation in sports, any task accomplishment, even washing or shining a car, feelings when their favorite team won an event. Creativity and flexibility are the keys in these difficult situations.

If clients can't identify a time, ask them to imagine they were someone they respect, or a movie, TV, or book hero, and have them imagine what it would be like if they were that individual.

2. Positive Treatment Goal

The ultimate goal of therapy is to help clients overcome difficult concerns and restore self-sufficient functioning. The latest trends in therapy have been to tailor treatment to the client's needs rather than mold the client to the treatment program (Hanna, 1994). The important factor in the success of treatment is the appropriateness of the goal for the individual. Given the differences among individuals, no one treatment can be appropriate for all clients (Lewis, Dana, & Blevins, 1994). Abstinence or controlled using is *not* a treatment goal, but the afterproduct of a successful treatment plan.

The concepts of visualization, focus, and concentration on positive feelings have been around for quite a while. It is important that the treatment goal be defined and owned by the client. It is their therapy, therefore their goal. Abstinence, although very highly desirable, is not required as a necessity in the definition of the positive goal (PG). The PG should be attractive and achievable, one that has a strong magnetic pull on which the client can easily maintain focus. If clients formulate their own treatment goal, they may be less resistant and more motivated. Client motivation is central to effective outcome results (Luborsky, Crits-Christof, Mentz, & Auerbach, 1988). The client's PGs are their definition of how they would feel coping and functioning in a positive, successful manner.

Studies in alcohol show so much natural remission that investigators call alcoholics who recover on their own "the silent majority" (Edwards, 1977). There are many stories of women giving up smoking and drinking because the attraction of having a happy, healthy child was more appealing than the need or compulsion to use. Their goal aided them to maintain their focus. There are also stories of veterans that were shooting heroin while in Vietnam and were able to walk away from the addictive component when they returned stateside. Other things became more important; enjoyment and functioning successfully became their focus.

I find it useful to help clients identify their positive treatment goal. *What do they want? What would it get them? How would they know when they got it? What would they be seeing, hearing, feeling, tasting, smelling?* Guide them through the specifics until they can create a clear image of how they would look being successful and fully functional, having attained their goal. Their goal does not have to include abstinence. It will be implied. Although abstinence is requested, it should not be part of the goal. Many treatment centers in other countries (Canada, Norway, the UK) offer controlled drinking programs. Only in the United States is abstinence treated as the universal treatment goal. It is impossible to concentrate on *not* doing something.

It is important that their goal must be achievable within a reasonable not-too-distant future, not a fantasy. I have my clients imagine seeing a picture of them having already achieved their goal, although initial descriptions are often stated in the negative, e.g., "I won't be . . ." or "I won't have to . . ." My next question then becomes *If you won't be . . . , or won't have to . . . what will you be doing instead?* It can take considerable effort guiding them to the right path and maintaining them on track. Remember, it is difficult to "not" do something (don't think of a pink elephant). The challenge is to guide them to describe their PGs in positive, concrete, and sensory-based terms. After assisting them in building their picture, check to confirm if this is really what they want. *Does it have a strong attraction or pull to it?* Make any adjustments to make it more appealing. *Does it feel better if you make the picture bigger (clearer, brighter, bring it closer, add sounds)?* If clients are smokers worried about gaining weight, be sure that they see themselves looking the way they want to look, perhaps in a special outfit (the same for weight-loss clients; inches are more important than pounds). When the picture has the strongest attraction and feels best to them, use BLS to make the goal more compelling and attractive. This positive goal is their positive treatment goal, the focal point of the treatment plan. It should be

- stated in positive terms
- time related—within a fairly close time period, not too far in the distant future

- reasonable—not a pie-in-the-sky dream
- achievable—not out of the individual's reach
- descriptive of coping and functioning successfully in their terms
- attractive, magnetic, compelling

3. Positive State

Since clients are seeing themselves in a situation, they are dissociated from the actual experience. The next step is to have them fully associate with their goal. Give them the experience of how it would feel to successfully achieve their goal, and then, using associative representation, anchor the experience into their physiology.

Anchoring installs the positive state (PS) into their physiology. Anchoring is a process of replicating the physiological experience associated with an emotion or state by linking it to a physical, visual, or auditory representation. I prefer to use a physical anchor. After obtaining permission, I exert slight pressure on a knuckle as the representation. I choose the knuckle of the little finger since it seems to be the least intrusive.

The client is directed: *Step into your picture of your positive treatment goal, into that body posture* (as-if state). *Notice and experience the positive feelings, breathe into these feelings, move around in them, experience being successful. Notice what you see, hear, feel, smell, and taste. Notice what it's like to function successfully* (the physiology of success). Then apply slight finger pressure to the knuckle (anchor). After that, lead them through the positive experience again and increase the good feelings.

Visual adjustments: *Make adjustments to the visual components. Change the brightness, the focus, the contrast, the tint, the size, distance. Report on the change in internal feelings.* Increase pressure slightly to that same place on their knuckle as the feelings peak. While I am utilizing the anchor, touching the knuckle, I simultaneously perform BLS. This strengthens the mind-body link through the representative touch.

Auditory adjustments: Repeat the same process using sounds. *Listen to the positive words or sounds you are saying to yourself and the positive words others would be saying to you. Adjust the auditory components: the volume, the tone, the tempo, and the balance.* As the association with success peaks, apply the anchor touch, and simultaneously BLS to further anchor the feelings of success into their physiology. Test the positive state by having the clients touch their knuckle and notice the results. They should report a pleasant experience.

It is important for the client to have a strong, positive, sensory-based experience of having successfully achieved their goal anchored into their physiology.

4. Identify the Known Triggers

During this step we want to identify the triggers that bring up the urge to use. These triggers are what are preventing the client from becoming successful. How do they know when to engage in the dysfunctional behavior? These triggers bring up their urges to use, whatever learned adaptive responses relieve the discomfort and anxiety associated with earlier traumatic episodes, and allow them to cope with life. These triggers could be places, people, times, emotions, smells, tastes, events, actions, or objects that are linked to the biological envelope surrounding the trauma(s). These triggers are associated with whatever the clients are noticing at those times they get the urge to use.

How do you know when to . . .? Guide the client through the process to pinpoint the specifics of each trigger and then label them $t_1, t_2, t_3 \ldots t_n$. for the next step in desensitization. For example, if clients who smoke report that they get the urge with morning coffee, after meals, and with drinks, I will mark the triggers $t_{morning\ coffee}$, t_{meals}, and t_{drinks}. For those with weight problems, the triggers should represent those times when they eat larger portions, the wrong types of foods, and unnecessary snacks.

After compiling the list of known triggers, prioritize triggers in the order of what seems to be important, from the weakest to the strongest. If you begin with the weakest trigger, client ego-strength will build as the triggers are desensitized and the positive state installed. Desensitization of some triggers can generalize to others.

5. Desensitizing Each Trigger

- I have the client identify a picture representative of the trigger. I ask them:

  - *Bring up the picture, along with any words, tastes, smells that go with it.*
  - *How strong is the Level of Urge (LOU), right now, from 0 to 10, where 0 is lowest and 10 is the strongest?*

○ I then have them associate the LOU with a body location. *Where are you feeling that number in your body? Hold the picture along with all the associated words, tastes, smells. Notice what and where you are feeling the urges in your body.* Begin BLS.

- After each set of BLS I ask: *What are you getting now?* or *What's coming up now?* or *What are you noticing now?*
- I record their answer and reply: *Go with that* or *Concentrate on that* or *Think about that.* Do BLS again.
- This is repeated until the desire drops to 0 (LOU = 0).
- When the client reports a LOU = 0: *Go with that.* Do another set of BLS.

This can be thought of as cutting the wire between the stimulus and the learned dysfunctional response (see Figure 7.3). If the client's answers seem to be looping or going off track, I will return them to target trigger and ask for the new LOU. I then have them tie the number to a body location and begin BLS again.

After each 12 BLS passes or when I notice changes in client physiology I will say "yes" or "that's right," acknowledging to the client their internal observations. Some clients report they appreciate the acknowledgment since they are not sure they are doing it right.

If clients abreact, continue the BLS until they calm down. If driving up a hill you take your foot off the accelerator, the car will slide back to the bottom. However, if you keep your foot on the accelerator, over-the-top momentum will keep the car on track. Also in abreactions, it is useful to tell the clients, *It is in the past, a long time ago,* and *Let it go where old stuff goes.*

If the client reports no change between sets, the therapist should try the following moves until the client again reports changes:

- Increase the width or distance of the eye movement
- Increase the speed (especially if they are intellectualizing)
- Increase the number of movements
- Change direction; change to taps or sounds.

If a thread opens up leading back to core issues, follow it through to completion, sometimes switching to the more standard 8 phase EMDR protocol.

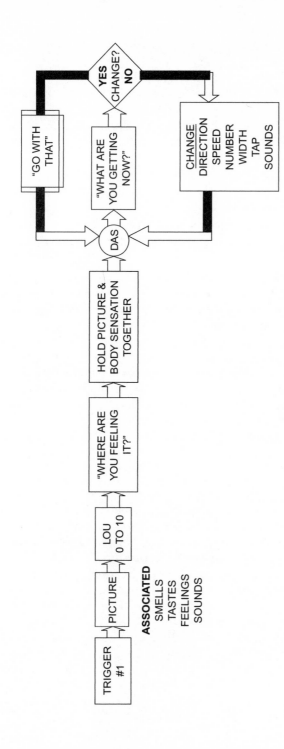

Figure 7.3 Desensitizing Triggers

If the clients dissociate, I will keep them in their body with statements like *Notice where in your body you are feeling it and any change, even the smallest.*

If the clients intellectualize, I increase the speed of the BLS, as they cannot move that fast and think at the same time. Thinking and pontificating stop the process.

The therapist should go back to target triggers:

- After long conversations
- When client is lost or confused
- When therapist feels that the LOU is 0 or close to 0.

It is during this desensitization process, where the therapist's individual styles and skills are required, that the clients get stuck, loop, or abreact, or other nodes open up. The therapeutic interweave, as taught in the Level II training, is the therapist's best tool to aid the clients during this desensitization or reprocessing phase. The therapist's style, training, and experience, along with client-specific information, should be used to create the therapeutic interweaves—that is, reframes, metaphors, and choices—to assist the client's situations at the appropriate times. They can be administered either between sets or during the set while the clients do the BLS.

6. Installation

This step installs the PS to the triggering urge (see Figure 7.4). Similar to the stimulus-response mechanism, this is replacing the "using" response with the positive response that has been anchored and set into the individual's physiology. Whenever the stimulus is activated, the response of positive-state-of-being comes up. It seems that this step allows the process to take place out of the level of awareness and enables the clients to be more withdrawal-free.

Have the clients *bring up that triggering incident again* and apply slight pressure to the knuckle while doing a set of DAS. Whatever positive feelings or statements the clients report after the set, have them hold them and do another set of DAS. If the client's reports are negative, then most likely another channel has opened up and needs to be addressed.

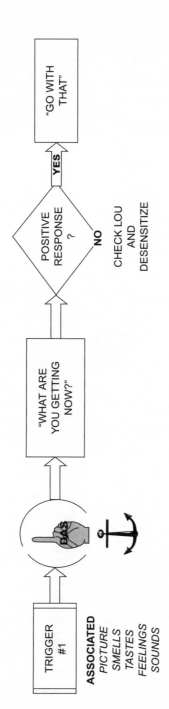

Figure 7.4 Installation

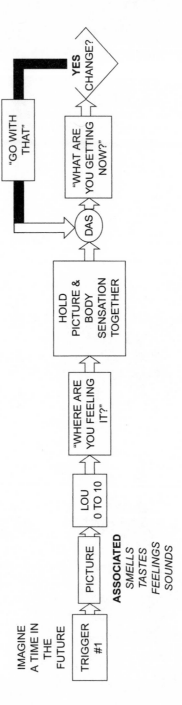

Figure 7.5 Test and Future Check

7. Test and Future Check

To test the installations, have the clients bring up the trigger again and ask for the LOU (see Figure 7.5). If there is any remaining urge, repeat the desensitization process. If the LOU = 0, have the clients imagine a time in the future and check the LOU again. If the clients report LOU = 0, have them *think about it* and with the anchor do another set of DAS.

8. Closure and Relapse Prevention

At the close of each session I explain to my clients that the process continues after they leave and they may or may not experience additional changes. I ask them to call me if necessary. I say, *If uncomfortable urges arise, pick a spot on the wall and move your eyes rapidly back and forth till the urge subsides and then touch your knuckle* (anchor of the positive state). *If the urge remains, call your sponsor. If you do use [the substance], make a note of what triggers are present.* I reframe relapse as new targets of opportunity to address next session. This seems to lower the shame involved with relapsing. Since I'm from California, I use the analogy of an artichoke, peeling away the leaves to get to the heart of the matter. I also introduce the tapping of EFT and give them the chart of spots to tap.

9. Follow-Up Sessions

At the beginning of each session check for:

- New targets of opportunity (relapse triggers)
- Any new information
- Previously desensitized triggers

If previous triggers have not brought on any urges, do BLS to install any or all successes. This helps build ego strength on the successes noticed to date. If clients report relapse, work on the newly emerging triggers that brought up the urge to use. In cases where clients have experienced new stressors, these stressors may have to be targeted with BLS.

CASE STUDIES

These case studies cover client sessions and utilize different adaptations of the DeTUR and EMDR protocol. The slash (/) separates the sets of

BLS. The asterisk (*) denotes return to target. The numbers represent either the LOU or SUDS, depending on what protocol was being used.

#1 Marijuana and Methamphetamine

Client was a white 33-year-old divorced male with two children. He had not been able to test clean in his drug and alcohol program. His wife was assigned custody of the children and she left the area with the children. He paid support to the courts and hadn't seen his children in several years. He was an out-of-work lineman. He had been using methamphetamine for 13 years, approximately $1/4$ gram a week, and had been smoking marijuana since 9th grade ($1/4$ ounce a week). He claimed that when he quit for 8 days he experienced headaches and nightmares.

Client identified his PG as having a better job and spending time fishing, with his children. After resource accessing, we built and installed a strong representation of his PS. We then identified his smoking triggers (t) as: t_1—wakeup rolls and smoke, t_2—in parking lot, t_3—on way to the job in his truck, t_4—setting up work, t_5—10 to 11 am, t_6—lunch, t_7—after work w/ friends, t_8—watching TV w/ friends, t_9—whenever he sees or smells marijuana, t_{10}—working on car, t_{11}—when fishing. For the first trigger (t_1) he felt a LOU of 5. After a set of eye movements he reported the LOU as 0. T_2—LOU = 5 went to 0, t_3—LOU = 3 to 0, t_4—LOU = 0. With t_5—LOU = 2, feeling in gut/emptiness/lonely/big abreaction/memory as a kid in school/kicked out of house/mom let her boyfriend kick him out/she didn't stick up for him/doesn't feel bad about self/ he then began to get angry. I switched to the EMDR protocol. His negative cognition (NC) was, "Something is wrong with me." His positive cognition (PC) was, "I'm okay, it was them." His emotion was anger. Subjective unit of disturbance (SUDs) was 8. The validity of cognition (VoC) was 5. After one pass /uptight jumpy/more at ease/calmer/relaxed/*, SUDs = 2/abreaction/relaxed/SUDs = 0, VoC = 7/Installation. Closure. I collected a urine sample for base level testing.

Next visit 1 week later: Client reported feeling really good, happier, at peace, with no urges, no nightmares or headaches. He reported that he wanted to work at seeing his children and pursue an education. We worked through the rest of the triggers, some generalized to 0. He also reported some fear about retraining for a new occupation. His NC was, "I'm incompetent." His PC was, "I can learn." SUDs = 3/0/Installed the PC and closed. Urine tests showed his level of use was down.

The next session was 2 weeks later. The client reported that he was clean, had not experienced any urges to use, and felt good. We did BLS on his feeling good. His tests were negative for methamphetamine and his marijuana level much lower.

The next session was 1 week later. Client reported he was enrolling in trucker's school and searching for funds for tuition. He had no headaches or nightmares. His tests were negative for methamphetamine and marijuana. Client tested negative throughout the remainder of the program.

#2 Marijuana

Client was a 28-year-old Hispanic divorced male with an 11th grade education. His ex-wife and four children were living in Texas. He and a son were living with his present girlfriend. He was referred to me because he was unable to test clean. He had been smoking marijuana for 15 years, about $\frac{1}{8}$ ounce a week. He claimed that his girlfriend used coke and all his friends in the neighborhood used. He reported that it relaxed him. He was then unemployed. He identified his PG as having a better relationship with his son and girlfriend, taking them to the park and sports events, looking thinner and in shape, and working as a car mechanic. His triggers were: t_1—friends next door at bar-b-que, t_2—in front of his garage with another friend across the street, t_3—when offered, t_4—late at night, t_5—at parties with grass, then cocaine, t_6—after a six-pack of beer, t_7—traveling alone or with his brother. He tested positive for marijuana.

On the next visit he reported he was angry with his girlfriend and the present living situation, and claimed he was experiencing stomach pains. Medical examination showed nothing wrong. We targeted the pain using the standard EMDR protocol. His picture was being stuck and not having the freedom to move out. The picture was anger at his girlfriend. His NC was, "I have no rights." His PC was, "I have rights." VoC = 5. Emotion was anger. SUDs = 10 /fight with ex-wife over child support/I'm a bad father/I'm improving/*0. He reported his stomach to be more relaxed and the pain to be gone. We then started targeting the urges using the DeTUR protocol, installing the PS for each trigger after LOU was 0. T_1—LOU = 6/0/, t_2—LOU = 7/0/, t_3—LOU = 0/, t_4—LOU = 3/0/, t_5—LOU = 5/0/, t_6—LOU = 5/0/, the remaining triggers generalized to 0. He tested positive again. On his next visit, he claimed he did not use, that his neighbor offered him a joint and he was able to turn it down. He felt good about it. We did BLS on the positive feelings. He tested lower. The next visit he reported he was clean and was interested in checking out junior college. He tested clean throughout the rest of the sessions.

#3 Marijuana, Cocaine, and Nicotine

Client was a 30-year-old white married male with a teenage son. He was a high school graduate and was laid off because of the recession in Silicon Valley. His wife was then supporting the family. He had been smoking crack cocaine for 10 years, approximately ½ ounce per week, and smoking marijuana for 20 years, approximately ⅛ ounce a week, 1½ packs of cigarettes a day for 20 years. He supported his habit by selling on the side. He was arrested for possession and being under the influence. His inability to support his family and the lack of trust and respect from his wife and son contributed to his low self-esteem. Previously his main outside interest was officiating at bicycle races. He stated that the last time he used was 4 days before our first session. His PG was feeling better about himself, noticing a renewed attitude of trust and respect from his wife and son, and enjoying the weekends at the races with his family while his son raced. He identified his triggers as: t_1—bored, t_2—when he would think about using, t_3—mornings, t_4—late at night, t_5—when he wanted money, t_6—when he received a call to supply one of his customers. We started with t_1, in the morning. He identified his LOU = 8/argument with his wife/didn't care about himself/why the desire?/it's stupid/I feel stupid doing it/LOU = 0. T_2—LOU = 0/I can't identify with it. After installing the PS and closure we ended the session. The client tested positive for cocaine.

Next week the client reported he had a good week. He was offered crank, felt the urge to use, but turned it down because feeling wanted and needed by his family was more important. This made him feel good about himself. We did BLS about feeling good and he reported, "I don't want it." We worked through the rest of the triggers. The remainder worked through fast. Others generalized to 0. He tested clean.

On the next visit he claimed he had not experienced any urges, had attended six AA meetings and that he wanted to stay clean. We reinforced his feelings with BLS. He tested clean again.

His next visit was 2 weeks later. He claimed that he had no urges and was proud of the fact that he was rebuilding his relationship with his family. He was also going out on job interviews. He tested clean throughout the remainder of the program.

#4 Methamphetamine

Client was 36-year-old Hispanic male, divorced, with one child, and living with a woman, using 3 grams a week for 10 years. He was arrested under the influence. He entered the program and then terminated for poor attendance. He was readmitted and referred to me by another therapist. His PG was to be there for son, working driving a diesel rig, and to be motivated and physically fit. Triggers were: t_1—boring things to do, t_2—get things off mind, t_3—mid afternoon watching TV, bored, t_4—if I have things to do. Again, I started with RA, PG, and PS. T_1—LOU = 4/0, t_2—LOU:8/0, t_3—LOU = 9.5/lazy/0, t_4—LOU = O. The rest of the triggers generalized to 0.

On the next visit he reported he got a job at a car agency, had no urges, and felt good about it. Performed BLS on feeling good.

Next visit he reported no urges. We did BLS on feeling good to enhance his good feelings. He tested negative throughout the remainder of the program.

#5 Methamphetamine

Client was a 28-year-old white divorced female. Her parents were also divorced. Her father was an alcoholic and her brother used. At 11-years-old she went to live with father. She claimed he let her down, remarried, and made her leave the house. Her brother was nonsupportive and offered her grass. Her husband threw her out after the second son was born. Children were 1- and 4-years-old, and wards of the court. The mother had the 4-year-old and the other was in foster care. Her husband was an alcoholic, physically abused her, and didn't see the children. A friend of family sexually abused her at 7. Her mother was very critical. She had a poor work history, was very intelligent, and extremely co-dependent. She started drinking at 14, using crank at 15, and taking LSD in high school.

Client complained about problems giving up crank. The client's PG was playing with her children outside her house. We identified her triggers. LOU was taken on each trigger and BLS until LOU was 0. Client was put into a hypnotic trance and triggers were future-paced. She was told to open her eyes and follow my fingers if any urges or desires to use drugs emerged. BLS was performed two times. Client was then given positive suggestions and the trance removed. Final body scan was performed and then closure.

Second visit, the client reported no urges to use speed. She was offered grass and had strong desires to smoke. We identified and desensitized the pot triggers to 0 and performed installation. A body scan and BLS brought up anger at her brother, father, and abuser. We switched to EMDR Standard Protocol and desensitized to a SUDs of 0. Performed installation and closure.

Third visit, the client reported no urges for speed or grass. We reviewed family history.

Fourth visit, client reported no urges for either speed or marijuana and tested clean.

Client missed last session. She moved in with her 44-year-old AA sponsor. She claimed he was going to teach her how to feel. Her codependency emerged. However, treatment was ended.

#6 Sexual Behaviors

Client was a divorced 39-year–old white male with a 15-year-old son who lived out of state with his ex-wife. He owned his own house and computer business, and lived with his twin brother. Both brothers were sexually, physically, and emotionally abused. Client was caught exposing himself, was classified as a sex offender, placed on Megan's List, and put on probation. He was referred after he relapsed and was ordered back to court. In order to keep him out of jail, I went to court with a stack of documents on EMDR research and convinced the district attorney and judge to keep him out of jail and instead assign him to a work furlough program so he could keep his business open and attend therapy with me. If jailed, he would lose his house and business, and both he and his brother would be homeless, without jobs, and wards of the system. If cured, it would be a win–win situation for them and the county. Client was overwhelmed with the thoughts that his customers, neighbors, and ex-wife would find out he was a sex offender and he would lose his business, his house, and rights to visit his son. We began with resource accessing to reduce the anxiety of being discovered (although that theme continued throughout therapy). His PG was to be happy and free-spirited, surfing with his son and brother in Santa Cruz. Working through his history for triggers, I discovered that he had two sequential triggers that had to happen fairly close together. The first trigger was having heavy arguments with his ex-wife regarding control over his son's life. These were arguments he couldn't win. The second trigger occurred when he saw a woman that resembled his ex-wife. Even telling himself, "No, I don't want to expose myself," he still exposed himself. The work was focused on desensitizing the triggers to expose and clearing the anxiety of being found out. We worked for about 6 months without any signs of relapse. As of 2 years ago, he had maintained himself, still had his house and business, and was still living with his brother. His son had moved in with him. He had experienced no relapse.

RESEARCH: TREATING SEXUAL COMPULSIVITY USING EMDR AND DeTUR

In this pilot study by Alex Spence (see Table 7.1) and Charles Walker, the preliminary research appears to demonstrate that both EMDR and DeTUR provide a set of effective clinical interventions in treating sexual compulsivity.

TABLE 7.1
RESEARCH RESULTS

RESEARCH DESIGN

Control Group	# of Subjects	# of Sessions	Tx Modality	Tx Modality	Tx Modality
Group A	6	10	Talk therapy		
Group B	6	10		EMDR	
Group C	6	10			DeTUR
Group D	6	10		EMDR	DeTUR

The subjects in Group B (EMDR treatment) reported a significant decrease in their SUDS, VOC, and trauma profile, and an increase in their healthful living scale. They also reported struggling with relapse issues.

The subjects in Group C (DeTUR treatment) reported a significant decrease in their LOU level, but did not report a significant decrease in their trauma profile or an increase in their healthful living scale.

The subjects in Group D (EMDR and DeTUR treatment) reported a significant decrease in their SUDS, VOC, LOU, and trauma profile, and an increase in their healthful living scale.

These preliminary findings appear to indicate that the combined use of EMDR and DeTUR is an effective means of treating sexually compulsive behaviors.

The DeTUR protocol has been presented at three EMDR International Association conferences, many EMDR Institute Level II trainings, and several one-day workshops. Over 500 therapists from all over the world have requested copies and are finding successes with their patients over a wide range of addictions and dysfunctional behaviors.

SUMMARY

The DeTUR protocol works with a variety of addictive and compulsive behaviors. It begins with empowering clients by accessing internal resources (RA), then helps formulate their positive goals (PGs) of coping and functioning in life, anchors the PG into their physiology (PS), identifies the triggers, t_n, uses the level of urge (LOU) to process triggers for compulsive or addictive behavior, with hypnotic interweaves and anchoring. It uses future rehearsal to test the work and teaches self-use of BLS and EFT for relapse prevention.

REFERENCES

Craig, G., & Fowlie, A. (1995). *Emotional freedom techniques, the manual.* Marin, CA: Author.

Edwards, G. (1977). Alcoholism: A controlled trial of "treatment" and "advise." *Journal of Studies on Alcohol, 38,* 1004–1031.

Hanna, F. J. (1994). A dialectic experience: A radical empiricist approach to conflicting theories in psychotherapy. *Psychotherapy, 31*(1), 124–136.

Lewis, J. A., Dana, R. Q., & Blevins, G. A. (1994). *Substance abuse counseling: An individualized approach* (2nd ed.). Pacific Grove, CA: Brooks/Cole.

Luborsky, L., Crits-Christoff, P., Mintz, J., & Auerbach, A. (1988). *Who will benefit from psychotherapy: Predicting therapeutic outcomes.* New York: Basic.

Shapiro, F. (1995). *Eye movement desensitization and reprocessing.* New York: Guilford Press.

Chapter 8

Targeting Positive Affect to Clear the Pain of Unrequited Love, Codependence, Avoidance, and Procrastination

Jim Knipe

IT HAS BEEN OBSERVED IN 16 PUBLISHED CLINICAL TRIALS THAT THE EMDR method is highly effective in assisting clients in resolving post-traumatic symptoms (Maxfield & Hyer, 2002). Many clients worldwide have benefited from Shapiro's simple observation in 1989 that if an individual holds in mind many aspects of a disturbing experience, while engaging in bilateral stimulation, the disturbance tends to diminish.

Most clients who enter therapy, however, do not have a simple problem of a single disturbing memory. More typically, clients come to therapy with a mixed presentation, of not only emotional disturbance, but also a history of conscious or unconscious choices about how best to soothe, contain, or avoid that disturbance. Thus, the initial presentation of most clients is complex and often ambivalent. Consider the following quotes: "When my husband wants sex, I get so nervous and it is easy to get angry with him. I know this is connected with what my stepfather did to me. I know it would help to talk about and resolve these old memories. But it is so hard to think of doing that. I *want* to want to, but I don't want to." Or take another example: "I realized the other day that my son doesn't ask me to play catch with him anymore.

I guess he just got tired of asking. I don't feel good about it, but it seems that when I get home from work, all I want to do is plop down and watch something on TV." Or, the woman in therapy who says, "I know I should be over my ex by now. He was really a jerk. It's stupid, but the truth is, I still think about him all the time."

In each of these examples, the client has a problem that includes positive and negative affective components. In the language of the Adaptive Information Processing Model (Shapiro, 2001), we could say the chain of experiential associations—the dysfunctionally stored memory network—has positively valued experience at the entry point into the network and disturbing material at other, less accessible places. Clients often experience this situation as one of conflicting ego states (Watkins & Watkins, 1998). Specifically, one ego state may be positively emotionally invested in an outcome that is an obstacle to the person's larger life goals. When this happens and the usual EMDR method of targeting negative affect is stalled, it may be useful to target the positive side of the issue, that is, an image that has a *positive* emotional valence. Such clients are asked to hold in mind the enjoyable aspects of a problematic wish or identity while engaging in Dual Attention Stimulation (DAS). In this way, they can process these positive aspects, "disinvest" from the problem, and go on to resolve the conflict.

Several session transcripts, below, illustrate how this approach can work in practice. The general steps are as follows:

- For clients who express ambivalence about their goals in therapy, identify the two or more sides to the ambivalence. Some examples:

  - the client who wants to heal an old disturbing memory but feels that the memory is too frightening to think of
  - the person who wants to be honest with others but doesn't want to say anything displeasing
  - the client who wants to have an important conversation with his parents but "never gets around to it"
  - the addict who wants to stop (e.g., alcohol, drugs, shopping, Internet porn, TV) but "can't stop" engaging in that problem.

Generally, the ambivalence will be either an issue of avoidance or one of an unrealistic positive emotional investment (e.g., in a certain image of self or of another person). Sometimes, for such clients, there is a hidden "blocking belief" that must be identified and addressed in order for therapy to proceed (Knipe, 1998a).

- Sometimes, even in these situations, the straightforward use of standard EMDR (i.e., targeting the origins of negative affect) can be very effective. However, if this approach stalls, it can be beneficial to shift to the positive pole of the conflict. In many instances, this can be done with a simple question:

  ○ *What's good about being able to just sit down and watch TV and not have to help your spouse in the kitchen?* or
  ○ *What's good about not thinking of that old memory?*

In other cases, more preparation is needed to clarify the positive pole. For example, a client might be asked,

- *When was the first time you really got away with telling a lie? Get an image that represents the good feeling of getting away with that. When you think of that good feeling, with that image in mind, how intense is it, 0–10? And where is that ("number") in your body?*

In my notes, I refer to this number as the client's initial Level of Positive Affect (LOPA) score. It is important for the client to know that the therapist is asking this question in a dispassionate way, neither judging nor endorsing this side of the ambivalent dilemma. In setting up this procedure, I generally ask for a representative visual memory, a 0–10 score for the positively felt emotion, and the location of that "number" in the body. However, I don't typically ask for a self-referencing cognition, since this is likely to bring up feelings of shame.

- Then, with the client's full permission, the positive element can be held in mind and combined with DAS. The likely outcome in these situations is a weakening of the positive affect, particularly those aspects of the positive that are, in some sense, self-defeating or antagonistic to the person's preferred, realistic life goals and sense of self. As this occurs, there may be an emergence of disturbing memories that the positive material was "covering," so clients should be advised in advance that this may happen, and the therapist should always be sure that there is ample time in the session for processing before targeting what may be a psychological defense. If disturbing material does emerge, it is then accessible for targeting using the standard EMDR procedural steps.

- Sometimes, when both poles of an ambivalent dilemma are intensely felt, it is useful to utilize Robin Shapiro's Two-Hand Interweave (Chapter 6), asking the client to put one side of the conflict in the right hand, one in the left hand. Then with DAS, it is typically the case that the intensity of emotion in each hand will shift, in the direction of adaptive resolution of the conflict.

Each of the following illustrative transcripts was taken from either a video or a written recording of dialogue within a session. Identifying information has been changed to protect the privacy of the clients, but the sequence of what was said and what occurred is unaltered. I am grateful for the generosity of these clients in allowing segments of their sessions to be presented. When *** occurs in the text, that indicates that I have said to the client, "*Stay with that*" or "*Think of that*" while initiating another set of eye movements.

GETTING OVER A FORMER LOVER, AFTER THE RELATIONSHIP HAS ENDED

Cora was previously in therapy with me to treat depression that originated in severe situational stresses, as well as childhood experiences of emotional abandonment within her family of origin. She had successfully finished a course of therapy 6 months prior to the session but was returning following an unexpected setback in her life. This is her second session after her return. Three weeks earlier, her partner had broken off their romantic relationship and had continued during the subsequent weeks to call this client and berate her. In the previous session, Cora used EMDR to work on her helplessness and anger regarding the loss of this relationship, and as a result her Subjective Units of Distress Scale (SUDS) level went from a 9 down to about a 4. It remained a 4 at the beginning of the current session because, in the client's words,

"I still love her; I want to hang on to her." The session then continued as follows:

JK: *After everything that's happened, would you like it if there were a way for you to no longer love her and be able to let her go?*
Cora: I'd like if I could do that, but I don't see how that's possible. I think of her all the time, all the good times we had. Even though it hurts, I can't stop thinking about it.
JK: *Does it go like this? You start to think of the good times, and then it turns to a painful sadness?*
Cora: Yes, that's what happens over and over again.
JK: *Would it be okay if we worked on this today?* ["Okay."] *Right now, can you get a mental image, a picture of the nicest time with her? A time that really represents the loving feeling, the positive feeling you still have for her?* ["Yeah."] *You don't have to tell me what it is but just hold it in mind right now. Is there a positive feeling connected with that?*
Cora: Yes. It's like a good feeling in my heart that then turns into a heartache.
JK: *When you hold that picture in mind right now, here's a question. Using numbers 0–10, with 10 the most, when you hold that picture in your mind of that loving time, how much right at this moment do you still love her and want to hang on to her?* ["It's a 10."] *So just hold in mind that picture, and those feelings in your heart, and follow my fingers. *** And what do you get now?*
Cora: It isn't just the times in bed, but we used to go out to eat. We used to have good times; we used to joke. *** I feel like I was blind. She described herself as caring, honest, and open. She was always on the phone with someone else trying to help them. That wasn't right. *** That's codependent. *** She's stuck working in a dead-end job. It would have been a barrier. *** I still care for her though. *** But in the future, things would have been a problem. *** And her breaking up with me because she says I was too dependent—that bothers me—like breaking up with someone because they have a cold or the flu. *** Part of me wants to call her up and chew her out. *** But that wouldn't be right, that would be hurtful. *** I'm mad at her for being so cold. *** There's other fish in the sea. *** I'm not crazy! I'm a healthy person who just happens to be under stress right now *** I gotta

get back on my feet. I took a shower yesterday for the first time in days. ***

This appeared to be the end of a channel of information, and so I then asked her to go back to the original image.

JK: *Go back to that picture we started with, the one that represents all of your positive feeling. When you think of that right now, using the numbers 0–10, how strong is that positive feeling now, that feeling of loving her and wanting to hang on to her?*

Cora: It's down to a 5. I can see how hurtful and immature she is. She is just diving into another relationship now. ***

JK: *Does it feel better now that it's a 5, and not a 10?*

Cora: Yes, that feels much better.

JK: *But it's not a 0. What makes it a 5?*

Cora: When I think about the good times, it was fun. *** I miss that kind of fun. *** I can't believe she is with ____. I feel better now, I am starting to realize that she wasn't the one; she is too much work!

JK: *Go back again and think of that picture that represents your love and good times together, 0–10, what number do you get now?*

Cora: A 3 or 4. I hope when she breaks up with the new one, and wants to come back, I can say no. *** She never even apologized for all the mean stuff she said. *** My heart still feels crushed but it will only be for a little while. *** I'm feeling hungry again right now! I haven't eaten in two days. *** I'm going home to get something to eat and I have a list of things to do by Saturday. ***

JK: *Go back again now and think of that picture. What do you get now?*

Cora: It feels like a 2 or 3. I'm starting to think I can have those nice things with someone else. *** I'd *rather* have those nice things with someone else. *** I'm feeling pretty good now. *** She said those things over the phone because *she* feels guilty. *** I will have a chuckle when they break up. I'll be long gone. ***

JK: *Go back to it again. What do you get now?*

Cora: Just a sliver. I don't have that pain in my heart right now. When we were together, I know that her feelings were true. *** She just got scared of getting too close. *** I can let her go now and just move on.

In the next session, Cora reported that she was no longer suffering from even a trace of the love-pain she had previously felt. I asked her to think back to the session 2 weeks prior when her grief, helplessness, and anger had been a 9, and her response, with a laugh, was "Why?!"

CODEPENDENCE

Sometimes, in a similar way, a positively felt urge can be the beginning point for processing. For example, a woman in her 30s was frequently frustrated by a repeating interaction pattern with her mother. Her mother would call her on a daily basis and want to talk for an hour or more. These calls would always be one-sided, with the mother listing complaints about her life, with little reciprocal interest in the daughter's life. Through EMDR, the daughter became less anxious and more effective in her use of assertion and limit-setting behaviors, but this outcome was not entirely satisfying. Her previous codependent behavior had been part of her identity, and, in addition, it had been her lifelong way of connecting to her mother. For this client, useful processing occurred following the question, *When you think of the phone call today, how much, 0–10, do you just want to go over to your mother's house and mop her kitchen floor, talk to the neighbor about the barking dog, and fix the wobble in the dining room table?* (that day's list of problems). The client said, "It's a 10!" After the 10 was located in her physical sensations, we started sets of DAS, and the scores went down, little by little, to a 4, at which time the client said that she was acutely aware of a lingering fear of losing her mother's love. This fear originated in specific events of childhood, and was targeted directly with the EMDR Assessment steps and continuing DAS, with the result that the client was able to define and comfortably carry out appropriate limit-setting, within her values of respect for both herself and her mother.

OBSESSION WITH SELF-DEFEATING
BEHAVIOR

As another example, a man had been arrested for violating a restraining order regarding his ex-wife. His self-concept was one of a law-abiding citizen, and he felt both regret and remorse at having violated the law by walking onto his ex's property. In spite of these feelings, however, during a subsequent session, he felt a strong impulse to "just drive by her house" to see if another man's car was in the driveway. He knew this would be unwise, but, nevertheless, he felt a strong impulse to do it anyway, regardless of the consequences. For him, processing began with the question, *How much, 0–10, do you want to drive by her house tonight?* As this urge decreased with sets of DAS, he became aware of the connection between this impulse and feelings of inadequacy he had felt in this relationship, and these issues could then be directly addressed.

IDENTITY AND ENTITLEMENT

This approach can also be effective with the more complex issue of a self-defeating identity. If a particular behavior or state of mind is often utilized to soothe intense childhood stresses, then that response may become incorporated into the individual's identity, that is, the particular way of thinking may be experienced as essential to the person's survival in the world. For example, a self-concept of narcissistic specialness and entitlement is often a defense against early experiences of abuse or neglect (Kohut, 1971; Manfield, 1992). In a previous article (Knipe, 1998b), I described a case that illustrated targeting the positive affect associated with a narcissistic "false self." A method was described of targeting the LOPA associated with defense. One could think of this method as the mirror opposite of the procedural steps used in the EMDR targeting of disturbing posttraumatic material, that is, narcissism is conceptualized as a kind of postindulgence entitlement disorder in which the person's irrational, distorted, and dysfunctional cognitions reflect a positive, not a negative, sense of self. If such an individual has a high degree of trust in the safety of the therapist's office, as well as a clear understanding of the therapist's positive regard, it then may be possible to identify a positive and valued visual image, which is representative of the client's unrealistic and self-defeating sense of entitlement. Then, with therapeutic caution, the positive affect associated with that image may be assessed, 0–10, and then combined with DAS. The likely result is that the image and the associated narcissistic concept of self are likely to become less positive, revealing the negative experiences that made this defense necessary. These experiences, then, can be the focus of EMDR standard processing. This type of "neutralizing" of the client's defensive structure does require a very solid, working therapeutic relationship, since the underlying trauma may carry with it intensely disturbing feelings. Clients going through this process generally do not experience the removal of their defense as a loss; rather it is usually seen as a release of a crutch that is no longer needed. As one client said, after resolving a problem with his impulsive, destructive temper, "I'm glad I got over feeling good about that!"

Why does this work? We can speculate that DAS, when combined with an individual's distorted and inaccurate perceptions of self, has the effect of removing the distortion. This seems to be true whether the distorted affect is positive (e.g., narcissism) or negative (e.g., anxiety when there is no real danger). In each case, the distortion is likely to diminish as channels of information are processed with eye movements, hand taps, or alternating sounds. If a client has a blocking belief, or ambivalence about a therapeutic goal, or secondary gain issues, or so-called resistance to the therapy process, it may be because there are elements to their presenting problem that are positively valued. If this is the case, and if these elements can be identified, the positive emotional investment in these obstacles can be directly targeted.

AVOIDANCE

A particular example of this phenomenon is avoidance, which can be psychological or behavioral. Many clients come to therapy with avoidance issues as part of their presenting problem. Avoidance can be conceptualized as a type of positively valenced dysfunction, that is, while it is clearly unpleasant to consciously remember an unresolved traumatic event, it is pleasant, with the emotions of relief and comfort, to be able to successfully avoid or suppress that memory. Anderson and colleagues (2004), in an experiment of memory suppression using SPECT Scan imaging of the brain, show that suppression may occur through an identifiable pattern of increased activation in the frontal lobe and decreased activation in the hypocampus. Whatever the neurological mechanism, if an unpleasant memory experience is repeatedly shut off, and that shutting off is reinforced, over and over again, by the affect of relief, an entrenched habit of suppression or avoidance is likely to be created. Thus, for some individuals entering therapy, the urge to avoid may be the predominant affective element of the initial presenting clinical picture, in spite of the person's true desire for help with a problem that is disturbing in a larger sense. Thus, for many, the best point of access into the neural network holding the overall dysfunction may be to actually target the *urge to avoid* thinking about or confronting that dysfunction.

An example will illustrate how this approach can work. A woman in her 40s, who had previously benefited from EMDR with some present-day relationship issues, expressed a strong interest in "seeing if EMDR could help" to heal a previously unmentioned incident of childhood sexual trauma. However, at the next session, and over the course of several subsequent sessions, she would "inadvertently" behave in a way that prevented this work. She would begin a session by saying, "I know we planned today to work on what happened with that neighbor, but before we do that—something important just happened at work. Could we just talk about that for five minutes?" The 5 minutes would become 40, leaving insufficient time to shift to the childhood incident. Or, for another session, this client would be 25 minutes late. Over the course of 4 weeks, the client and I both became increasingly aware that there was an avoidance issue. Moreover, she was increasingly frustrated with herself, wanting very much to resolve this disturbing memory, but caught in an intense impulse of avoidance whenever an opportunity for this work was possible. Given this pattern, it seemed clear that her avoidance urge would have to be understood and processed before we could directly address the memory. So, at the start of a session, I said, *When you realize we have 90 minutes in front of us, and plenty of time today to work on what happened with your neighbor, how much, 0–10, do you not want to? I know that intellectually you really wish to do this work, because you think it will help. But what I am asking is, how much is your gut-level urge to talk about something else, to just get away from it?* She said it was a 10, and she could feel that 10 in her stomach and chest. With her permission, I began eye movements with her holding in mind her strong urge to "not get into it." With each set, information emerged, relating not just to her avoidance impulse, but also to the trauma itself, such as, "If I think of that, I'll feel the feelings!" and "I never could tell my parents." When it appeared that we had reached the bottom of a channel, I went back to target with the question, *When you realize we now have _____ minutes left in our session, and we could use that remaining time working with this old memory, how much, 0–10, do you not want to, right now?* The numbers diminished with continuing sets, until, when the number was 4, the client said, "It's easier to think of it now." We then directly targeted the incident using the EMDR Standard Protocol, and over the remainder of this session, and the next three sessions, this client was able to experience significant resolution of the disturbance associated with this specific event.

In session notes, I refer to this paradoxical method as the Level of Urge to Avoid (LOUA). It should not be used with those clients who truly do not wish to access a disturbing thought or memory. But for many other clients who are frustrated in their ambivalence, the most accessible point of entry into effectively using EMDR to process a problem may be the feeling of relief associated with avoiding that problem. These procedures were partially derived from Popky's (1994 and Chapter 7) protocol for using EMDR to treat addictive disorders. This protocol is complex, but one element of his procedure is the use of what he calls the Level of Urge (LOU) Scale, a means of assessing, 0–10, the intensity of a client's urge to use an addictive substance in certain specified trigger situations. Popky's approach fits into the model described here, in that, generally, addictive behaviors tend to be maintained and reinforced by the stress relief associated with using. The LOUA method is simply extending Popky's approach to those individuals who habitually use mental (i.e., not substance-assisted) avoidance to contain disturbing material.

The LOUA is illustrated in the following transcript, which is taken from a video recording of the fourth session of therapy for a 44-year-old man. Carl had previously had a course of brief and incomplete EMDR therapy. He had successfully worked on some present-day frustrations, but had been reluctant to address issues originating in his childhood. In these earlier sessions, he had said enough for me to know that during his growing-up years his father's drunken rages had been a constant stress in his family situation. Carl frequently had suffered physical and emotional abuse. But what had been even more troubling to him was his repeated helpless witnessing of his father's physical abuse of his mother and his younger sister. In our previous work, he had been very reluctant to talk about these things. He was reentering therapy while on a forced leave of absence from his job as an Emergency Medical Technician with an ambulance service.

His employer had insisted that he take time off following a "breakdown" Carl had experienced while responding to a fatal accident. At the crash scene, the driver was drunk but relatively unhurt. However, a young boy was dead, a woman was badly injured, and a 6-year-old girl in the backseat was frightened, though uninjured. When Carl saw the situation, he "lost it" and walked away from the scene. At the time of the recorded session, 10 days following the accident, he still was experiencing intense feelings of shame, and also fear that he no longer could trust himself to perform adequately on the job. His previous work record had been very good, and he was strongly motivated to continue in his profession. But he was distressed and self-critical because he did not understand the origins of his emotions during this incident.

Carl had experienced EMDR before, and he wanted to use it again to help with his acute stress. Among all the troubling images from the crash scene, the most disturbing was the face of the frightened little girl. His negative cognition (NC) was "I can't help anyone; I am worthless." His positive cognition (PC) was, "I have the ability to help others, and my best is good enough," which had a validity of cognition scale (VOC) of 1–2. When I asked him what emotions were connected with thinking about the girl, he said, "I don't *want* to think of that little girl! That really was a failure on my part!" It was apparent that he was frustrated. He wanted to benefit from our appointment, but an impulse to avoid this memory was overwhelming his intentions. The transcript continues from this point in the session.

Therapist: *Carl, here is a question that might help. When you realize that we could work today with your feelings associated with this accident and this little girl, how much, 0–10, do you want to get away from thinking about this image? How intense is that feeling or urge to not look at her, using those numbers?*

Carl: It's an 8 or 9. I don't want to think about that.

JK: *Where is that 8 or 9 in your body right now?*

Carl: Right here (puts hand over solar plexus). Actually, I feel it all over.

JK: *Would you be willing to stay with that feeling while you follow my fingers?* (Carl nods yes.) *Just stay with the feeling of how much you don't want to think of that little girl.* ***

Carl: There is no point in thinking about that. *** I failed. *** I keep saying, it's okay, it's okay, and then I say, it's not okay, it's not okay. *** It feels a little better.

JK: *What's your number now, 0–10?*

Carl: It's about a 6. I still don't want to think about it. That night, I was just like my father. It was my job [to stay at the accident scene] and I didn't do that. And Dad's job was to protect me and he didn't do that. *** There were lots of times he was drunk with all of us in the car. I remember one time, looking at the speedometer at 95 miles per hour, and thinking, "I guess my life isn't worth much." [with much emotion in his voice] Dad failed in his responsibilities, and I failed in mine. *** I'm thinking I'm no different, but then I think, I *am* different, in most ways. ***

JK: *How much do you not want to think of it now?*

Carl: It's a 2 or 3. I can think of it. *** There was a 10-year-old boy. I couldn't help him. The girl got help and the mom got help, and she made it. Everybody made it. It's just . . . I didn't. *** It's okay. *** And I'm really okay.

JK: *Carl, can you stay with that?*

Carl: I hope I can stay with that. *** I think I'm ready to try. *** Most of the tension in my body is gone. *** I'm okay. Dottie [Carl's younger sister] is okay. Mom's okay. I mean, Mom's dead now—she died a few years ago, but it's okay. And that little girl in that car that night is okay. She *was* taken care of. Not by me, but she was still protected.

Carl was able to continue from this point in using standard EMDR, directly accessing the memory of this incident, resolving his disturbance and seeing a connection between events of his childhood and his behavior the night of the incident. Although, as before, he did not wish to target additional traumatic childhood memories, it was my sense that he had worked on an important theme of his childhood by way of this present-day situation. During the week after this session, he was able to resume his work as an EMT, and in a 10-month follow-up phone call, he related that he was feeling confident and able in his work, and that this incident was no longer troubling to him.

PROCRASTINATION

A pattern of recurring avoidance behavior will often resemble an addictive disorder, even if there is no substance involved. Procrastination is a behavioral difficulty that can be conceptualized as a type of addiction, an addiction to putting things off. That is, the procrastinator consistently chooses the short-term gratification of delay and avoidance of work, and thereby foregoes a long-term result that might, in the end, be more gratifying. There are also other commonalities between procrastination and substance addictions. The procrastinator suffers ongoing erosion of self-esteem, which then, in turn, can lead to a vicious cycle of continued procrastination. Also, like substance abuse, procrastination behavior may function as a defense—a means of avoiding other life issues that are disturbing. This type of addictive behavior typically does not bring an individual's life to ruin, but is often highly damaging in more subtle ways. The intervention that follows borrows heavily from Popky's (1994) method of using EMDR with addictive disorders.

"Isabel" had been in individual psychotherapy with me for approximately 2 years at the time of this session. During this time, therapy had occurred on an as-needed basis, sometimes weekly, sometimes with intervals of 2–3 months between sessions. Initially, our focus was on her posttraumatic stress disorder (PTSD) resulting from an injury, as well as ongoing chronic pain resulting from that injury. Both the physical and the emotional disturbance were responsive to EMDR. We also targeted issues of self-esteem relating to dysfunction in her family of origin. And we targeted Isabel's loneliness and anger following the breakup of a long-term live-in relationship. As therapy was successfully winding down, I asked, *What's left?* she replied that one remaining issue was an ongoing problem with procrastination in many areas of her life. We focused on a representative example of this problem. The transcript begins about 10 minutes into a 55-minute session.

JK: *I am going to ask you some questions and you just answer whatever is true. If you get over your problem with procrastination, what "goodies" would you have in your life, that you don't have now?* (Client starts to have tears.)
And Isabel, this is bringing up some feelings. Notice what that's about.
Isabel: I don't know what it's about. It feels like some kind of anxiety. The question was . . . ? What would be good about *not* being a procrastinator? It seems like if I just got done what I needed to do . . . I always wait until the last minute. I've had a couple times in my life when I haven't done that and that feels better. It feels better to get it done when you are supposed to get it done.
JK: *So, if you didn't have a problem with procrastination, do you think you'd feel better?*
Isabel: Yeah. Maybe I wouldn't overeat. Maybe I'd feel better.
JK: *What would be the connection with not eating so much? I think I can see what you are saying, but what would be the connection?*
Isabel: I think the procrastination causes me some anxiety, so then I think, "I have to eat." Or, I'll say, "I guess I'll eat. I'll make some

food," and that will distract me from paying my bills or getting my lesson plan ready, or something like that.

JK: *So that would be a bonus, actually, if you solved the problem with procrastination. You wouldn't have to eat to soothe yourself anymore. You'd eat when you are hungry but not to soothe yourself.*

Isabel: I just remembered why I do it. I guess I'm kind of an alternative person. I'm not sure why people think that about me. I guess it's because of the radical things I say. . . . If I pay my bills on time, I'll be like everybody else. I mean, I have a desire to be like everybody else, but I guess I also want to be different. So it's a problem.

JK: *Okay, so if this is a problem that gets handled somehow, what would you like your attitude to be?*

Isabel: Well, what I'd like to be true is that if I got all the little things done every day it would open up the space to do the things I like to do, the things I am interested in, or get out more. But I procrastinate, so it gets bigger and bigger and bigger.

JK: *So if you were able to do all those things you like to do . . . get a picture in your mind of a day in the future when you really no longer have any problem with procrastination. The space has been opened up, you feel good about yourself. You don't have anxiety. Just think of this day in the future. Get a picture of it. What are you doing on this day in the future to enjoy your time? Make it as positive as possible.*

Isabel: I'm at home and it's a beautiful sunny day and I have the door to my deck open. I have some lemonade, and some friends are going to stop by, and my house is all clean and everything is put away. And I feel comfortable, and they come over, and we have fun and talk and laugh.

JK: *Okay, just do this right now, just enjoy your friends coming in the door, really good friends, and it feels so good to know your house is cleaned up and the bills are done. Is this a nice image for you to think of?* ("Yeah.") *Just hold that picture in your mind and make it bright and clear, with colors, get an image of it. It really feels good. Add in anything else that makes it feel even more positive. Just notice how good that feels.* (Isabel closes her eyes and appears to be accessing this positive image.) *Does that feel good right now?* (Isabel nods.) *Notice where that good feeling is in your body.* (She places her hand on her chest.) *Good, now just continue thinking of that, and enjoying that, and follow my fingers* (a slow set of eye movements *** begins while the therapist continues talking). *That's right . . . just enjoy that. Just enjoy being there, and now . . . step into the picture. That's right.* (eye movements stop.) *How is that?*

Isabel: That's good.

JK: *Just continue to think of that. *** And while you are enjoying that, take your right hand and tap on the top of your left hand, noticing those feelings in your body, the nice feelings of enjoyment, while you think of your good friends coming in the door. Good.*

This step, of Isabel tapping her hand while enjoying this pleasant image, is an important element of Popky's protocol for addictions. A positive resource—the positive emotion of a procrastination-free day in the future—is being strengthened with eye movements. In this way, Isabel can become more clear about what she stands to gain, in return for giving up the short-term relief she derives from procrastination.

JK: *Okay, now let's shift gears a little bit.* ("Okay.") *You said you have a problem with procrastination—and it's tied in with this thought: "If I pay my bills on time, I will be just like everybody else—ordinary." And the attitude you'd like to have is: "If I get all the little things done, I'll have more space in my life to do the things I really enjoy." Now, bring to mind a really clear example—a representative example of what is really problematic to you about being a procrastinator.*

Isabel: I cleaned out my basement. I was looking for something actually. I moved out all these boxes, and they are still there at the bottom of the staircase, because when I was trying to lift them, I hurt my back and I needed someone to help me. I really need someone to help me. I live alone, and it brings all that up. (Isabel starts crying.) Because I don't have anybody to help me, I feel overwhelmed sometimes. And, if you came to my house you'd say, Isabel, you really don't have any messes that need to be cleaned up, but these little things really bother me, like these boxes at the bottom of the stairs.

JK: *So, when you think of these boxes at the bottom of the staircase, what's the emotion you are feeling right now?*

Isabel: They are too heavy, and who is going to move them for me?

JK: *It sounds like you have a good reason to not move them. Are you sure this is a problem with procrastination? You don't want to throw your back out. Or, maybe it is a problem with procrastination.* ("Yeah. Maybe.") *Maybe there are a couple different problems that are intertwined. One is you'd like to have someone to share your life with. The second is these boxes are kind of in the way, and you'd like to get them out of the way.*

Isabel: It's a reminder that I have to do everything by myself, and it's a lot. Like, right above the boxes, the lightbulbs are burned out, and I have to change the lightbulb so that I can see where to move the boxes to. And I haven't changed the lightbulbs because I need four lightbulbs there, and I only have two lightbulbs. (She starts to laugh.) It seems like to get one thing done I have to do another thing and then another thing and I have to do it all by myself, and it seems like more than a person should have to do.

JK: *So this problem with procrastination is part of it, but it's linked to other issues. But if you were to simply solve the problem of the boxes when you go home today . . . What if you really got it in your head, with a sense of determination, today is the day I am going to solve this problem of the boxes. What would you do?*

Isabel: I could push them with my foot into the storage unit.

JK: *So that would be possible to do and would solve the problem?*

Isabel: Yeah, except that I'd have to look at all the boxes. I'd have to go through what's in each of them. But maybe I could get that high school kid across the street to help me lift them. That would be a good idea. My neighbor has offered for her son to help me, if I need to move things around, and I don't let him.

JK: *Okay, so here's a question. Think of the boxes at the bottom of the stairway and think of those numbers from 0 up to 10. When you look at those boxes right now, and you are aware of those feelings of being sad because you are living by yourself, how much, 0–10, do you want to just go do something else?*

Isabel: You mean . . . does 10 mean I want to go do something else? ("Yes".) It's a 10.

JK: *And where is that 10 in your physical sensations right now?*

Isabel: In my chest, and in my neck a little bit.

JK: *Can you hold those boxes in mind right now, as if you are standing right in front of them? And, you haven't decided yet . . . maybe you are*

*going to do something with the boxes, or maybe you are going to do
something else. And just be aware of that urge to go do something else,
and follow my fingers. *** And just be aware how strong the urge is to
go do something else. That's good.* (Eye movements stop.) *Just think
out loud.*

Isabel: The reason I haven't moved them is because I'm not sure
what's inside those boxes. *** Because I don't even know what is
in those boxes, and maybe it's all stuff I don't want, or maybe
there's things in there that I need to find. I don't know. *** I was
thinking that they've been there quite a while, and it's just been
one excuse after another. I'm kind of mad really that life is . . .
that life has caught me up so I haven't been able to do it.

JK: *Okay, now, take a deep breath. Now, go back to the image we started
with. You are standing in front of the boxes. What do you get?*

Isabel: It's not so much the boxes. It's that I have been too busy to
deal with them. *** And that makes me think of all the other
things that I have been too busy to mess with: legal issues, problems at work, friends and family and responsibilities, and my
house is the last priority. But my house is really important. *** It's
like a sanctuary for me to go to and get reenergized. ***

JK: *Okay, go back again, and you are standing in front of the boxes, and
what do you get now? You could clean up the boxes or you could go do
something else. What do you get right now?*

Isabel: Well, the first feeling is that I could really deal with them
today, but the second feeling is that before I do that, I have to
change the lightbulbs. But I have to move the boxes in order to
get at the lightbulbs. (Client laughs.) And I wish I had a son or a
husband who I could yell at, go change the lightbulb! So instead
I yell at myself.

JK: *Okay, given all this, go back and stand in front of the boxes and what
do you get?*

Isabel: I get that the most important thing is to first put in the
lightbulbs because it is so dark, and then I can move the boxes.
That's just something I need to do whether I want to or not. ***

JK: *Go back again. You are standing in front of the boxes. How strong is
the urge right now to go do something else, 0–10? It might not change.
Or, maybe it has changed.*

Isabel: It's gone down to maybe about a 5.

JK: *What's different from when it was a 10?*

Isabel: It's just not that big a deal. Maybe I'm stubborn or silly or whatever, and it's only going to take 10 or 15 minutes to do it, at the most. *** I don't have to let everything in my life be symbolic of something. I can just get things done. ***

JK: *It was a 10. Now it's a 5. That's good, but it's a 5, not a 0. What makes it a 5 right now? I'm not trying to talk you out of it being a 5. Just talk about that 5.*

Isabel: It's a 5 because there's parts of me that like the place I live, but it feels too big for me to live there by myself, and I have too much space. I'm afraid I am going to fill it all up. I'm in a transition. I don't know whether I should throw things away or save them. *** Because when I have lived in small places in the past, I got by having very little and it was fine. I didn't need all the stuff I have now.

JK: *So given all this, go back now and stand in front of the boxes, and what do you get now?*

Isabel: I really need to go through each of the boxes and look and see what's in them before I throw them away, or even before I push them back into the storage room. *** And maybe make every two boxes into one. *** I'm thinking of when I can do that. *** I need a wife! That's my problem . . . somebody who will do all these things for me. (She laughs.)

JK: *Go back again. You are standing in front of the boxes. How strong, right now, 0–10, is your urge to go do something else?*

Isabel: It's a 4 now. ["Okay."] I'm going to look through those boxes and see what's in there, and also some other stuff, see what there is to give to Goodwill. ***

JK: *Okay, Isabel, talk about that 4. What's that about?*

Isabel: I'm at 4 because I have other things I have to do today, but I really do want to get it done. So it's a 4. *** If I clean up the boxes, there are other things I'd want to move on to. But it's okay because I want to get this done. I want to do it. *** This is good.

JK: *Go back again to it, and see if there's any urge left, even a trace, any urge to do something else instead of taking care of the boxes.*

Isabel: It's down, moving in a positive direction, it's not a big deal. The urge isn't a 0. . . . . Let me think. [Long pause] I guess it's that even if I do all that, there'll always be something else to do—domestically. It's like you are never done and it's just kind of boring. *** It's amazing to me how one person has so much stuff. I just get overwhelmed by that. I don't want all this stuff. *** I've had a lot of interesting experiences in my life, and maybe these day-to-day things aren't things that hold my interest very much. It helps to realize that. It's okay. It's just who I am.

JK: *Here's another question: Would you like it to be a 0?* ["Yeah!"] *Okay, now go back and look at the boxes again and what do you get?*

Isabel: That I have to do it by myself. *** I just keep thinking there ought to be an easier way to live if you live by yourself, but there's really no role model for that. I have to find my own way and I . . . sometimes I just don't like it.

JK: *The issue of living by yourself . . . can you see the connection with procrastination?* (Isabel nods.) *Does it help to see that connection?* (She nods.)

Isabel: It helps to see that connection. If I clean up these boxes then it's going to be easier to invite someone into my house.

JK: *Okay, with all this in mind, go back to this simple image of looking at the boxes, the way they are at your house, right at this moment as we are talking, and they will be like that when you go home today. What do you get now . . . when you think of that?*

Isabel: If I go home today and get really busy, it's like I'm zooming around—doing everything. And I don't like that feeling. *** I'd rather just leave them there. At this point, Isabel paused for about 10 seconds, with a troubled look on her face. Because we were nearing the end of the session, and nearly out of time, I introduced a cognitive interweave.

JK: *Could I offer a suggestion? What if you did these things, but you didn't zoom around? What if you took your time, stopped in the middle of getting things done, and had a cup of tea, and enjoyed doing it at your own pace?* (She nods.) *Can you imagine that?* ***

Isabel: That feels better. ***

JK: *So again now, go back and look at the boxes. What do you get?*

Isabel: I want to go home and move them right now. ***

JK: *So is there any trace of urge, while you are looking at those boxes, to go and do something else?*

Isabel: No, it's a 0 now.

JK: *Think of that. Just realize that.* (Client nods.) *And as you realize that, reach over and tap your left hand with your right hand* (in order to strengthen this work by activating the positive emotions associated with giving up procrastination). ***

When Isabel came back 2 weeks later, she reported that on the day of her session, she went home, moved the boxes, paid her bills, did a number of other tasks, and felt energized and good about doing these things. And in addition, during the intervening weeks, she had signed up to take a class, with the hope that she might be able to make some additional contacts with potential dating partners. It appeared that that she had been able to make significant progress on her procrastination problem, as well as seeing some connections with the issue of loneliness. Our work with the boxes had generalized and helped her restructure her attitude toward doing routine, mundane tasks. At a subsequent session, 1 month later, she said that she no longer would call herself a procrastinator.

CONTRAST WITH RESOURCE
DEVELOPMENT AND INSTALLATION

How are the methods described here different from the widely used approach of Resource Development and Installation (RDI; Kiessling, 2003 & Chapter 2; Leeds, 2002)? Both target images and memories that have associated positive affect, but in the situations described here, positive affect is *reduced* on the way to the client achieving resolution of a disturbing life problem. RDI, in contrast, is intended to result in the *enhancement* of purely positive experiential resources. In practice, this distinction may often be blurred, in that an image that serves as a resource may, in fact, also be functioning as a defense or express a thought that is unrealistic or idealized. For example, a client might identify "Aunt Susan" as a positive resource: "I always knew she loved me. She was always so kind. I knew I could tell her anything. It feels so good to think of being with her." However, if the warm feelings associated with Aunt Susan are paired with repeated sets of eye movements, the client may come to realize that part of the positive valuation of Aunt Susan derives from the contrast with the coldness and aloofness of Mother. Proponents of RDI recommend that resource installation proceed with short sets, possibly for this reason—that many positive resource images have the potential to "go negative." The therapist can be aware of this issue, using short sets when the positive image is to be used as a resource and longer sets when the goal is to get to the unresolved trauma beneath the defense.

THE IMPORTANCE OF A STRONG THERAPEUTIC RELATIONSHIP

In many instances, the methods described in this chapter are best used late in an individual's therapy. Letting go of an overly idealized image, or a defense, is a very vulnerable act for a client, and therefore it is something that should be attempted only when the person has experienced good results from the prior therapy, is comfortable with the therapist, and is able to glimpse the benefits that would be attained by giving up the defense. Sometimes the client's experience of an unrealistic emotional investment or of a defense will be restructured in a single session. In other instances, many sessions, focusing on a variety of different examples, will be needed. Some clients simply "use" a positive image or defense. For other clients, the pattern of thinking and feeling may be part of their very identity or core definition of self. In the latter case, of course, much more preparation will be necessary and a clear therapy contract will have to be in place in order for therapy to proceed successfully.

SUMMARY

The purpose of this chapter is not to present a specific formula for intervention but rather a general concept that can then be applied flexibly for the client's benefit. And, of course, the response of each client is unique and often surprising. For example, occasionally it has happened that a client, when asked "How much, 0–10, do you not want to think of that?" has paused and then replied, "0! I want to think of that, and work it through." It seems that in these instances, the LOUA question has had the effect of increasing the client's determination to continue bravely with some difficult work. In other cases, DAS processing of the urge to avoid specific behaviors has brought to light, with increased clarity, some true dangers of the avoided situation, resulting in the positive outcome that the client was able to proceed with appropriate and realistic caution. I have not collected data systematically on how often these approaches are successful in resolving a therapeutic impasse. However, since first using the LOUA method (Knipe, 1995), I have found it very useful and, at times, essential, with over 70 clients.

EMDR originated in 1989 as a set of procedures for treating disturbing memories, and many therapists continue today to regard the method as useful primarily for clients displaying posttraumatic symptoms. If EMDR is used only in this narrow way, a phenomenon of "practice shift" is likely to take place, that is, the nature of the therapist's caseload will change, over time, toward an increasing proportion of clients with complex presentations. The methods described here provide a partial solution to this problem, by allowing the treatment of a wider range of client issues, while still adhering to the Adaptive Information Processing model of psychotherapy.

REFERENCES

Anderson, M. C., Ochsner, K. N., Kuhl, B., Cooper, J., Robertson, E., Gabrieli, S. W., Glover, G. H., & Gabrieli, J. D. (2004). Neural systems underlying the suppression of unwanted memories. *Science, 303* (5655), 232–235.

Kiessling, R. (2003, June). *Integrating resource installation strategies into your EMDR practice.* Paper presented at the EMDRIA Conference, Denver, CO.

Knipe, J. (1995). Targeting avoidance and dissociative numbing. *EMDR Network Newsletter.* August, 7.

Knipe, J. (1998a). A Questionnaire for assessing blocking beliefs. *EMDR International Association Newsletter.* Winter, 12–13.

Knipe, J. (1998b). It was a golden time: Healing narcissistic vulnerability. In P. Manfield (Ed.), *Extending EMDR* (pp. 232–255), New York: Norton.

Kohut, H. (1971). *The analysis of the self: A systematic approach to the psychoanalytic treatment of narcissistic personality disorder.* New York: International Universities Press.

Leeds, A. (2002). A prototype EMDR protocol for identifying and installing resources. In F. Shapiro (Ed.). *Part 2 training manual* (pp. 45–46). Pacific Grove, CA: EMDR Institute.

Manfield, P. (1992). *Split object/split self: Understanding and treating borderline, narcissistic, and schizoid disorders.* Northvale, NJ: Jason Aronson.

Maxfield, L., & Hyer, L. A. (2002). The relationship between efficacy and methodology in studies investigating EMDR treatment of PTSD. *Journal of Clinical Psychology, 58,* 23–41.

Popky, A. J. (1994, February). *EMDR protocol for smoking and other addictions.* Paper presented at the Annual Meeting of the EMDR Network, Sunnyvale, CA.

Shapiro, F. (1989). Efficacy of the eye movement desensitization procedure in the treatment of traumatic memories. *Journal of Traumatic Stress Studies, 2,* 199–223.

Shapiro, F. (2001). *Eye movement desensitization and reprocessing: Basic principles, protocols and procedures* (2nd ed.). New York: Guilford Press.

Shapiro, R. (2000, September). *Two hand interweave.* Paper presented at the EMDRIA Conference, Toronto, Ontario.

Watkins, J. G., & Watkins, H. H. (1998). *Ego states: theory and therapy.* New York: Norton.

Chapter 9

The Reenactment Protocol for Trauma and Trauma-Related Pain

James W. Cole

AFTER A TRAUMA, AN INDIVIDUAL IS OFTEN TORMENTED BY THE IMAGES of the tragic incident. These recollections return as nightmares, intrusive thoughts, and flashbacks. Physical pain related to the trauma triggers recollections of the trauma. These images reinforce the victimization. Those who take flight or who fight back during a trauma hold images of being active while those who freeze have more passive images. The Reenactment Protocol (RP) is a process of developing a new active image that reflects control, safety, and efficacy that is then associated with the trauma to allow the client a new set of meanings. I've never seen an abreaction, or reexperiencing of the trauma, arise during the RP. After the RP, clients report feeling in control. Their Subjective Units of Distress Scale (SUDS) have significantly lowered. Their physical pain has often lessened or disappeared. Clients often laugh at the point of reenacting their story, and the positive affect remains for the rest of the session. In therapies that have relied heavily on the RP, many clients gain a sense of control and sureness and increase their assertive behaviors.

WHEN TO USE THE REENACTMENT PROTOCOL

Many victims of trauma reexperience it as if they are spectators who are powerless, helpless, and inactive. When these clients transform their orientation to a physical experience by imaginally asserting themselves and gaining control of the traumatic memory, it can reduce the symptoms of trauma including depression and chronic pain.

- When clients were *inactive* during the traumatic event, they are active during the reenactment process. This seems to mobilize them and change the event from something endured into something empowering.
- When the trauma was *physical* in nature, they can imagine taking charge and changing the outcome of the situation or creating a new ending that has a different meaning. Many clients create an ending that is humorous and spontaneously begin to smile or laugh. At this point the client's perspective of the trauma makes a dramatic shift that continues beyond the therapy session.
- When *helplessness* and depression are part of the presenting symptoms, the images of physical activity help to overcome that depression and activate different emotions. Clients often demonstrate new strengths after reenactment processing.
- When *chronic pain* is related to the trauma, a reduction in the pain and its related disability is possible by encouraging a stronger internal locus of control and by reducing the pain catastrophizing and pain vigilance. While it may not reduce the actual pain, it seems to reduce the need for pain medication and the level of disability related to the pain.
- With a *single physical trauma* some therapists have reported a fast response using the RP. Sometimes transformation occurs within minutes.

THEORY

Trauma provides powerful evidence of one's lack of control, helplessness, and loss of safety. Trauma memory reinforces feelings of being unsafe and fearful. As Peter Levine (1997) portrayed it, reenactment of the traumatic event is something that one is drawn to as an unfinished event. His therapeutic process, Somatic Experiencing, encourages the clients' impulse to reenact, giving clients permission and support to finish the process in a productive way, while creating their own more resourceful ending and integration.

In EMDR, responsibility, safety, and choices are foci for most cognitive interweaves (Shapiro, 2001). A sense of control and responsibility for oneself is fundamental for healthy people and instrumental in a person's ability to cope with pain after a trauma. Women who blame themselves immediately after a rape have a better prognosis than those who don't (van der Kolk, 1989). While this initial blame is a mistake, it reflects the person's own sense of self-control and personal responsibility. The freeze response during a trauma predicts future pathology (Ehlers, Mayou, & Bryant, 1998; Ozer, Best, Lipsey, & Weiss, 2003), and this frozen state provides a target for therapy. Reworking this freeze response and encouraging the client to visualize physically acting out a powerful superhuman self-expression seems to free the client to recover. The RP creates a new set of associations by rewriting the traumatic memory and changing the negative reflections on the individual's identity.

After developing the RP, I discovered that Barry Krakow was already using similar therapeutic components in an effective treatment for posttraumatic stress disorder (PTSD) that he called imagery rehearsal therapy (Krakow et al., 2001a, 2001b). In one study, imagery rehearsal therapy reduced nightmares in PTSD clients by 71% in a 1-month period. This method and the RP share some therapeutic components, and the RP has a few more that, I believe, make it stronger. In the RP the therapist works with the client to create a new outcome that does not involve avoidance and emphasizes control over the situation in the fantasy. There is focus upon the body and the memories in the body of the pain or of the feelings of the trauma. Traumatized body parts are relied upon and central in the re-creation of the dream or trauma. Bilateral stimulation during a slow-motion reenactment process seems to enhance the integration. Directing the client's attention to his strong body posture and facial expressions of control strengthen the therapeutic process. Finally, in the RP, in addition to the behaviors, a newly developed client identity is installed and rehearsed.

THE PROCESS

After getting a SUDS rating I ask the clients to create a fantasy image that changes the trauma incident. It might be presented in the following way:

Fantasies and dreams seem to have a powerful influence. You have likely had some dreams where you woke up with a strong feeling and recalled having things happen in the dream that weren't physically possible. Even when these things were clearly not possible, you still experienced the feelings. Let's use this process with bilateral stimulation in order to have more access to some emotions and recovery.

Imagine yourself being unlimited by the laws of the physical world. You are able to do superhuman things. Imagine that you can reach long distances, exert great forces, move with lightning speed, and generally do any superhuman task. With these powers, go back to the time of the trauma or just before the trauma and create a new story with a positive outcome. In doing this, take note of the pain you have experienced and imagine yourself fully using that part of your body in this superhuman fantasy with powerful physical strength in that part of your body. I want you to decide what you will do, then share it with me.

During the reenactment fantasy every description or reference needs to be in the present tense, using a personal and active voice. It is not something that has happened or will happen or could happen. It is something the client is doing and experiencing now.

Clients need to have the following elements in their imagery:

- The clients take control of the situation.
- The clients feel safe within the situation.
- The clients are active, not passive.
- The clients do not escape in any way but dominate the situation.
- The clients use the limb or body part that was hurt or that holds the sensation of the trauma, when possible or appropriate.

It is important to:

- Give the clients time.
- Listen to the new story.
- Ask clarifying questions if needed.
- Be supportive of the new superhuman story. Never be critical.

I make suggestions if the clients do not include all of the above elements. For example, I might say, *Taking another street on your way to work would not be helpful for this fantasy. I want you to see the oncoming car and then take charge with your actions so that you dominate the situation.*

I encourage physical involvement and then focus upon the physical sensations during the active process.

Okay, now that you have re-created the incident with you having superhuman powers, I want you to go slowly through this process while we do some bilateral stimulation. I will give you all the time you need. You let me know when you have finished your fantasy.

I then start the bilateral stimulation and continue until the client signals that the fantasy is finished. (I have found no difference in the process using eye movements, tapping, or audio stimulation. However, many people find they are better able to follow a guided imagery if their eyes are closed.) As the story unfolds, I periodically direct the client's attention to the physical sensations and encourage positive feelings of self-appreciation and self-efficacy. I do this by simple reflective statements that direct the client's attention.

Let yourself feel the strength in your arm as you reach out and stop the oncoming car. Or as it was with one client, *Let yourself feel the strength in your arms, shoulders, and back as you resist those who hurt you and take charge of the situation.* With another client I suggested, *Focus on the strength in your back as you lift that SUV and throw it into orbit.*

While the client is receiving bilateral stimulation I make intermittent comments. *Feel the power in your arms (or whatever part of the body is involved), Enjoy the perspective as you take charge of what is happening, Feel yourself being in complete control. Experience the freedom of being able to decide everything without any threat.*

During the reenactment process clients often start to laugh and enjoy their imagery. As one female who had been working as a firefighter expressed it, "It is enjoyable to imagine comforting those supermacho guys while they are crying and to do it with my arm that had been hurt." I support these lighter expressions that seem to come with the relaxation of the body tension. As one therapist related to me, her client spontaneously reported that "the cars were now going past her and waving to her instead of colliding with her car" (Judy Webb, personal communication, 2002).

I then direct the clients to focus on the meaning that the superhuman fantasy might have on their self-perception or identity. One client imagined herself beside the freeway with the driver of the other car and her own passengers expressing their deep appreciation for her actions. They were grateful for her preventing the accident that seemed certain to happen had she not acted with superhuman speed and power. As a way of completing the process I have the clients focus on the way they were seen by others in their superhuman fantasy and upon the self-perception that came as a result of it. These perceptions are generally positive, and I encourage the clients to view themselves in this way. They created the imagery and the action reflects their nature. This image of the self then becomes a positive cognition that is referenced in response to the reworked superhuman fantasy. While focusing on this self-perception I do a few sets of eye movements, or other form of bilateral stimulation, until the feelings seem more true or believable. I often suggest that the client wanted to do those powerful and positive things, and the desire for that good really does reflect their true nature. Following this, I will do a few sets of bilateral stimulation to install this new positive cognition.

A client who processed a freeway accident reported feeling sensations in her left arm during the reenactment fantasy process. Her left arm had been hurt and it was this arm that she used in her fantasy to reach out of her car window and stop the other car before it hit her from behind. After the reenactment, the pain in her left arm seemed to be diminished.

At the conclusion of every reenactment fantasy I check the SUDS level. Unless the SUDS is already 0, the process needs to be adjusted and repeated.

I have had some clients work a traumatic memory down to a SUDS of 0 using the standard EMDR protocol followed by the RP. The Standard Protocol took away the discomfort and the RP freed the clients, leaving them giggling and empowered.

Sandra "Sam" Foster (2001) suggested that clients maintain a strong proud posture during the positive installation. I have found it effective to do the positive installation after this interweave while the clients are standing, feeling grounded and strong, focusing on their physical strength and clarity of purpose. I often have clients stand and place their feet apart in a strong stance with shoulders held in a proud strong way. In addition to the posturing, it seems important to have them express the feelings on their faces (Ekman, 2003).

With difficult cases, where there seems to be a commitment to helplessness or some other blocking dynamic, I make relaxation audiotapes including the clients' reenactment fantasies. I have the clients listen to a guided imagery tape that focuses on the fantasy and, repeatedly, on the positive body sensations in their fantasies. These tapes include images of relaxation, control, and confidence. I suggest they listen to this guided imagery tape at home while doing butterfly hugs.

AGGRESSION

It surprises me that the images are rarely revengeful. The most revengeful fantasy was portrayed in a caring way by a woman who had been raped with a knife to her throat by a man with a record of sexual offenses. He was never charged with her rape. In her superhuman fantasy she threw him off of herself and then blew flames from her mouth until he simply floated away as a bit of ash. As she expressed it, she felt a strong need to stop him from hurting other women.

Sometimes the anger is expressed as aggression. Shortly after engaging in a fantasy of aggression, clients usually switch spontaneously to another emotion and continue with the process. Aggressive fantasies have generally turned out to be superficial feelings that are safer to express, and as soon as they are, the clients move to something stronger and less aggressive. When we talk about how behavior is an expression of one's identity, the clients' aggressive fantasies usually seem to evaporate. I sometimes talk with the clients about the difference between real power and aggression. For example, aggression is a compensation for the lack of power, as in an aggressive small dog. Then we compare the disposition of larger dogs, which are more relaxed and more powerful.

CASE EXAMPLES

The applications of and reactions to this protocol can be illustrated with a few case examples.

- Reenactment as resource: One client who had been profoundly neglected as a child (locked out of the house and frequently ignored by his single mother) wanted to be so strong at eliciting nurturing that his mother couldn't resist nurturing him. We set up the reenactment imagery and I suggested that he imagine himself as that young boy eliciting all the love and nurturing that he needed. I started to tap his hands with a wand and made short statements about his feeling her love and attention. Since I had told him to take all the time he needed, I stayed with him, tapping during his lengthy period of silence. I made unobtrusive statements to help him focus his attention on the physical feelings and feelings of being important and valued. After 50 long minutes, he opened his eyes and reported that his fantasy mother had provided a pizza party and sleepover for his friends. He had had the experience of being nurtured. The session was later referred to as a breakthrough. Prior to this session, his wife had had plans to leave him because of his lack of affection. Now they are back together and he is able to give and receive affection.

- One client who has memories of organized abuse wrote the following about reenacting a memory of abuse where she was tied down:

"I imagined growing very long and thin and slippery so I could slip out of the ties. Then I pretended I was VERY strong and I stood up on the bed with my back to the wall and I shouted very loud STOP!! And I kept shouting STOP till all the grown-ups in the room got very small. Then I scooped them up and put them in a little wooden box and gave them to the police to take care of. This pretending helped me to change my memory. Now, whenever I think of that bad time, I see myself getting very big and strong and making the bad men STOP, and I remember putting them in the box. This bad thing isn't something I want to think about, but if it pops into my head, I have a way to make it not so bad and I have a way to be strong and stop the hurting. I have a HOPEFUL way to look at it instead of a weak, trapped way. So this was very good for me and I like it a lot!"

- Sometimes clients choose to repeat the process on their own. After using the RP to work with the images of a rape, one client wrote the following:

"I then decided to apply this imagery to other men who have assaulted me: my husband; a friend who had rubbed his erect penis against me in the presence of my husband when I was two months pregnant; a jealous boy who had knocked me unconscious and caused a brain injury when I was 16 years old."

Later in the same letter she wrote:

"I have noticed a difference with my ability to control my crying. I usually sob during the domestic-violence support-group meeting. This week, I did not, and I spoke about the trial in positive terms instead of focusing on my fears. I have recently questioned two people who I knew were lying to me; whereas, I have not commented about the lies in the past."

CAUTIONS

Often the client's primary approach to stress and trauma will interfere with therapeutic process. Whether the client's approach is one of avoidance, dissociation, helplessness, "victim" identity or something else, if it conflicts or prevents the process, it needs to be addressed.

- Clients who have tendencies toward dissociative responses might create fantasies where they leave their body or split in some other way. In such cases I suggest that they need to be totally present to carry out this fantasy as one person.
- With clients who tend to create escape fantasies in which they are suddenly flying away or disappearing, I bring them back and suggest that, without retreating, they cope with the issues and solve the problem directly and actively.
- The client must be clearly and fully in control within his or her own fantasy and to imagine having unlimited power or strength in the reenactment process. The outcome needs to be clear, quick, and decisive, never a prolonged unclear struggle. Once I did not stress a good outcome. After a long period of time I checked with the client (a volunteer for a workshop demonstration). I discovered that in her fantasy she was digging her fingernails into the tires of a truck and trailer rig on the freeway trying to stop it. In her trauma the truck had hit her and then left the scene of the accident. In her reenactment her fingernails smoked from the friction of clawing the tires of the truck, in an unsuccessful attempt to stop the truck.
- With those who see power and control as evil, I question them about powerful people they respect and admire. I have them imagine those powerful and good people in their situation. Then I have the client imagine that admired person going through the reenactment. This seems to make the guided imagery doable, and often makes it possible to complete the guided imagery as themselves.
- For others who equate power with evil, it seems critical that the therapist not accidentally suggest that the client become evil. For example, while some clients might be very comfortable in a

controlling fantasy, others may have a negative association with a word like *dominate*. The needed adjustment might be as simple as the therapist talking of "being in charge," "conducting the action," "being in the driver's seat," or "having total control."

TABLE 9.1
ELEMENTS OF REENACTMENT FANTASIES

THE LEAST EFFECTIVE		THE MOST EFFECTIVE
Passive	→	Active
Victim	→	Victor
Catastrophizing about future	→	Optimistic about future
Controlled by environment (external locus of control)	→ →	Controlling their environment (internal locus of control)
Feeling anxious and fearful	→	Feeling relaxed and calm
Self-doubting	→	Self-confident
Abstract in focus	→	Physical in focus (focus on body sensations)
Fearing others or environmental conditions	→	Trusting in one's ability to cope with anything that might come along
Suffering pain and yielding to the pain	→	Going beyond pain and not yielding
Focus on pain and vigilant of pain	→ →	Focus on life Only slightly aware of pain

---

DEALING WITH TRAUMA-RELATED PAIN

For clients who have experienced a trauma resulting in chronic pain, look for the psychological dynamics that affect the pain and weave these issues into the reenactments.

- Listen for subtle clues of the psychological dynamics while gathering the history. These clues might be expressed as catastrophizing thoughts, helplessness, fear of pain, pain vigilance, an obsessive focus on the unfairness of the traumatic event, repeated statements of "If only," unrealistic dreams, high levels of anxiety, or many other strong expressions.
- Acknowledge the feelings and empathize with the discomfort while avoiding any validation to the dynamics that support the pain. These psychological dynamics seem to insulate these people from directly engaging the reality of their condition. This failure to accept one's own reality along with the fear of future pain creates a disabling posture and maintains the level of the pain.
- Gently test the strength of the beliefs about pain, blame, victimhood, and fear of pain. Explore the strength of these dynamics and the level at which the clients will defend these positions.

  ○ Precede the reenactment process with a short session of progressive relaxation if the rapport level has been well established and the anxiety is still an issue.
  ○ Suggest the reenactment process without defending it or pushing it. I might say, *Since dreams aren't reality and dreams do seem to impact emotions, then let's create a dream that has positive emotions. I will help you make the dream as vivid as possible and then you can practice that dream.*
  ○ Give clients a great deal of permission and support to allow them to create their own reenactment fantasy. The clients' involvement encourages greater commitment and allows them to become more involved.

Whereas the pain and memory of the traumatic incident may be the most overt targets of the therapy, the underlying orientation toward and belief about the pain is just as critical. During the clients' reenactment, it is helpful to use gentle suggestions to focus on the beliefs that clients have about the pain. The therapist can suggest a reduction in the "fear of pain" or encourage a stronger "internal locus of control" or encourage a "reduction in helplessness." The therapist can subtly encourage the reduction in "pain catastrophizing" while the clients are experiencing the bilateral stimulation and going through their reenactment fantasy. The therapist can also do this with beliefs about "pain," "pain anxiety," and "self-efficacy." Using the clients' own vocabulary or more personal terms (not words like *locus of control* or *self-efficacy* or *catastrophizing*), the therapist can help clients focus on their own power and control and experience the reenactment without fear.

In the standard EMDR session, a therapist might say to a client, *Go with that* or *Good*. In the reenactment session the therapist will say, *Be aware of your strength and control* (locus of control); *Let yourself feel yourself dominating the situation* (fear of pain and locus of control); *Experience yourself being in charge, Feel the strength in your arms and shoulders* (targeting related neurons in the motor cortex); or *Experience the control and power in your back* (locus of control and targeting the neurons of the motor cortex).

These suggestions are made while the client is slowly going through the reenactment process. I will sometimes suggest that the clients do this reenactment process in slow motion in order to feel all of the muscle groups involved. This slow motion allows time for the therapist to make suggestions to help the clients focus on the physical sensation of strength, control, and calm.

USING THE TRAUMATIZED MUSCLES

It's important that the guided image be related to the specific body parts that were involved in the original trauma. The best images are the ones that the clients identify with most easily. For example, I was working with a woman who was beaten frequently during a marriage. Later in her life she had nightmares of a fist coming toward her face in the way that she had experienced many times. We looked at a number of images. She tried using her hand to wipe the image away as if it were really on a screen that she could simply wipe clean. This process seemed to have little value. She was using her hand but she was doing something that was somewhat abstract. Later we talked of her using the facial muscles that had experienced the pain in the original trauma. She imagined opening her mouth and simply chewing the fist or blowing a quick puff of air that would cause the fist to disperse like dust. These images had more power than the wiping image and seemed to reduce the fear related to the image of the fist coming toward her face. As she worked with this image I had her picking up the fist and biting it or blowing it with air that would cause it to disperse. With each of these images she became less fearful and seemed to enjoy the process, even to the point of a smile. She felt more in control and less like a victim.

Scaer wrote of his understanding of myofascial pain: "the proprioceptive memory of the protective movement of the body in the accident generated by stretch receptors are immediately and indelibly stored in the brainstem motor centers. Thereafter, they will be resurrected time and again in situations of perceived life threat, leading to recurrent regional patterns of myofascial pain" (2001, pp. 75–76).

Scaer also wrote of the chemical cycle of trauma and reenactment (Scaer, 2001), asserting that the biochemistry of trauma may condition the person to the repetition of the reenactment process. It might be that the RP breaks that cycle by having the client create a drastically different conclusion in the reenactment. I have had a few clients spontaneously tell me that each time the old trauma images come to mind, they now have the new endings.

Physical pain and emotional pain have often been related to the common idea of a "broken heart" or "pain in the neck," yet only recently have Eisenberger and others (Eisenberger, Lieberman, & Williams, 2003) started publishing papers showing the deep neurological similarity between physical pain and emotional pain. This same connection is demonstrated in the Body Scan part of the standard EMDR protocol. In the RP, it is critical to cope with trauma and related physical pain together. It seems that the factors that are central to the experience of physical pain are also central to recovery from psychological trauma.

Clients who have trauma histories have more chronic pain (Green, Flowe-Valencia, Rosenblum, & Tait, 1999). Those with histories of childhood sexual abuse have more painful body areas, diffused pain, diagnoses of fibromyalgia, surgeries, hospitalizations, and physician visits (Finestone et al., 2000). The interaction of this pain and the psychological factors related to trauma demands our attention.

Within the RP, attention is given to the same motor centers that were involved in the original accident or pain incident in order to stimulate the same motor centers and both create new strength associations and weaken existing pain associations. For this reason, use the same muscles in the reenactment fantasy that originally generated the signals to the brain stem motor centers. Thus we replace what was "the victim's attempt to survive messages" with "the client's confident, safe assertion of control messages," in order to make these associations in the same brain stem motor centers and the same stretch receptors.

OUTCOMES

From my own experience and verbal or written feedback from 150 RP-trained therapists, I see that

- The RP is effective with physically based trauma.
- It can relieve some trauma-based pain.
- It can transform a PTSD response to a giggle, often in less than 10 minutes, sometimes in less than 5.
- It does not create abreactions (reexperiencing of the trauma).
- It can complete processing for clients who were looping, abreacting, or moving very slowly with standard EMDR processing.
- Most clients can do RP.
- Clients with multiple traumas, who were treated primarily with RP, gained feelings of control, strength, and sureness while exhibiting more assertive behavior.
- It is often enjoyable for the client and the therapist, creating little secondary trauma in the therapists.

SUMMARY

The RP is the installation of feelings of responsible power grafted upon a painful memory of being a victim. While it does not change what has happened, it provides a restructuring of the individual's identity with regard to the memory. The client is building an image of responsible power, security, and control upon the memory of trauma and victimization. As a result, PTSD and chronic pain symptoms often lessen or disappear after treatment with the RP.

REFERENCES

Ehlers, A., Mayou, R. A., & Bryant, B. (1998). Psychological predictors of chronic posttraumatic stress disorder after motor vehicle accidents. *Journal of Abnormal Psychology, 107*(3), 508–519.

Eisenberger, N. I., Lieberman, M. D., & Williams, K. D. (2003). Does rejection hurt?, an fMRI study of social exclusion, *Science, 302*, 290–292.

Ekman, P. (2003). *Emotions revealed.* New York: Henry Holt.

Finestone, H. M., Stenn, P., Davies, F., Stalker, C., Fry, R., & Koumanis, J. (2000). Chronic pain and health care utilization in women with a history of childhood sexual abuse. *Child Abuse & Neglect, 24*(4), 547–556.

Foster, S. (2001, February). *Using EMDR for performance enhancement*. Workshop, Vancouver, British Columbia.

Green, C. R., Flowe-Valencia, H., Rosenblum, L., & Tait, A. R. (1999). Do physical and sexual abuse differentially affect chronic pain states in women? *Journal of Pain & Symptom Management, 18*(6), 420–426.

Krakow, B., Hollifield, M., Johnston, L., Koss, M., Schrader, R., Warner, T. D., Tandberg, D., Lauriello, J., McBride, L., Cutchen, L., Cheng, D., Emmons, S., Germain, A., Melendrez, D., Sandoval, D., & Prince, H. (2001a). Imagery rehearsal therapy for chronic nightmares in sexual assault survivors with post-traumatic stress disorder: A randomized controlled trial. *Journal of the American Medical Association, 286*(5), 537–545. Available at http://www.nightmaretreatment.com/

Krakow, B., Sandoval, D., Schrader, R., Keuhne, B., McBride, L., Yau, C. L., & Tandberg, D. (2001b). Treatment of chronic nightmares in adjudicated adolescent girls in a residential facility. *Journal of Adolescent Health, 29*(2), 94–100. Available at http://www.nightmaretreatment.com/

Levine, P. (1997). *Waking the tiger: Healing trauma*. Berkeley, CA; North Atlantic Books.

Ozer, E. J., Best, S. R., Lipsey, T. L., & Weiss, D. S. (2003). Predictors of posttraumatic stress disorder and symptoms in adults: A meta-analysis. *Psychological Bulletin, 129*(1), 52–73.

Scaer, R. (2001). *The body bears the burden*. Binghamton, NY: Haworth Medical Press.

Shapiro, F. (2001). *Eye movement desensitization and reprocessing: Basic principles, protocols, and procedures* (2nd ed.). New York: Guilford Press.

Simonton, O. C. (1978). *Getting well again*. New York: Tarcher.

van der Kolk, B. A. (1989). The compulsion to repeat the trauma: Reenactment, revictimization, and masochism. *Psychiatric Clinics of North America, 12*(2), 389–411.

Wilson, S., Tinker, R., Becker, L., Hofmann, A., & Cole, J. (2002, September). *Treating phantom limb pain with brain imaging (MEG)*. Paper presented at the EMDRIA, Toronto, Ontario.

Wilson, S., Tinker, R., & Cole, J. (2000, April). *Phantom pain*. Presentation at EMDR Conference, Vancouver, British Columbia.

Chapter 10

EMDR with Cultural and Generational Introjects

Robin Shapiro

EMDR, A THERAPY PRIMARILY KNOWN FOR THE TREATMENT OF TRAUMA, can root out destructive cultural or generational introjects. It can target the cultural transmission of racism, sexism, class expectations, and the increasingly narrow parameters of acceptable appearance, interests, and personality. It can also transform the effects of the generational transmission of destructive beliefs, identities, and emotional states. Some facts about a person, such as sexual orientation, race, class, level of success, or appearance may never be acceptable to many of those around them, including their families. We can help people accept themselves even when they are bombarded with external messages that they are unacceptable.

Cultural expectations may be clearly negative: "Working class people are stupid." "Indians are lazy." "Blondes are ditzy." Positive expectations may also have negative effects: "Women should be slender and cute." "Big boys never cry." "Asians should be brilliant." "Everyone should be young and beautiful."

When exploring internalized race, gender, cultural, ethnic, or class-based introjects I use the Standard Protocol, often in conjunction with two other techniques, to explore and clear the split between a client's self and negative or positive cultural expectations.

THE STANDARD PROTOCOL

The EMDR Standard Protocol can be successfully used to target the trauma, emotional states, or deeply held beliefs that stem from the experience of a lifetime of racism, sexism, or difference from some cultural norm. The Standard Protocol can be aimed at one particular incident of racism or a culturally induced cognition (i.e., "I must be anorexic, tall, athletic, blond, or white to be acceptable"). Some culturally induced traumas are simple to target and simple to clear out. In Phase 1, the history-taking phase of EMDR, it's easy to collect trauma targets with their appropriate negative and positive cognitions for later EMDR processing. Targets include experiences of violence, ostracism, or shaming for being in a certain group or for being different. Here are some examples:

- Event: Gay-bashing incident

  - Negative Cognitions (NC): I'm helpless. I deserve it.
  - Positive Cognitions (PC): It's over. I'm strong. I deserve respect.

- Event: Being repeatedly beat up by neighborhood kids for being Jewish

  - NC: I'll always be under attack.
  - PC: My life is different now. I can confront anti-Semitism. I'm safe. (If true!)

- Event: Being ostracized or humiliated in junior high school for being fat, smart, from the wrong social class, race, religion, or any other difference

  - NC: I'm unacceptable.
  - PC: I'm acceptable. I'll never be in junior high school again! It's over.

- Event: Coming out to somebody, especially family members or close friends, and receiving a negative or shocked reaction

- o NC: I'm unacceptable.
- o PC: I am acceptable, even if people don't approve.

- Event: Becoming a new "dot-com millionaire" and fearing alienation from middle-class or working-class friends and family

  - o Future template: Imagine inviting your family to your big new house.
  - o NC: I'm too different to be acceptable.
  - o PC: I can handle their reactions.

The Standard Protocol works well for clear-cut and time-limited events. Sometimes it isn't enough. Clients may move through node after node of distressing memories without completely clearing the traumas and distress related to their difference. They may have difficulty pinpointing the generational transmission of the familial beliefs that haunt them. They may leave our offices and face the same discrimination and disapproval every day, making them subject to constant retraumatization. In these cases the Standard Protocol may be interwoven with other techniques to bring the client to self-acceptance and resilience in the face of ongoing disapproval.

When I think about internalized oppression, I borrow the idea of introjects from object relations theory, in which introjects are defined as psychic objects that are unconsciously taken in by a person. These objects may be emotional states, ideas, or even an ego state of another person or group (Ogden, 1991). Michael White's (1995) narrative therapy described personal, familial, organizational, and cultural/ historical narratives from which people create their reality and sense of self. In narrative therapy, problems are externalized, disowned, and conquered. Generational and cultural traumas, narratives, and ego states can be externalized and consciously disowned with the help of the Standard Protocol and the Two-Hand Interweave. I found that by using narrative questions, introjects, and the Two-Hand Interweave, I was able to create quick and relatively painless ways to move entrenched cultural distress. Some time later, I found that the same techniques work well with familial and generational issues. It's no surprise to note that cultural and familial issues are often intertwined.

THE TWO-HAND INTERWEAVE

The Two-Hand Interweave (see Chapter 6) can delineate the difference between the client's "true self" and the negative or positive cultural projection: *Place the stereotype of how fat people/working-class people/blind people are in one hand and who you really are in the other hand. Go with that.* (Dual Attention Stimulus [DAS].) After a few rounds the clients will spontaneously grasp the ways in which they don't fit the internalized stereotype. They may even begin to know that they don't have to fit the cultural expectation in order to be acceptable to the self. In that case, install the spontaneously created variation on "I'm acceptable the way I am" and move on.

Often after a few sets of the Two-Hand Interweave the client spontaneously floats back to the heart of her distress. You already have the NC. Grab the PC, move through the rest of the setup of the Standard Protocol, and commence DAS. The processing will take you to events from which the negative belief arose. "My older brother called me fat." "I got beat up for being Jewish since I was 8 years old." "Those Gap ads! I can never look like that." Keep clearing until all the nodes are gone. People often move from shame, to anger, to grief, to acceptance of self within one long round of EMDR.

A Japanese-American young woman, 21, thought that she should either be tall and blond or else she should be the "perfect" Japanese girl, demure, with long straight hair (her hair was rough). In both cases she thought that she should be long-waisted and slender. (She had little body fat, but a short and wide build and a major binge-and-purge eating disorder.) Eighteen months into therapy, we used the Two-Hand Interweave to find targets for the Standard Protocol.

In one hand, hold the tall, blond, blue-eyed girl you should be. In the other hand hold the person you really are. (DAS.) Enormous shame arose. We set up a Standard Protocol Assessment to find where it lived in her body and the cognition: "I'm fine the way I am." Her Subjective Units of Distress Scale (SUDS) was 9. In five sets of EMDR, her SUDS fell to 0. She said, "I'm better than fine."

We installed that, then went on to: *In one hand hold the long-haired demure perfect Japanese daughter you should be. In the other hand hold the person you really are.* (DAS.)

Immediately a picture of her mother frowning at her arose. We kept tapping on that. "Mom" moved through and the client said, "It's okay. I don't have to be who she wants me to be. I'm not!"

After we installed that, I asked her: *So in one hand hold the tall, blond, blue-eyed girl. In the other hold the perfect Japanese girl.* (DAS.)

She giggled. "They're fighting! They're so not me. I'll let them fight it out on their own!"

Go with that! (DAS.)

Her eating disorder abated after this intervention. She accepted her body and her personality. Her mother's frown no longer had the power to get her to binge, purge, or starve.

Here's another example of the Standard Protocol and Two-Hand Interweave helping to clear a lifelong experience of racism: When discussing relationship issues, Joe talked about never acting angry around white people, including his boyfriend, for fear of scaring them. Joe, a total sweetheart, is very aware that his presence as a black, tall man is intimidating to nearly everyone on the street. He had experienced others' flinching, "hate stares," and avoidance, over and over. We used the EMDR Standard Protocol to clear his reactions (shame, frustration, and inhibition) to the fear response in others. We imagined him getting the fear reaction in the future. PC: "It's not my fault, it's not my problem." We used the two-handed approach: *In one hand, put the way that strangers perceive you. In the other hand put the way you really are.* He felt a huge discrepancy between the "mean, shiftless, dangerous guy" that strangers see and the intelligent, gentle, cultured person that he is and familiar people know him to be. We then used the Standard Protocol's Future Template to imagine him assertively telling off his partner: *Imagine telling him everything you feel about what he's been up to.* SUDS: 8–0. NC: "I'm too scary." PC: "I am assertive, not abusive." He cleared it down to 0 and was able to feel good about imagining telling the truth to his partner.

After our work, he is less bothered by people's reactions to him on the street. He no longer takes it personally. He finds himself laughing at the weirdness of it: "If they really knew me, they'd know how funny their reactions really are." And he's resolved some previously unspoken issues with his partner. In fact, Joe and his partner took their first vacation together in years, after clearing the air with some good (and loud) conflict resolution.

NARRATIVE THERAPY

Narrative questions within a modified EMDR protocol help clients with especially pernicious introjects. While clients are considering each question, I use short sets of DAS to help them along. Ellen Fox (personal communication, 1999), a Narrative and EMDR therapist in Seattle, suggested some of the questions to me. I use these questions in clear steps:

1. Identification and etiology of the introject
2. Separation of self from the introject
3. Disowning the introject
4. Resource Installation
5. Inoculation

I'll interweave answers from a composite 30-year-old woman who thinks she's fat and ugly, when she's in fact an attractive size 14 (not tiny, not obese).

1. To identify the introject as coming from outside, I ask one or all of these questions:

RS: *Where did you learn that?* (DAS.)
Client: First from my mom. She was always dieting and afraid that I'd get fat. Then at school it's all we talked about. All the people on television, in movies, and in all the media don't look like me.
RS: *How did that idea/feeling/way of seeing get inside you?* (DAS.)
Client: My mom's fear and all those millions of images just took over my head!
RS: *How does the culture put that inside your head?* (DAS.)
Client: Repetition! Kate Moss! My mom!

   (There are often great EMDR Standard Protocol targets here: Racial/gender/appearance taunting, the hate stare, put-downs, or Gap ads. With this client, we use the Standard Protocol to clear out her experience of her mother's fear. The SUDS goes from 9 to 5, and doesn't drop lower. It's time to go after "culture" to clear the rest of the introjects.)
2. To separate the client's self from the cultural introject, I ask three more questions:

RS: *Is that what you want to know/feel?* (DAS.)
Client: No! I'm tired of it!
RS: *Is that how you want to see yourself?* (DAS.)
Client: No!

RS: *Where in your body are you holding that idea/feeling?* (DAS.)
My stomach. It's disgust.

3. Now it's time to disown the introject with two questions and an
    instruction:

RS: *Are you ready to pull that idea/feeling out of you?* (DAS.)
Client: Yes!
RS: *Where do you want to send it? (Outer space, back to the culture,
blow it up, etc.)* (DAS.)
Client: I want to send it back to all the clothing designers, ad exec-
utives, and mean eighth-grade girls in the world.
RS: *Pull it out.* (Continual DAS.) *Physically, that's right. Is it all out?
Not yet? Keep going until it's completely gone.*
Client: It's gone! That has been inside me for a long time. I don't
even know who I am right now, without that.

4. Resource Installation:

RS: *What would you like to think/feel/see instead?* (DAS.)
Client: Self-love. And appreciation.
RS: *What embodies that new thought or feeling?* (DAS.)
Client: A rose pink feeling.
RS: *Bring that into every cell of your body.* (DAS.)
Client: Okay, I'm doing it.
RS: *Does any part need an extra dose?* (Turner, 2003) (DAS.)
Client: My thighs and my butt.
RS: *Bring in more of that new feeling.* (DAS.)

5. Now it's time for Inoculation, a variation on the theme of
    EMDR's Future Template:

RS: *The culture will keep trying to put this idea inside of you. How do
you recognize when that's happening?* (DAS.)
Client: If I feel that self-disgust feeling.
RS: *How are you going to stay free of this feeling?* (DAS.)
Client: I'm going to tell it to F***-off, I'm okay the way I am. And
then I'll pull it out of my body and send it back to the mean
girls.

RS: *Imagine encountering the strongest possible intrusion of this idea/feeling into you. How will you keep it out of you?* (DAS.)

Client: I'm trying on clothes. Even worse, with my mom, and she looks at me "that way." I'm going to talk about how I like my body, and I like not being afraid of it. I can feel myself sticking my chin out. It feels good.

RS: *Go with that.* (DAS.) *How will you move it out of you if it creeps back in?* (DAS.)

Client: I'll pull it out like we did today, and think of how much those ad executives get paid.

RS: *Imagine doing that.* (DAS.) *Can you fill up again with that new thought* (positive cognition) *about yourself?* (DAS.)

Client: All right. I'm acceptable the way I am, and I'm pulling in rose pink acceptance, especially to my butt.

RS: *So imagine you're with your mom, and you're trying on clothes and she says something negative about your appearance.*

Client: Who cares!

FAMILIAL AND GENERATIONAL
INTROJECTS

Generational issues are introjects that have been handed down for one or more generations. They can consist of anxiety (sometimes a sense of existential danger), shame, impossible expectations, ego states, or complex ideas about who the family and its members can be or should be. Issues of family loyalty, identity and survival are often strongly imbedded within familial introjects. For instance, a son may feel disloyal to his father if he lets go of the family legacy of "failure." A client could feel that both she and her mother won't survive if she lets go the introject of her narcissistic mother's internal child. If "all Joneses go to Yale," who is Betty Jones if she doesn't? Maureen Kitchur's genograms (see Chapter 1) are an excellent place to spot familial trends or introjects. Recurrent family roles ("the failure," "the savior," "the neglected middle child") may pop right off the page.

Here are useful questions in different cases:

What would be the effect of you letting go of "failure"?

What does your most adult part think of pulling that piece of your mother out of you?

What would happen if you gave her back to herself to care for?

What would need to happen for you to pull this family anxiety out of you?

Think about what it would be like to . . .

Use the EMDR Standard Protocol to target

1. The transmission of the introject
2. The beginning of the family issue (if known), for example, when the Cossacks raped Great-Grandma and burned our house. (PC: *It's over, I'm safe now.*) or when we were starving sharecroppers in Mississippi. (PC: *It's over. I have enough.*)
3. Fears of letting go of the introject. (PC: *I will survive.*)

Use the Two-Hand Interweave to help differentiate between then and now. *In one hand, hold those times when vigilance was mandatory for the survival of your family. In the other hand, hold your current life.* or *In one hand, hold your father's feeling of failure. In the other, hold your capabilities and your situation. Just notice . . .*

Here are some examples of using the Standard Protocol, narrative questions, and the Two-Hand Interweave:

SELF-SACRIFICE

Ellen's grandparents were immigrants. Her father owned a small business and made an adequate but small income. Ellen's mother, grandmother, and great-grandmother were very responsible caretakers. There is a strong ethic of self-sacrifice in her family. As a child, she was shamed for reading books and for sitting down to rest. One of the family narratives was that women must sacrifice everything for their families. Ellen had done exactly that in both marriages. Despite marrying into wealth, she refused to hire help in her home or to pursue any of her myriad interests. In each marriage she had zealously taken over most family functions. In each, she had "given herself away," then had withdrawn in disgust from her husband. Her commitment to providing a stable home for her child kept her in the current marriage.

1. Identification and Etiology: Ellen's ancestors were poor Eastern European Jews, subject to severe difficulties in basic survival. Sacrifice of self for the good of the family and the community was necessary for survival. This narrative was transmitted to Ellen by example, by shaming when she was "selfish," and by many sayings and directives.
2. Separation of self from narrative: We cleared shaming incidents with the Standard Protocol. We did the Two-Handed Interweave. While tapping, we noted her family's former situation. *Hold your great-grandparents' reality in one hand and your current reality in the other. Notice the difference. Do you have enough money? Are people trying to kill you? Are you surviving? Thriving?*
3. Disowning the introject (with DAS): *Think back through the history of your people. All the generations in Diaspora. All the generations being chased from country to country, trying to survive hunger, hatred, and new situations. Think back all the way to the slaves in Egypt. Notice how each generation of women gave the gift of survival to the next generation. Notice how your mother and your mother's mother, and her mother, and all the generations back to the beginning gave the gift of survival, and how to ensure survival to each generation. How happy would they be to know that you no longer have to sacrifice yourself in order to survive, in order than your child survives? They have been striving for 3,000 years to create a generation that is safe; that can make it through without constant struggle. Can you thank them for the gift of self-sacrifice? Can you show them that it is no longer appropriate for you? Can you feel their jubilation, that one of theirs finally gets the luxury of knowing what she wants, and taking care of herself? Is it time to thank them for the gift and let them know that you will use it, only if it is appropriate for the survival of your daughter?*
4. Resource Installation: *What part of you would you prefer to expand?* Ellen's fun-loving, adventurous, creative, younger self.

Feel her inside of you. Bring her into every cell of your being. How would she live your days? What would she do differently?
5. Inoculation: *Think of what situations will bring out that self-killing sense of overresponsibility. How will you combat that?*

After this session, Ellen was able to give her husband more responsibility for the house and child care. She hired house-cleaners. She began some creative projects. She was more able to know what she wanted and felt less guilty when she did what she wanted. When shamed by her nasty and narcissistic mother-in-law for not knuckling under about a family issue, Ellen was able to "hold on to herself" and keep her sense of goodness and entitlement. She was more able to tell her husband exactly what she wanted. She began to feel closer to him and to her daughter. Her depression lifted perceptibly, but not totally.

RAGE AND ABUSIVE BEHAVIOR

We'd discussed in the last session that Bill's rage at his family was enacted exactly like his father's rage toward his mother, and his grandfather's rage at and abuse of Bill's father. This session was planned to be an "abusectomy" of the generational rage in Bill's family. We surmised that it might have been passed down for many generations, passing from man to man in the family. Bill wanted the abuse to end at his generation. He wanted to be a good husband and a good father. (Continual DAS.) *Think of the last time you blew up at Irene. Where do you feel that in your body?* Upper Chest. *Think of what you said and how you said it. Notice that you were "going for the kill."* (Pause) *Feel your father's abuse, and your grandfather's abuse and all the generations of hatred and humiliation of loved ones. Do you want to continue this family tradition? Good, then physically pull the thoughts, sensations, and emotions out of you. Keep going. Good, keep going. That's right. Let it go. Clear it out. It's gone? What do want there in its place?* He didn't know. I suggested his wonderful maternal grandfather's equanimity, generosity, and self-containment. He thought that was a great idea. We did a resource installation of his maternal grandfather's character traits. Then we imagined Irene doing the most triggering behavior she does and Bill responding to it post-abusectomy and post-Resource Installation. He reported a SUDS of 2, which we cleared with the Standard Protocol. When he thought of Irene again, he could feel his beloved grandfather's strength and sense of humor in him. Both Irene and Bill reported that Bill showed much less rage and abuse toward all members of the family. Bill reported that he was "hard to provoke anymore."

"MOMECTOMY"

With a 30-year-old depressed and anxious woman, in the setup for a session with a particular ego state, we started DAS, found the Internal Adviser, and began to make contact with her 3-year-old part. A 6-year-old part popped up. She was terrified and chaotic and made it impossible to stay in contact with the 3-year-old.

Client: That's my mother! She's inside of me. I have to take care of her and it's too much.
RS: *Do you want to keep trying to take care of this part of your mother?*
Client: NO!
RS: *Has your mom grown up since you were a child?*
Client: Yes.
RS: *Are you ready to do a Momectomy?*
Client: Right now!
RS: *Then pull that 6-year-old out of you and send her to the competent mother you have now.* (DAS.)

Five minutes later, a beaming Melanie declared that a huge, good space had opened up inside of her. She reported that her mother had filled up all the space in her and that she had room for herself now. She filled the space with "the light of self love" and the positive cognition, "I am lovable."

SUMMARY

It's helpful to examine a client's family, subculture, and the culture at large as possible creators of negative cognitions and destructive identities. Once you've identified and delineated the destructive introjects,

EMDR can be used by itself or in combination with other therapies to clear the effects of destructive cultural and familial introjects.

REFERENCES

Ogden, T. H. (2001). *Projective identification and psychotherapeutic technique.* Northvale, NJ: Jason Aronson.

Turner, E. (2003, April). *EMDR weekly class, level II.* Children's Unit, Seattle, WA.

White, M. (1995). *Re-authoring lives: Interviews and essays.* Adelaide, Australia: Dulwich Centre.

Chapter 11

Exiting the Binge-Diet Cycle

Susan Schulherr

EVERY SO OFTEN YOU RUN INTO A CLINICAL EPIPHANY THAT PERMA-
nently changes the way you organize experience. For most of us, EMDR
was one such reorganizer. For me, another epiphany, more localized,
occurred in the late 1980s at a symposium on alcoholism (Berenson,
1988). A family therapist, Berenson illustrated how families with an alcoholic member tend to cycle between "wet" and "dry" phases, the former characterized by chaos and acting out, the latter by a tense surface
order organized through tight controls. Berenson called on the work of
Fossum and Mason (1986) to present the view that these cycles of control and release occur across the spectrum of addictions and are princi-
pally driven by a family's attempt to manage unbearable shame.

Around the time I attended the alcholism symposium, I was given the
chance to work with hundreds of weight-loss clients as a group leader.
Although binge eating disorder (BED) was not yet a part of the clinical
nomenclature, bingeing was clearly a part of the experience of a number
of the program's members. Repeatedly these clients reported the enormous relief they felt within the structure of the program. They viewed it
as saving them from their own overwhelming urges to eat 'til it hurt.
Most of them talked about the all-or-nothingness of their experience and
the boom-and-bust cycles of trying one diet after another, only to find
themselves time after time back in the land of no limits.

I connected these experiences to Berenson's model. I began to invite
clients to do the same. As they described their personal experiences
through each step of the binge-diet cycle, they confirmed for me the

prominence of underlying shame and the desperate attempt to contain it through rigid behavioral controls.

My early interest in sharing the model with clients was primarily that they use their own experiences to make a case against dieting. Research had already made that case on a physiologic basis. If you place normal eaters on starvation diets, they become bingers when again allowed to eat what they want (Johnson & Connors, 1987). Undereating induces overeating in anyone. Fossum and Mason's model made the case on a psychological basis. I developed what I call the Binge Cycle Exercise to help clients see it for themselves. I'd like to walk you through the first part of it now with my composite client, Ericka, to give you the lay of the land from a client's perspective.

ROUND 1 OF THE BINGE CYCLE EXERCISE

I begin by placing the word *BINGE* on the left side of a blank sheet of paper and the word *DIET* on the other side (see Figure 11.1). Each word stands for the period of time Ericka is in that phase of the cycle.

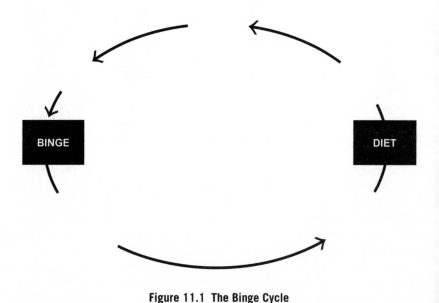

Figure 11.1 The Binge Cycle

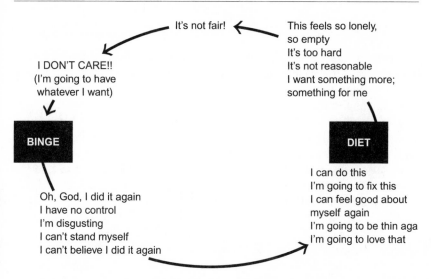

It's not fair!

This feels so lonely,
so empty
It's too hard
It's not reasonable
I want something more;
something for me

I DON'T CARE!!
(I'm going to have
whatever I want)

BINGE

DIET

I can do this
I'm going to fix this
I can feel good about
myself again
I'm going to be thin aga
I'm going to love that

Oh, God, I did it again
I have no control
I'm disgusting
I can't stand myself
I can't believe I did it again

Figure 11.2 Erika's Responses to the Binge Cycle Exercise

I then tell Ericka that we won't actually be talking about bingeing or dieting today. Instead we'll focus on the transition points in which she is moving out of or into one of these two phases of the cycle. I like the advantage of focusing on something Ericka is not used to thinking about (obsessively); at least I have her attention!

I ask Ericka to start by telling me the thoughts and feelings that come up for her at the time when she knows the binge to be over (Ericka and all BED clients know exactly when that is). Ericka pours out a litany of self-loathing: "I'm a pig. . . . I hate myself. . . . I can't believe I did it again. . . . I'm disgusting. . . . I'll never be thin. . . . I can't stand this. . . . It's hopeless. . . . I'm so gross!"

I duly record each response just beneath the BINGE stage (Figure 11.2). When Ericka is finished, I stop to appreciate with her just how truly awful this aftermath of the binge is. I then ask Ericka to take me to the moment when she has committed to the next diet. Maybe she's selected a diet she saw in a magazine. Or she plans to return to a commercial program she's tried in the past. Whatever it is, I'm looking for that moment in which she's decided what she's going to do. Again, I ask for the thoughts and feelings that come up at that point. Ericka's responses are typical: "I'm in control again. . . . I'm really going to do it this time. . . . I'll be thin. . . . I feel hopeful, excited. . . . I'm going to feel so good."

I now stop to compare and contrast the two sets of responses with Ericka. You may wish to take a minute to do the same right now. I notice with genuine awe how the decision to go on a diet completely transforms Ericka's experience: from truly wretched and despairing to hopeful, upbeat, even euphoric; from feeling helpless and out of control to feeling once again in control, resolute, and certain of a happy outcome; from a sense of profound unworthiness to a sense of being on a path that will restore her to a feeling of worth. It's better than magic! I hope Ericka will begin to look at this old familiar place with some of the amazement that I do.

I now ask Ericka to take us to that point of the dieting phase when it's not so exciting anymore. This is probably a time in which the pounds are coming off slowly, if at all. It feels like the effort required is so disproportionate to the outcome and that desired rewards are unbearably far off. I call this transition "The Thrill Is Gone." Ericka's thoughts and feelings at this stage are: "This is too hard! . . . It isn't worth it. . . . This isn't working. . . . I'm tired of this!" Ericka's next response is almost universal and, to my mind, marks a shift to the next transitional stage. You can almost hear her foot stamping as she protests: "This isn't fair!"

I take a detour at this point with Ericka. I ask her if there is any other place in her life where it feels like the demands are so great compared to the rewards or that she's so far from her goals. Ericka thinks of her job. She's widely respected in a high-profile position. Yet she always feels defeat and exposure of her inadequacies are just around the next bend. She's never living up to her own vision of how she should be performing. She's in a constant state of exhaustion from the stress, much of it self-induced.

This detour is a preview of work to come in which the symptoms of Ericka's eating disorder will be connected to underlying beliefs that govern much of her life. These beliefs will have to shift if she is to resolve her eating symptoms.

I now ask Ericka to tell me what she is thinking and feeling in the moment right before she enters the binge phase. She hasn't yet had a mouthful but has committed psychologically to the binge. Ericka's response is a resounding and colorful version of Heck with it! And even more resoundingly: "I DON'T CARE!" (If a particular client doesn't spontaneously say "I don't care!" I report that that response comes up for a lot of people at this point in the cycle. I ask if it does for her? It always does.) In this circumstance, "I don't care" means "I don't care about the consequences; I'm going to have whatever I want."

"I don't care" is the gateway into the binge. It's a telling moment. We can understand it best with another compare-and-contrast, this time with the responses to the "Thrill Is Gone" transition. That's where Ericka's perfectionistic standards and her sense of measuring up badly are visible in sharp relief as she reacts to the stringency of her diet: "It's too hard. . . . I'll never get there." You might say these responses represent caring too much. As Ericka journeys through the diet phase, it's as if a coil of tension begins to tighten between spontaneous desire on the one hand and the imperatives of thinness, perfection, and control on the other. The tension increases dramatically as Ericka's best efforts stall out. She experiences a chasm between what she feels she's supposed to do and what she can or wants to do. The coil tightens to the limits of Ericka's bearing; she revolts against the rigid regime by throwing off all restraint. I point out to her that caring not at all seems like the perfect antidote for caring way too much. I say it seems very much like going on strike against unfair working practices. If asked, most binge cyclers will tell you that the moment of "I don't care" is really what they prize, more than the food itself.

Of course, at this stage "I don't care" is just pretend. The underlying perfectionistic demands and beliefs haven't shifted; Ericka is just taking a breather. She enters an "as if" world in which the rules are temporarily suspended, like a weekend pass from prison. She knows this and binges all the more for knowing the return to prison is coming.

At some point during the binge Ericka inevitably comes back into connection with her implacable standards for herself and the loathing begins . . . again.

CLINICAL USES OF ROUND 1 OF THE BINGE CYCLE EXERCISE

I prefaced the story of Ericka's journey with the comment that I originally used the Binge Cycle Exercise to interdict dieting. Now that you know the steps of Round 1, let's consider how these can be put together for diet interdiction and a few other purposes as well.

I point out to Ericka that enacting one pole of the cycle will inexorably lead to the other: if she binges, she will be drawn to dieting to "cure" the self-hatred and despair that follow bingeing; if she diets, she'll eventually revolt against the self-denial and deprivation of her stringent regime. Put another way, bingeing is a trigger for dieting and dieting is a trigger for bingeing. This is big news for Erika and all binge-cyclers who regard dieting as their salvation.

I also point out the human phenomenon that we tend to correct for extremes in one direction with extremes in the other direction. Such self-corrective cycles can take on a life of their own, independent of original causes. It can be useful to find a place to put a wedge in the cycle to interfere with the self-correction engine. The work Ericka and I have just done together provides that wedge. First of all, we have just dethroned dieting. Second, Ericka, like the majority of cyclers, is a bit shocked and awed to see her familiar experience in this new light. She is now more amenable to a direct suggestion that she stop dieting.

For some clients this is a good time for a referral to a nutritionist. For Ericka it is sufficient to spend time in our sessions talking about discovering a nondiet way of eating that suits guidelines of health and her own taste. She understands that a crash course of change is going to feel like a diet and thus risk triggering bingeing. So she works on a wholly new approach, an incremental one, with the aim of gradually developing a way she can eat for the rest of her life.

Ericka, again like most cyclers, is well aware of her black-and-white, all-or-nothing approach to eating and to life. Working on incremental development of a personally right, nonextreme way of eating is a great practice arena for discovering what middle ground can be like.

I mentioned other purposes for Round 1 of the Binge Cycle exercise. Two are most important in my experience. First, this shared work can be a powerful engagement tool with new BED clients. It helps the clinician gain rapid entry into the very personal terrain of the client's symptomatic experience. Furthermore, by bringing new awareness to such familiar ground, the clinician establishes expertise and along with it a little sorely needed hopefulness.

Secondly, it's de-shaming to do just this much of the exercise. Consider your explanations for bingeing compared to your client's. Your client's explanations for her bingeing can be found in her responses after the binge: "I'm a slob; I'm disgusting; I'm weak." In contrast, you've shown how understandable the binge is as a response to a stringent dietary regime, not to mention the stringent and overwhelming life demands that go along with it. In the same vein, you've defined self-corrective cycles such as binge-diet as broadly human phenomena.

THE BINGE CYCLE EXERCISE IN A COMPREHENSIVE EMDR TREATMENT PLAN

Let's leave Ericka for the moment to consider how to integrate the Binge Cycle Exercise into a comprehensive EMDR treatment plan for BED clients. I think of three major domains of work that are going to be necessary for most BED clients. The first is the development of affect management skills. The second is the processing of targets related to the beliefs and dynamics underlying the binge-diet cycle. The third is the processing of all other targets of the particular client.

Within the 8-Phase treatment model (Shapiro, 2001), I include Round 1 of the Binge Cycle exercise in Phase 1, Client History and Treatment Planning. I like to introduce it early on for the reasons just outlined: (a) it offers an early opportunity to interdict dieting; (b) it's a valuable engagement tool; and (c) it tends to be de-shaming. As we'll see, the exercise also yields multiple targets for future processing specific to BED dynamics.

As with every client, you'll need a thorough history. Dynamics underlying the binge cycle tend to coexist with other issues that help maintain BED symptoms. Frequently eating disorder (ED) clients have trauma histories and attachment deficits, all of which will need to be addressed. You will also need to take a history of the eating disorder itself. Its onset will probably be an important clue to issues the client or her family were struggling with at the time. These will often involve the client's entering a developmental stage that is threatening to herself or other family members in some way, for example, adolescent sexuality or the approach of adulthood with implied separation from the family (Terry, 1987). The clinician should also inventory current BED symptoms—including diet behavior—to establish a baseline.

Phase 2, the Preparation Phase, can be lengthy for BED clients. I follow many others in believing that the eating disorder represents, among other things, a desperate attempt to self-regulate emotionally for people who haven't developed sufficient internal skills for doing so. Several excellent approaches for this work have been developed by members of the EMDR community, such as: (a) John Omaha's (2001)

Affect Management Skills Training (AMST), (b) Eileen Freedland's (2001) adaptation of Andrew Leed's Resource Development and Installation (RDI) for ED clients, and (c) "The Somatic Interweave" adapted from Somatic Experiencing by Victoria Britt and Nancy Napier (2002), Shirley Jean Schmidt (2002), April Steele (2004), Debra Wesselman (2000), and Roy Kiessling (see Chapter 2) all offer effective ways for working with attachment deficits. ED clients are likely to need these experiences to be sufficiently stabilized for the work ahead and to have the internal resources they'll need for it.

When the client is demonstrating reasonable capacity to self-soothe and to keep reactivity within a manageable range, she can start to process targets identified in the previous stage. I usually start with the ED-specific targets prior to processing more general ones. BED clients tend to be so overwhelmed with their symptoms, it's often hard to focus on much else until that arena has quieted down.

ROUND 2 OF THE BINGE CYCLE EXERCISE

In Round 2 of the Binge Cycle Exercise you and your client can generate ED-specific targets from her responses to Round 1. When I work with clients on this material, I am organized by the view that binge-diet cycling is sustained by an internalized belief system in which perfection and control are prized above all whereas personal needs are suppressed and suspect. Round 2 introduces what you might call preprocessing educational *interweaves* about these underlying beliefs as you work on developing targets. You will be teaching about families in which people never grew comfortable with the reality of human imperfection. As a consequence, they live with a lot of shame. Everyday living is a threat to self-esteem because any moment can lead to a revelation of one's flaws. A "cure" commonly attempted in such families or by certain members is rigid control of behavior to minimize the chances for shameful error and failing. Dieting is one such rigid control.

You will also be teaching about how the rigid control cure can make a person's personal needs seem like potentially troublemaking intruders. Selflessness will almost always be part of the perfectionistic ideal your client has internalized. So in Round 2 you'll be alert at every step to let the client's material illustrate aspects of these two key dynamics: (a) rigid control and perfectionism as the cure for shame; (b) suppression if not contempt for one's own needs. Let's see how that looks.

Starting again right after the binge, just as in Round 1, we find ourselves in a hotbed of shame responses. Explaining shame to the client is a first educational interweave. I tell the client that shame is an estimate of personal worthlessness implicating the whole self; it is an "I am" rather than an "I did." It is an implicitly social experience, a sense that one will and should be excluded from the herd. The impulse is to hide from exposure, to be swallowed by the very earth. It's a good place to stop and reflect with the client on how she experiences shame in her own life.

I will then generally select one of the "I am" phrases from the client's list of post-binge responses. A near-universal example is "I'm disgusting." Next I notice with the client that this "I am" of disgustingness follows from the "I did" of overeating. How is it that an act of overdoing it, even overdoing it big-time, becomes a sweeping estimate of her worth as a person? I ask this question on two levels. The first is rhetorical: I want her to be taken aback, a little confused. I want her to start questioning a reaction that has felt so natural and appropriate.

I give her plenty of time to think about it and us to think about it together. Then I'm going to ask the question again, this time looking for an explanation, a source, that is, looking for a target. Probably the way I'll ask it is: *How did you learn that an act of overdoing it results in personal worthlessness (or makes you disgusting)?* We are now transitioning to the development of BED-specific EMDR targets. We are looking for the familial underpinnings of a set of beliefs that help anchor the symptoms of BED.

INTRODUCTION TO CLIENT

Before we learn how Round 2 unfolds for Ericka, I'd like to introduce you a little more formally to her and her family. Ericka is 32 years old, white, Catholic, and single with an MBA. She is the youngest of three daughters. Ericka's father, who died when Ericka was 13, was a junior college professor. Her mother, now retired, was a librarian and is a devout Catholic.

Ericka went on a diet to lose 15 pounds shortly after she entered high school. She was highly successful, adhering strictly to a dietary regime her doctor gave her. Her binge eating began about 6 months later when she could no longer sustain the momentum of the early stages of the diet and when she was facing certain social pressures. Thereafter she

spent years following different diets, each of which she'd maintain perfectly for a few weeks, only to find herself bingeing again. Her weight
fluctuated over a range of about 30 pounds. At the time she entered
treatment with me she was bingeing 3–5 times per week. She was exer-
cising moderately, though occasionally increased her efforts to try to
compensate for a binge. Ericka reported no use of alcohol or substances.
She had been in therapy once for several years. It hadn't helped with
her eating disorder but Ericka found it useful in other respects.

ERICKA'S ROUND 2 WORK

By the time we completed sufficient Preparation Phase work, approximately 5 months, Ericka's bingeing was down to about once every 2
weeks. However, she was aware that she continued to eat in a rather
compulsive way when distressed or lonely. At this point we turned to
Round 2 of the Binge Cycle Exercise to target the familial dynamics
around shame and perfectionism fueling her symptoms.

It turned out with Ericka that the most fruitful response from the period after the binge (Figure 11.2) was "I have no control." Asked what this
meant about her, Ericka replied, "It's scary. I'm all alone with no guidance and no controls of my own." I asked Ericka to *float back* on this experience, which led to early family targets exemplifying several key themes.

Ericka's father, Joe, had periodic rage reactions. Though Ericka could
remember no instances of physical violence, his screaming tantrums
left the whole family trembling. No doubt mirroring this family experience that couldn't be discussed or resolved, Ericka developed her own
episodes of rage reactions. Her mother stood by as helplessly with Ericka as she did with her husband. Ericka felt profound shame about
her new behavior. As you'll see from her negative belief statements,
feeling out of control and feeling shamed had become fatefully intertwined in Ericka's experience.

Ericka's first target was raging at her older sister, Lisa, who knew
exactly how to get her goat. In this memory, Ericka's mother pleaded
helplessly with her to quiet down so the neighbors wouldn't hear.

Negative cognitions (NCs): "I'm sitting on a poisonous volcano; I'm contaminated."

"I have to hide my anger so nobody knows. They'll be disgusted."

Positive cognitions (PCs): "My anger was understandable. I deserved support and acknowledgment."
"I can be angry and still be loved, loveable."

Not surprisingly, there was also a tremendous amount of fear associated with expression of anger, her own and that of each parent. Though her father's rage stood out in the family lore, her mother's silent disapproval actually felt more malevolent. A target Ericka worked on for a number of sessions involved a particularly acid but characteristically passive-aggressive expression of her mother's hostility toward her father, this time about his beloved fishing. At one point in her processing, referring to her mother's barely veiled anger and disapproval, Ericka stated: "It feels like it connects us—the shameful secret that we both have this angry, venomous snake coiled in our guts." Of course, Ericka was full of what felt like unmanageable anger then and now. A large part of her processing focused on recognizing it, coming to terms with it, and finally being able to own and direct it in self-empowering ways.

Another prominent theme that emerged from this material was that of self-indulgence as another form of shameful overdoing. Ericka's mother, rigorously self-denying, was the arbiter of what was too much. It seems that most of what interested her husband fell into this category. The same target, mother on father's fishing, yielded:

NC: Self-indulgence is contemptible.

PC: Self-indulgence, in balance with other values and other people, is healthy and delightful.

(Of course, the issue of self-indulgence went into high gear when the family learned shortly before Joe's death that he'd been having an affair for several years.)

At the end of 12 sessions of successfully processing targets from the post-binge phase of the cycle, I asked Ericka what her bingeing meant about her. Ericka stated: "I'm trying to manage distress when I binge or overeat, but it doesn't mean I'm disgusting."

BACK IN CONTROL AGAIN

The main focus for educational interweaves in the transition preceding the diet is to make the client aware of her use of control and suppression of needs as a cure for shame. To this end, I ask questions about the client's excited anticipation of dietary restriction. The questions provoke awareness of the connection between shame about overeating and restriction as cure. At the same time they lead to targets about the origins of this strategy. For example, Ericka responds: "I can do this, I can fix this; I can feel good about myself again; I'm going to be thin again, I'm going to love that." I might have asked any of the following questions:

- *How did you learn to associate such good feelings about yourself with deprivation?*
- *How did you learn that control means deprivation?*
- *How did you learn that control is a cure for imperfection?*
- *How did you learn that imperfection has to be cured?*
- *If depriving yourself feels best, where does satisfying your own needs come in?*
- *What does satisfying your own needs mean about you?* (Typical NCs: I'm selfish. My needs are burdensome to others.) *How did you learn . . . ?*

I asked Ericka the question: *How did you learn to associate such good feelings with deprivation?* She came up with the following memory. When she was on her first diet as a teen, a friend with whom she regularly had lunch remarked, "I can't ever stay on a diet. I don't know anyone who stays with it like you." To work with this target and the inappropriately positive feelings that accompanied it, I adapted an approach I learned from Jim Knipe when he co-presented the workshop, "Narcissistic Vulnerability and EMDR." Knipe demonstrated targeting "positive emotional investment in a sense of self that is unrealistically entitled, superior, perfect or controlling" Knipe (1998) used what he dubbed the Level of Positive Affect (LOPA; see Chapter 8) 0–10 in lieu of the Subjective Units of Distress Scale (SUDS) to measure inappropriately positive affect associated with aspects of narcissistic grandiosity or other defenses.

Ericka reported a LOPA of 7–8 in her chest for the pride and strength she felt when thinking of her friend's comment. After the first set,

Ericka said, "I am a superior being because I am able to deny myself things others can't." Then, after each new set:

"I thought about my mother's self-denial. It doesn't seem superior. It seems cramped and tiny and miserable."

"My friend's comment feels less appealing."

"If I don't indulge myself, then I'm not those disgusting things my father was."

Interweave: *Do you have any models for indulging needs that don't involve hurting other people, that don't seem disgusting?* Ericka included examples of real people she admired and an "improved mother" who gave her guidance and a more balanced approach to food and living. Ericka reached a LOPA of 0 for the target and generated the PC: "I can lose weight but I have to do it like a human."

Ericka had already worked successfully in the post-binge phase with targets about her mother's self-deprivation as a seemingly safe container in comparison to her father's self-indulgence. Processing the foregoing target about her dieting seemed sufficient for the aims of the pre-diet phase.

"THE THRILL IS GONE"

There are two potential dysfunctional belief sets I wish to elicit and target during the phase when "the thrill is gone" from the dieting: (a) those related to the pressure to live up to expectations in order to be valued or valuable; and (b) those related to making mistakes or failing to achieve goals.

Ericka's responses to this phase are typical (Figure 11.2). What she and others are expressing is the sense of an intolerable gap, first between where they are versus where they think they are supposed to be and, second, between what they think is required of them versus what they actually want to do. It is both crushing (consciously) and enraging (not so consciously). When I ask for words that describe the mood, I get responses like *overwhelmed, beleaguered, oppressed, trapped,* or *burdened.* If I haven't asked in Round 1, I ask now where else in the person's life they might feel like this. In Round 1, Ericka thought of her job. Others might experience these feelings in relation to family obligations or in friendships. Virtually any arena in which others might hold expectations, or, more likely, in which the client can project her expectations onto others carries potential vulnerability.

Looking at Ericka's reactions to this phase of the binge cycle, I asked her to float back on "This feels so lonely, so empty." She recalled a handful of experiences from high school and college. Ericka also realized she'd taken it on herself to make her unhappy mother's life better, to make it seem worthwhile. So the internal pressure to excel increased sharply.

Ericka's first target was "thinking of all the fun things other kids were doing while she felt tethered to a weekend of particularly hard studying." In what was to turn out to be typical of work on targets from this sector, we spent about five sessions processing to resolution.

NCs: I can only have fun when all my work is done (but the work is endless).
There isn't enough of me to do this. I'm inadequate.

PCs: I can decide how much I take on. I can choose to balance my life.
I'm fine as I am.

Ericka then worked on two similar targets from college, each involving her feeling trapped, beleaguered, and isolated with her studies while others were able to play and relax.

NCs: I'm all alone because I'm not good enough.
You have to endure and struggle through whatever gets handed to you.

PCs: I don't have to struggle endlessly to prove my worth.
I can stop for fun, support, or connection whenever I want to.

Throughout her processing Ericka made ample use of resource people, real and imaginary, who supplied her with messages that had been missing in her childhood about her worth, the importance of balance and fun, and the correct apportionment of responsibility in her family.

In many sequences, one or more of these resource people would step in to tell her it wasn't okay for her to be so miserable. In a crucial moment of clarity Ericka recognized tearfully, "It isn't only important that I perform; it's important that I'm okay."

We then turned to the second dysfunctional belief set characteristic of BED clients that shows up in this sector, those about making mistakes and not achieving goals. Ericka discovered that her parents' marriage had provided a profound cautionary tale about the consequences of mistake-making. Specifically, she perceived that the marriage had been her mother's Waterloo and that it had destroyed her. Reworking this perception was a key point in her processing.

We began a search for targets with my question: *What did you learn from your mother about making mistakes?* Ericka had an image of her mother collapsing in tears over a cooking error with company on the way.

NC: Mistakes reveal how fundamentally flawed and inadequate I am.

PC: Mistakes are part of living, even for really competent people.

Ericka processed unexpectedly high activation in relation to her mother's distress. It was during the processing of this target that she recognized her perception of the marriage as the *über* mistake. She was at first enraged with her mother for having put the teachings of the Catholic Church about divorce before her family's well-being (not to mention her own). The family had suffered terribly and Ericka had a problematic model for personal entitlement. But in subsequent sets she slowly started to notice all the strengths her mother had shown in putting her life back together after Joe's death. Processing included the recognition: "Mostly my mother's mistakes all seemed so tragic and unfixable. I was thinking maybe some mistakes are, but mostly they're not."

An image emerged at this point in which Ericka saw herself and her mother and sisters washing up on shore after a shipwreck—battered and bruised, but having survived. She repeated several times, as if first realizing it: "We survived; I survived." Ericka reported starting to feel embodied.

Ericka then realized that she had attached the same calamitous appraisal to several experiences with peers in high school:

NC: My mistakes are so bad, they can't be forgiven or fixed.

PC: My mistakes are no worse than other people's.
People care about me even if I make mistakes.

Work on these targets led to awareness of how many people besides her mother had pinned their hopes and expectations on Ericka to perform at a consistently excellent level. There were coaches, teachers, guidance counselors, and peers. Mobilizing her anger about this was crucial, especially as it helped her begin to get perspective and establish boundaries. She laughingly dubbed her new position: "I don't need your stinking expectations."

PC: My skill set isn't what makes me worthwhile.

"Worthwhile," nonetheless, remained an elusive quality for Ericka. We turned to work on targets having to do with how her family responded to her mistakes. Ericka described a contemptuous tone of voice and facial expression displayed by her mother. When she accessed it, it felt so toxic she could barely tolerate it at first.

At the same time Ericka thought about a way her father had of inflating the family's worth compared to other people. She was surprised to find she'd carried around, unintegrated, conflicting views of being both better than and worth less. She targeted some extremely painful experiences she characterized as being "taken down a peg" resulting from going public with her father's inflated views. She then realized why "worthwhile" felt not only elusive but also dangerous: she couldn't distinguish false compensatory pride from the healthy version.

Work in this sector was for Ericka and most BED clients v-e-r-y slow going. It challenges rules for living that seem necessary to make them safe. When Ericka could think of making mistakes with a SUDS of 0 and could feel safe when taking pride in herself, we had accomplished the goals of this sector.

Having completed Round 2 of the Binge Cycle exercise, we turned to working with urges to binge, using Popky's Level of Urge to Use (LOUU; see Chapter 7) protocol. Urges no longer felt overwhelming. Ericka was able to combine EMDR processing with a few behavioral techniques to essentially stop bingeing.

CONCLUSION

I have presented a tool I use with BED clients to gather information about enactment of binge-diet cycling and to link it to underlying beliefs learned in the family regarding the management of shame. I have shown how this information can be incorporated into an EMDR treatment plan.

I wish to emphasize that working with this material is just part of a comprehensive treatment plan for BED that necessarily includes development of affect-regulation skills, behavioral and nutritional input, attention to the quality of relationships, and processing of "big T" and "little t" traumas besides those related to shame. The treatment of eating disorders most often requires attention to every level of the person's experience: body and body image, intrapsychic, intrafamilial, interpersonal, and societal/cultural. Ericka, for example, had to develop skills for negotiating with her mother and to work through some considerable fears about partnering with men. Preoccupation with her ED had been a safe place to avoid both of these. We also spent extensive time talking about the impact of cultural messages about women and their bodies that only serve to reinforce shame and perfectionism.

APPENDIX: THE BINGE CYCLE EXERCISE
AT A GLANCE

ROUND 1 develops client awareness about the cyclic relationship between bingeing and dieting.

1. Place the words *BINGE* and *DIET* at opposite sides of a blank sheet of paper. Explain that you'll be focusing on transition states in and out of these two phases of the cycle.
2. *Transition 1.* Begin after the binge. Elicit client's report of thoughts and feelings.
3. *Transition 2.* Ask about client's thoughts and feelings when she's decided to go back on a diet.

4. Compare the two sets of responses to demonstrate how your client is attempting to "cure" shame, self-loathing, and despair with the plan to diet (i.e., be in control).

5. *Transition 3.* Ask for thoughts and feelings at the point when "the thrill is gone."

6. Ask about other aspects of client's life in which she might have similar feelings (e.g., job, family).

7. *Transition 4.* Elicit client's thoughts and feelings just before entering the binge phase.
   Look for "I don't care" response.

8. Point out:

   that one pole of the cycle invariably leads to the other.

   that humans tend to correct for an extreme in one direction with an extreme in the opposite direction.

   that discontinuing the extreme of dieting removes one significant trigger for bingeing.

ROUND 2 uses client responses from Round 1 to generate BED-specific targets for EMDR processing. (You will be targeting a belief system that fuels the binge-diet cycle. The core of this belief system is that shame can be cured with perfectionism and rigid controls.)

1. *Transition 1.* Begin after the binge as in Round 1. Main focus: challenging shame-based beliefs. Explain "shame." Demonstrate its presence in client's responses. (Preprocessing interweave.) Notice the shamed response to an act of overdoing (the binge). This is an NC for the current target of bingeing. You may return to this after processing historic targets.

2. Ask: "What experience did you have growing up that taught you that an act of overdoing it makes you disgusting? (client NC; e.g., "I'm disgusting.") This will be your first EMDR target memory.

3. Ask for the other elements of the target memory: NC (if different from original post-binge statement), PC, emotions, SUDS, body location.

4. Process according to standard procedure.
5. Elicit and process as many of the early targets giving rise to this aspect of the belief system as needed to generate solid new PCs.
6. Return to original NC (e.g., "I'm disgusting") in relation to target of bingeing. Generate PCs; apply DAS.
7. *Transition 2*, deciding to go on a diet. Main focus: making client aware of control and suppression of needs as a cure for shame. Preprocessing educational interweave is embedded in target-eliciting questions (e.g., *How did you learn to associate such good feelings about yourself with deprivation?*)
8. Process targeted memories according to standard procedure.
9. *Transition 3*, "The thrill is gone." Two main areas of focus are beliefs about:

   (1) Living up to expectations in order to be valued, valuable

       (a) Help clients give words to the emotional experience in this transitional stage (e.g., beleaguered, oppressed, burdened).
       (b) Ask about other areas in client's life in which she might have similar feelings.
       (c) Ask client to float back on the feeling to elicit early targets.
       (d) Process according to standard procedure.

   (2) Making mistakes; failing to achieve goals

       (a) Ask target-eliciting questions about how making mistakes was handled in client's family

           How did members of your family handle their own mistakes?

           How did members of your family handle others' mistakes?

           How did members of your family handle your mistakes?

(b)   Ask for related targets in realm of peers and school.
(c)   Process resulting target memories using standard procedure.
(d)   Repeat above steps for issue of failing to achieve goals.

Transitions 1–3 represent the bulk of the processing work. You may wish to work with Transition 4, before the binge, by allowing the client to devise new meanings for the signature statement, "I don't care." As gateway to the binge, it means, "I don't care about the consequences; I'll eat whatever I want." PCs might include statements about client respecting her own needs and having choices about how to express or satisfy them.

10. Process targets related to cultural reinforcers of the dysfunctional belief system if relevant for a particular client.

APPENDIX: A BED-SPECIFIC EMDR TREATMENT PLAN USING INFORMATION FROM THE BINGE CYCLE EXERCISE

Phase 1: Client History and Treatment Planning

• Take a thorough history.
• Evaluate the bingeing symptom.
  Include the Binge Cycle exercise (Round 1)
  List remaining triggers for binge behavior.

These two sources of information about bingeing triggers will be the basis for ED-specific preparation, targeting, and processing.

• Defer identification of targets related to the binge-diet cycle until after the Preparation Phase

Phase 2: Preparation
An ED signals lack of adequate affect regulation skills. Depending on the degree of deficit, there could be significant work to do in this

stage. Use your approach of choice (e.g., RDI, AMST, relaxation techniques, guided imagery). Include attachment repair work as needed.

Return to Phase 1 Treatment Planning for development of targets related to the binge-diet cycle. At this point a more complex level of information can be elicited from the Binge Cycle exercise. Development of targets is mediated by the therapist's understanding of the self-image-regulating belief system underpinning the client's responses. ED-specific target development is interwoven with educative material and insight-producing questions and framings ("preprocessing interweaves").

Complete Phases 3–8 (Assessment through Closure) with each ED target.

Phases 3–8: Non-ED-Specific Targets

Assess and process remaining targets, following the Standard Protocol.

RESOURCES

Britt, V., & Napier, N. (2002, June). *The somatic interweave.* Paper presented at the EMDRIA Conference, San Diego, CA.

Freedland, E. (2001, June). *Using EMDR with eating disorders.* Paper presented at EMDRIA Conference, Austin, TX.

Omaha, J. (2004). *Affect management skills training protocol.* Available at http://www.emdrportal.com/2004/2004-5-19a.htm

Schmidt, S. J. (2002). *Developmental needs meeting strategy for EMDR therapists.* San Antonio, TX: author.

Steele, A. (2004). *Developing a secure self: An approach to working with attachment in adults for EMDR therapists* (2nd ed.). Gabriola Island, B.C.

REFERENCES

Berenson, D. (1988, May). *Alcoholism and the family.* Paper presented at the LifeCycle "State of the Art" Addictions Symposium, New York.

Fossum, M. A., & Mason, M. J. (1986). *Facing shame: Families in recovery.* New York: Norton.

Johnson, C., & Connors, M. (1987). *The etiology and treatment of bulimia nervosa: A biopsychosocial perspective.* New York: Basic.

Knipe, J. (1998, July). *Narcissistic vulnerability and EMDR.* Paper presented at the EMDRIA Conference, Baltimore, MD.

Shapiro, F. (2001). *Eye movement desensitization and reprocessing: Basic principles, protocols and procedures.* New York: Guilford Press.

Terry, L. (1987). Ordering a therapeutic context: A developmental interactional approach to the treatment of eating disorders in a college counseling center. In J. Harkaway (Ed.), *The family therapy collections* (vol. 20; pp. 55–62). Aspen, CO: Aspen Publications.

Chapter 12

Utilizing EMDR and DBT Techniques in Trauma and Abuse Recovery Groups

Carole Lovell

MARSHA LINEHAN'S (1993) DIALECTICAL BEHAVIOR THERAPY (DBT) IS A wonderfully effective treatment for people with borderline personality. It is a nonblaming, compassionate, therapeutic approach, based solidly on research data about what borderline personality disorder (BPD) is and how to treat it effectively. Her workbook, *Skills Training Manual for Treating Borderline Personality Disorders*, provides many effective tools for working with traumatized patients. I have used the techniques of DBT for the past 9 years in trauma and abuse recovery groups for women. DBT provides a solid foundation for the group. EMDR, adjunct therapies, and other trauma related resources complete DBT by including the treatment of trauma within the group setting. The groups are successful in that the intensity of symptoms decreases and the group members report feeling increased competency regulating their emotions.

Results are excellent using EMDR Standard Protocol, resource installation with Shirley Jean Schmidt's *Developmental Needs Meeting Strategy* (2002), and Roy Kiessling's *Integrating Resource Installation Strategies* (2002 & Chapter 2). Also included in the psychoeducational agenda for the groups are materials from *The Body Remembers*, written by Babette Rothschild (2000), and information gleaned from lectures by Bessel A. van der Kolk (2000) and other EMDR International Association (EMDRIA) approved presenters.

In her book, Linehan stated that DBT addresses the core issue of BPD: emotional dysregulation. The theory asserts that borderlines have difficulty regulating several if not all emotions (Linehan, 1993). Emotional dysregulation is viewed as a joint outcome of biological disposition, environmental context, and the transaction between the two during development. DBT provides the group members with effective tools to assist in regulating these emotions.

DBT teaches patients the skills necessary to calm the chaos in their lives. By staying in the moment and focusing on what is effective, they are able to decrease their anxiety level. They find that it is possible to self-soothe and practice methods of doing so. They learn to validate themselves and to accept validation from other group members as well as the therapist. They practice interpersonal relationship skills so they may improve their ability to trust their own perceptions rather than mirror the thoughts and feelings of others. Perhaps most important, they learn the skills needed to decrease self-harming and self-destructive behaviors.

DBT alone does little to address the trauma issues that are so much a part of BPD. Linehan leaves this for another phase of treatment. I find it effective to address skills and trauma at the same time. Talking about the traumas (both big T's and little t's) seems to normalize the experience of group members. It seems to remove much of the stigma that is frequently attached to the borderline diagnosis and helps to create a strong bond among members.

Ross (2000), van der Kolk (2000), and others have described a link between BPD and posttraumatic stress disorder (PTSD). Ross's book, *The Trauma Model* (2000), thoroughly described how trauma shatters the matrix of the personality, causing many of the symptoms of BPD. BPD never occurs without comorbidity. It is the most common personality disorder among psychiatric patients crossing all socioeconomic barriers. Ross stated, "I view borderline personality as a trauma disorder. It could be called the reactive attachment disorder of adulthood." Ross elaborated. "The trauma that gives rise to borderline personality disorder is a complex and variable mix of parental rejection and neglect, difficult infant temperament, inconsistent child rearing practices with harsh discipline, physical or sexual abuse, lack of supervision, early institutional living, frequent changes of caregivers, large family size, association with delinquent groups and certain kinds of family pathology" (2000, p. 206).

We are appalled when we hear of children who have been physically, emotionally, or sexually abused. We shake our heads when we see videos of babies and toddlers learning ambivalent or disorganized attachment styles. We see them at 38, 45, and even 60 years old labeled BPD. It is a tremendous breakthrough to offer genuine hope for reduced symptoms and recovery from the trauma.

Ross says that in his residency he was taught to have a belittling, demeaning attitude toward BPD clients. He says that he was taught that they are bad, manipulative, dangerous, highly prone to regression, and untreatable (2000, p. 206). Many people with BPD have a negative experience with therapists. The DBT therapist must use a tremendous amount of validation. It is helpful to teach these clients in the beginning to honor their experiences and to admire their ingenuity in surviving difficulties.

BPD clients are difficult to manage in or out of groups. In the beginning phases of the groups, they go from crisis to crisis and many of them actually have fears about how their recovery will affect their life and relationships. They cannot imagine life without chaos. As they begin to feel success within the group and the acceptance of others, they develop hope and some degree of confidence. They begin to rely on the acceptance of other group members and have the confidence to try new skills.

THE TRAUMA AND ABUSE
RECOVERY GROUP

In the trauma and abuse recovery group, all of the members are women. Members represent a wide socioeconomic range. Some of them are disabled and living on a fixed income. Others are actively engaged in various active and successful professions. They meet criteria for BPD and/or PTSD. They must agree to the rules of the group and be willing to make attendance a priority.

The format is 32 weeks with a minimum of 2½ hours per group. Homework is an important part of the group process. Group members are encouraged to share mistakes as well as victories when they learn to put these skills into practice. In doing this, they internalize their newly developed skills and extend their ability to access them far beyond the group sessions.

BEGINNING THE GROUPS

Group members are selected after a thorough completion of a diagnostic assessment. This assessment includes a profile measuring the severity of each criterion for both diagnoses. As the group progresses, the profiles are used to measure progress. Group members may be accepted on referral from other therapists for prescreening and the initial assessment. Their primary therapist must be familiar with DBT and with EMDR.

Group members remain in individual therapy, to process materials that they may not wish to disclose in the group setting. The frequency of the need for individual therapy varies with members and individual progress. In individual therapy, they work on their suicidal and parasuicidal thoughts, problems that they believe to be too personal to discuss in the group, and other issues that the therapist believes can be handled best in individual sessions. All of the members of the groups get EMDR for their trauma in individual sessions. For this reason they are comfortable when EMDR and adjunct EMDR therapies are used within the group setting.

The four basic modules follow Linehan's model. I alter the format a bit to fit my style of therapy and to meet the needs of the individuals in the groups. I incorporate some trauma theory as the members' interest and tolerance permit. I frequently experiment with new material as I am learning. On one occasion, I revised the group format to accommodate members who had diagnoses related to eating disorders.

EMDR IN THE GROUPS

It seems natural for me to incorporate EMDR into the groups. I do not present any new EMDR techniques or protocols in this work. I am experienced and comfortable with group therapy and EMDR. I do not advise therapists who are inexperienced with groups or just beginning to use EMDR to use EMDR in group settings. It is important to understand and become comfortable with group dynamics prior to adding EMDR.

STRUCTURE OF THE GROUPS

BPD clients need a tremendous amount of structure. The 2½-hour sessions are divided into several distinct parts. In the beginning the first portion of the session is spent allowing members to get acquainted, settling on group rules, and teaching about trauma. Once past the initial formation of the group, usually about four sessions, the first hour is spent reviewing homework assigned the previous week and completed prior to coming to the session. The homework section is essential. This is when members discuss what they have tried to do differently during the week.

The therapist and other group members provide validation for all efforts. When members are successful, this is encouraging to everyone. If they are not successful, they are asked to rewind the tape and describe how they would like to handle the situation. By identifying this, they visualize their success. This is one of the first places that many have found that it is all right to make mistakes. They feel that it is acceptable to share mistakes and to try again.

If members are not doing homework, other group members confront them. This eliminates some people from the group. (I begin groups with 14 members to allow for this. We usually end the 32-week session with 8–10 members).

The homework section is followed by a 15-minute break. The break is an important time. Group members talk with one another informally and begin to bond. I frequently tease them and tell them more therapy gets done in that 15 minutes that in any other section of the group.

After the break, new information regarding skills is introduced and members discuss how they can incorporate this into their lives. New information is threatening for borderlines and involves risks. Members are encouraged to proceed at their own speed. All movement is considered great progress.

Handouts are always given out with the new information. Homework assignments are made based on the new information. Some groups progress faster than others. How fast we go in providing new information depends on how members are using the information that has been given previously. A great deal of time is spent in review. Many scenarios and role-play exercises are incorporated into the new information section. Members do better when they see examples that they can understand.

It is important to keep members active and participating because borderlines and PTSD patients tend to dissociate if they do not stay involved. New information is always related to one of the four modules, described later.

The last 20 minutes of the group is a wind-down session. Members are asked to discuss what they experienced in the group for this session.

They are also asked to describe what they observe about others in the group. Sometimes they say something about what they believe they need that they are not getting. They are frequently impatient and desire instant cures.

Members' families are often critical. They complain that recoveries are taking too long or the members do not need group or any therapy. Group members encourage one another to resist family-directed sabotage. The group closes with everyone standing in a circle holding hands and repeating the Serenity Prayer. A genuine bonding is sensed at this time and the commitment to continue is strengthened.

PROTOCOLS APPROPRIATE FOR A GROUP SETTING

The EMDR Standard Protocol may be used within the group setting when a patient becomes stuck in some area. It is most likely to happen because they believe that they cannot do a homework assignment correctly. Group members are familiar with the process and know when to be quiet and when they can validate members. Standard Protocol, plus the Float Back and Float Forward techniques, can be used in any of the modules.

These are the adjunct techniques I find most effective in the different modules.

A. Module 1—use bilateral music for Dual Attention Stimulation (DAS)

    1. Safe Place
    2. Relaxation exercises
    3. Body work

B. Module 2—use bilateral music for DAS

    1. Positive circling—Shirley Jean Schmidt's work, connecting to the spiritual core self (Schmidt, 2002, pp. 9–10)
    2. Resource installation—Roy Kiessling, *Integrating Resource Installation Strategies into Your EMDR Practice* (a workshop & Chapter 2)

C. Module 3—Bilateral music, Two-Hand Interweave (see Chapter 6), and/or self tapping shoulder or knees technique

    1. Affect containment (Wilson & Foster, 2002, p. 32)
    2. Healing circle (Schmidt, 2002, pp. 11–13)

D. Module 4—Bilateral music, Two-Hand Interweave, shoulder taps

    1. Skill development
    2. Performance enhancement
    3. Grounding techniques to manage flashbacks

EMDR STANDARD PROTOCOL

The first time I used EMDR in the group setting was completely spontaneous. This occurred during the second module, Interpersonal Communication Skills, while discussing a member's struggle to complete the previous week's homework assignment.

Eva is completely stuck in misery because of her inability to tell her father that she no longer wanted to manage his rental property. Eva had a history of humiliating sexual abuse by her paternal grandfather. She is at this time 37 years old and recently disclosed her abuse history in individual therapy.

After a lengthy discussion of her perceived inability to be assertive with her father with other group members completely validating her efforts, she is unable to acknowledge her ability to change. She sees no hope. She is convinced that if she is honest with her father she will lose him completely. She cannot face this because her mother died recently. Her fear of abandonment is extreme.

The frustration of the group was growing into a negative experience. I simply rolled my chair over to her assuming the standard EMDR position.

1. Issue with her father
2. Picture—I asked her to picture her father giving her an assignment regarding his rental property. She said, "He comes over to my house and talks to me for a little while and then he tells

me about these horrible renters. He says that I am so much better than he is at talking to people. He also tells me that this property will be mine someday. He just gets his hat to leave, telling me to call him and let him know what happened."

3. *What's the worst part of that?*

4. "I am a teacher. I am busy with my life. I do not want to do this."

5. *What is your negative belief about yourself when you see this picture?*

6. "I am not good enough to have my father love me. I have to earn it."

7. *What would you like to believe about yourself when you think about this?* (positive cognition)

8. "I am okay. The way I am, without doing anything I do not want to do."

9. *How much do you believe that when you think about the picture you described on a scale of 1–7 with 7 being completely true and 1 not true at all?* Validity of Cognition Scale (VOC)–2

10. *What emotions are you feeling?*

11. "Fear, I am scared"

12. *How distressing is this to you on a scale of 1–10?* (Subjective Units of Distress Scale [SUDS])

13. "8 or 9."

14. *Where do you feel this in your body?*

15. "Chest and stomach." (Eva is bulimic.)

The first set took Eva straight to her grandfather. She said that she was never able to stand up to him. I was careful to guide her away from uncomfortable disclosure at this point. I asked her how her father reminded her of her grandfather. She said that she was afraid he would not love her if she did not do what he wanted her to do.

Go with that.

In the second set, Eva was able to remember that her father could not stand up to her grandfather either. She said that he always seemed intimidated by him.

Go with that. By the third or fourth set, Eva stated that her father was very proud of her because she was a teacher and he probably really did think she was better with people than he was.

The other members of the group had been very quiet up to this point. One of the members said that maybe her father needed to learn the skills. Eva responded to that and I simply said, *Go with that.*

Eva was then able to picture herself talking to her father and making suggestions to him about how to handle situations.

Her SUDS level went down to 1 within the group and she began to see her father as having the problem rather than this being because she was not good enough.

The group debriefed the session for about 10 minutes. The intervention worked because all of the group members in this session were familiar with EMDR. I had discussed the process in the group and had used EMDR with some of the members (including Eva) in individual sessions.

The group members seem to know when they can participate and when to remain silent and allow the member to work. It is similar to other times when the therapist is doing intense work with an individual within the group setting. Borderlines have an incredible ability to zone in on the feelings of others. By nature they are better able to "read" others than themselves.

I continue to use the Standard Protocol for individual clients in groups. I do it when the need arises, and it almost always occurs in the homework segment of the meeting. When we are stuck on an issue, the group members expect me to use EMDR. It provides a tremendous addition to already effective group therapy.

SPECIFIC GUIDELINES FOR USING EMDR IN THE GROUP SETTING

Here is a list of what you need to do before you begin EMDR processing in a group.

1. Be sure that all of the patients in the groups understand the EMDR process, including the risks and benefits.
2. Have signed documents and informed consent from everyone in the group before using EMDR in the group setting.
3. Candidates for whom the DBT group has been recommended are usually those I have seen for individual therapy. However, other agency providers who are also certified in EMDR refer some of them. As a rule the clients are familiar with the EMDR process and have been overwhelmingly positive about it.
4. Complete Blocking Belief and Dissociative Experience Scale (DES) assessments for each patient prior to trauma work. (This

is usually completed in the individual session and is already in the chart.)

5. Complete the Safe Place exercise in the group several times prior to any processing of traumatic materials.

6. Group leaders must be experienced in leading groups and in doing EMDR.

FOUR CORE MODULES OF GROUPS

The following is a description of the group modules with outlines for each session. This is ever changing. I am including some possible places to use EMDR. Most EMDR occurs spontaneously in my groups. This is much the same as in individual practice where therapists may use a variety of therapies in one session.

Each module builds on the others and there is always review and repetition.

Sometimes we merely use DAS to strengthen new skills.

A. "Living Consciously"—Eight sessions

Session 1: Introduce to the group welcome, hopeful statements regarding the possibility of decrease in symptoms, basic rules, expectations, consents signed, format explained, and "Log Story." The "Log Story" graphically describes a woman who holds on to behaviors long past their usefulness. The behaviors saved her life in the past, but are currently holding her in a negative behavior pattern. The moral of the story is that while we are grateful for what helped us to survive, it may need to be given up for us to learn more effective methods for the present.

Session 2: Explain the theory of trauma; discuss relationship between BPD and PTSD and the differences in these disorders and other types of emotional illnesses in order to normalize members' experience. This session usually entails a lot of questions from participants. Plenty of time is allowed for this. If members have difficulties verbalizing their questions, I provide them with a list of frequently asked questions. This alleviates a lot of anxiety related to the group and helps members to set realistic expectations.

Session 3: Explain the difference in posttraumatic stress (PTS) and PTSD. Rationale for validation is given and basic DBT methods are outlined. Patients are told that whatever their methods of surviving are, they have brought them to this point and should be honored. DBT attempts to enter into those experiences with them to seek ways to cope that are less destructive and more helpful to them. For the first time homework is given.

Session 4: Educate members about how trauma is felt in the body and explain triggers. The handouts are related to emotions as they are experienced in the body. Group time is devoted to increasing members' awareness of ways in which "The Body Bears the Burden." I introduce the concept of "body work," the physical sensations and signatures typically associated with various emotions. Members work on being able to identify this.

Following the break, I use the music of David Grand with a body awareness and relaxation meditation by David Wilson (Wilson & Foster, 2002, pp. 8–14). The group is asked to get quiet, as comfortable as possible, take everything from their lap, and close their eyes. I read the relaxation meditation while playing bilateral music. Speakers are placed at opposite ends of the room to achieve the bilateral effect. Following the meditation, members discuss the increase in body awareness and their overall experience. Their ability to fully participate varies. In this phase, do not be discouraged if some members are unable to report positive results. What we are going for is increased body awareness.

Session 5: Introduce Linehan's (1993) concept of emotional and rational mind and begin to move group members to "wise mind" by combining the two frames of mind (core mindfulness). We discuss the tendencies for family and friends to push our buttons and we look at the skills used to "step out of the circle" in order to observe this. Following the wind-down session, we introduce the safe place with bilateral music and the butterfly hug. Because members have been discussing how family members push their buttons, it's a good time to relax.

a. The therapist demonstrates the Judith Boel's butterfly hug technique (in Kiessling, 2000): "Cross arms so that the right fingers tap the left shoulders and the left fingers touch the right shoulder, or cross hands over the heart, and tap about 14 times. Do this several times until you are comfortable with the technique. Breathe as deeply as possible while doing this."
b. Dim the lights and members close their eyes.
c. Members find their safe place and tap as they visualize it.
d. *"Visualize someone trying to put you into an emotional mind."*
e. *"Tap as you visualize finding your safe place in the midst of this."*
f. *"Visualize the person trying to push your buttons."*

g. *"Draw an imaginary circle around yourself and the other person."*
h. *"Step backward out of this circle and tap."*
i. *"Bring your safe place where you are and tap."*
j. After completing the exercise, ask members if they feel less anxious about people trying to push their buttons. Some of them will and it will encourage others that the technique works.

Session 6: I facilitate a thorough discussion of the skills of core mindfulness: observe, describe, and participate. Sometimes I bring in objects and ask the participants to observe them and write down as many things as they can think of using their five senses. Other times I may bring one object and ask each member to make an observation that is different from any that have previously been made to describe the object. The focus is on using the five senses to become more aware of surroundings. We discuss preferred sense and discovering them becomes a part of homework. Other homework involves describing two or three observations using all five senses. Participation is encouraged using scenarios and role-play.

Session 7: Introduce new skills of focusing on what is effective, staying in the here and now and doing one thing at a time. Members are challenged to be nonjudgmental and a variety of scenarios are used. We also use a priority exercise deciding what characters get to go into a bomb shelter. This introduces the idea of values into the group. It is interesting to see the members as they begin to learn to differ with one another instead of needing to agree all of the time.

Session 8: In the last session, introduce the skill of "turtling" or "buying time." Members are not usually comfortable with not having to answer ever question asked of them or always being available because someone else demands it. We use the turtle to teach that it is all right to retreat at times until we feel more ready to meet the demands of others. Careful consideration is given to the fact that this does not mean avoiding. The module concludes with a discussion of using breathing techniques to center and meditation to relax. Bilateral stimulation is incorporated into this. As a celebration for finishing the module, members select a restaurant to eat at following the last session in each module.

B. *"Interpersonal Communications Skills"*— *Eight sessions*

Session 1: Identify four communication types: aggressive, passive, passive-aggressive, and assertive. Role-play is used in combination with the skills of observe, describe, and stepping out of the circle to identify each of these styles. A communication self-assessment tool is used. Patients are also requested to write their names with their non-dominate hand as a way to illustrate that new ways of relating are uncomfortable and may take time to learn. Homework is assigned to identify the communication styles of the people in their life and observe interactions this week.

Session 2: Participants complete a personality profile to identify their personal strengths and weaknesses. This is a fun group as everyone enjoys learning more about their own temperament. They are given extra assessments for any family member they might want to take it. This ultimately identifies emotional needs for each temperament and assists the patient to learn effective communication with each one. This also helps them to understand that different people respond differently to the same things. They become very familiar with the term, "it's not about me."

Session 3: Synthesis pulls together the things we have already learned so that patients have a good understanding of their own style of communication. We discuss how to set up an important conversation to ask for what we need. It sometimes takes time to overcome their belief that they do not deserve to ask that their needs be met. We introduce the idea of three components of making a request: objective, relationship, and self-respect. Homework involves identifying some of their needs.

Session 4: Introduce strategies for agreeing with one's attacker and making nondefensive replies to threatening situations. The ABCs of noncommunication are introduced along with a handout describing what does not work well. This comes from materials that I have developed over time in my practice. Most of the members have histories of destructive relationships and this is a difficult module. It is difficult to learn to ask for what we want when the people in our life have not really cared. To ask is to risk what little approval is there and to face the dreaded abandonment issue. This is where I introduce the healing circle work of Shirley Jean Schmidt. Using bilateral music I read the following meditation:

"Close your eyes and take a long deep breath. Get in touch with that part of you that is quiet, peaceful and still. And in this place it is possible that you will get in touch with the core of your being. It is the essence of who you are. It is you exactly as you are created to be. It is the essence of who you are and it has been with you since the moment of conception, purity innocence and truth. And your body knows

exactly how to connect you to this part of you. Notice as you connect
that you become less attached to the irrational fears and concerns of
the past and more fully present in the here and now. Notice as you
begin to feel quiet, rested, peaceful, warm, and safe. Allow these feelings to become stronger and stronger and you feel more and more relaxed" (Schmidt, 2002, pp. 9–10).

After the meditation we discuss what it means to get in touch with
the innermost part of ourselves. Most of the members find the concept
foreign. We do the meditation or a variation of it several times.

Session 5: Introduce the HELP model of communication. In this
model participants are taught to get information they need from others
without taking ownership of their problems. This is an empowering
tool because it allows members to safely show concern for others.

a) *What is **happening?***
b) *How do you feel **(emotion)** about it?*
c) ***Listen** actively and paraphrase what was said to you: I can see that
    you are giving this a lot of thought.*
d) *How do you **plan** to handle the situation?*

As participants learn these communication skills, they report victories in the homework segment. They are now discovering that some of
the people in their lives are not happy that they are getting stronger.
They are no longer easily manipulated and this takes some adjustment
on the part of family members. BPD clients tend to overvalue or un-
dervalue relationships. Therefore at this point it may become easy for
them to prematurely terminate some of their relationships. It becomes
a fine line to define which relationships really are abusive and which
people only need to be trained to relate to them in healthier ways. We
discuss this a lot as we review Linehan's concept of the three components of effective communication. Participants take the Relationship
Satisfaction Survey (Burns, 1992).

Session 6: Continue teaching self-nurturing skills using other meditations from Shirley Jean Schmidt's book, *Developmental Needs Meeting
Strategy for EMDR Therapists*. The therapist, with accompanying bilateral music, reads the meditations. Sometimes we also use the butterfly
taps. Deep breathing is always emphasized. Results of the meditations
are processed within the group discussion. Having little experience in
self-nurturing, patients find this to be an emotional experience. The

patients and therapists use a lot of validation to encourage one another in self-nurturing.

Session 7: Teach assertiveness skills. Linehan provides user-friendly tools for assertiveness skills development, "GIVE DEAR MAN FAST," described in detail in her workbook (Linehan, 1993). This entire session focuses on these skills. We use real patient situations of patients capitalizing on current interpersonal interactions and identifying things they need to ask or tell someone. Members practice role-playing with several of them participating. This is combined with the three components of effective communication. Homework requires members to generalize the new tool while they strengthen their skills.

Session 8: In the last session, review all of the aspects of communication skills covered in the module. Members describe how the application of their skills changes the context of their relevant relationships. Some of the members report positive results and others still have family members who are threatened by the change. Members are encouraged to continue to use the skills. By this point, they almost always report feeling more empowered and less like victims. The profiles for PTSD and BPD are repeated, as this is the halfway point of the group. This assesses progress and reinforces treatment gains when profiles are compared to entry data.

C. "Recognizing and Regulating Emotions Module"—10 Sessions

Session 1: In this session we use the Distorted Thinking Exercise (Burns, 1993). Burns provides an assortment of cognitive worksheets that work well with this population. I hand out a list of cognitive distortions. As part of the homework assignment, patients are asked to review this list and to identify five thought distortions that are problematic for them.

Session 2: I introduce the concept of primary, secondary, and tertiary emotions. Members are told that we will later introduce a 10-step plan to regulate emotions. We use material from *The Body Remembers* (Rothschild, 2000) to assist patients in identifying specific emotions. I provide the group members with lists of emotions to facilitate identification of their emotions that week. Most find identification of emotions difficult and state they feel a lot of anxiety. This is where we introduce another EMDR technique, discovered in the work of Roy Kiessling (2002 & Chapter 2).

Kiessling contends that the advanced use of EMDR requires strategies that are instinctive, natural, intuitive, creative and proactive (2002). I find this to be true in using EMDR in the group setting.

According to Kiessling, the use of "Cognitive Interweave" is a means by which the clinician is deliberately laying down new tracks or pathways for the client. The clinician is attempting to change the client's maladaptive perspective or referents to a more rational and adaptive perspective, therefore speeding up the reprocessing.

Because anxiety is frequently identified as an emotion in this phase of the group process I use the butterfly technique and a modified approach for cognitive interweave. I follow this process:

a. Therapist to group members: *Fold your arms across your chest, touching your left fingers to your right shoulder and your right fingers to your left shoulder. Tap your shoulders in alternating motion to see what that feels like.* (Demonstrate bilateral tapping so that everyone understands how to do it.)

b. *Close your eyes and think of a current situation that you feel anxiety about.* (Allow a few seconds until everyone indicates they have something in mind.)

c. *On a scale of 1–10, what is your level of discomfort about this situation.* (Allow a few seconds for this.)

d. *As you again think about your problem, think about how would you like to feel and what you would like to believe about yourself.* (Allow time to formulate thoughts.)

e. *While you think about this, tap in an alternating motion about 10 times, visualizing yourself in this positive manner.*

f. *See if you can think of two specific characteristics that you like about yourself. Allow yourself to remember two useful characteristics that you have noticed about yourself in the past.* (Instruct members to signal you with a raised hand when they are able to do this.)

g. *Think of an image that represents each of those characteristics.*

h. *Now think about the situation that is creating anxiety for you.*

i. *Think about how you would like to think about yourself and tap about 14 times in bilateral movement.*

j. *Continue to picture the anxiety and bring one of the two images into the picture of your anxiety and continue tapping in the bilateral manner.*

k. *Bring the other image into the picture and surround your anxiety with the two characteristics that represent your good qualities.*

l. *Continue tapping and repeat this a few times.*
m. *Ask the patients to assess their level of anxiety at this moment.*

There is always significantly less.

This is a wonderful way to teach them to self-regulate emotions. They become excited about using DAS to assist in self-regulation. It may be used in any of the sessions during the last two modules. I use it frequently, depending on the needs of the group.

Session 3: In this session I reintroduce the cognitive distortion log. Patients are instructed to keep a log of their distortions for the week to measure the expansion of their skill. Sometimes patients wish to repeat the EMDR process using another anxiety-producing situation. They are learning a new technique and repetition is vital to this learning.

Session 4: Discuss old tapes and survivor memories. We talk about how these memories are stored differently than other memories and require effort to change. During this session we define 10 Steps to Emotional Regulation. These are:

a) Physical response (where do you feel this in your body?)
b) Name the emotion accompanying the body sensation
c) Trace the thought behind the emotion

    1. Internal triggers—old tapes that we replay
    2. External—something distressing just happened

d) Identify the underlying distortion in the thought-check perception
e) Correct the distortion, if present
f) Reframe the thought, correcting misperceptions and distortions
g) Identify choices if the distressing situation is reality
h) Make a decision about what to do
i) Take a positive action
j) Experience relief of distress. Scan body for remaining distress
k) Evaluate current distress level and repeat cycle if distress continues.

Session 5: Most of this session is focused on homework and allowing members to process efforts they have made to use these skills to regulate emotions. We use the analogy: out-of-control emotions are much like sliding around on black ice without guardrails. Members sometimes come up with additional metaphors to describe their feelings. Metaphors can be quite creative.

Session 6: This session begins with what we refer to as "Wall Work." It is an exercise where we guide patients into free association and feeling words to tell their life stories. The group becomes much closer and a lot of healing takes place, providing for corrective emotional experiences. We are careful to tell the patients to disclose only what they are comfortable telling. However, most of them experience a genuine catharsis and tell their entire story. Members become bonded and are assisting in leadership, asking questions and providing validation at this time.

Session 7: Wall Work continues (it takes time for each person to tell her story).

Session 8: Wall Work completed.

Session 9: Linehan's section on Emotional Regulation skills is outstanding and a wonderful way to wrap up this module (1993, pp. 153–162). In this session, we acknowledge the value of emotions and celebrate the positive aspects of paying attention to them. Members are encouraged not only to listen to their emotions but also to use them to guide them to positive actions. This is amazing to some of the patients. They have been told what to feel or not to feel at all for most of their lives. This can be a very freeing experience. When time permits, I like to tell a story entitled "What a Woman Wants Most." This illustrates their feelings of freedom.

Session 10: In the last session of the module we talk about the strategies for regulating guilt, shame, and fear. We review concepts, answer questions, and pull together what we have learned in the module. A lot of time is spent in evaluating where people are in their recovery at this time. Time is allowed for questions. Termination is mentioned for the first time.

D. "Tolerating the Pain Module"—Six sessions

Session 1: *When we have done everything possible to alter our environments, and to become stronger, it would seem that situations would improve. This is the case most of the time. However, there are some challenges and difficulties in life that we cannot change even if we are strong and we do everything right. In these situations we must learn to effectively tolerate pain.* We read and discuss the story of learning to love the daffodils. Each member is encouraged to share a time past or present when she tolerated something because she had no choice.

Session 2: We watch a humorous tape entitled *The Joy of Stress.* We talk about learning to use some of Linehan's techniques like the half smile and evaluating pros and cons of a situation (1993, pp. 167, 169, 172).

Session 3: We watch a video entitled *Tongue Fu* by Sam Horne. This is a tape related to using more effective communication strategies to improve difficult moments. We discuss the purpose of our emotions and talk about the concept of radical acceptance. We are discussing termination of the group in three weeks.

Session 4: We watch videos by John Bradshaw called *Mystified Love* and *Self Love.* This encourages group members to use self-soothing techniques when they need to do so. This is an effective way to get through difficulties. Bradshaw emphasizes that self-love is healthy, self-validating, and an effective antidote to self-defeating behaviors.

Session 5: We watch a tape titled *Letting Go.* This encourages members to let go of the lies we believe, to let go of unhealthy practices, and to minimize the time we spend in negative relationships that rob us of the freedom to be ourselves. The profiles are taken again and the group makes plans for the last session.

Session 6: The last session is spent in discussing other available group sessions, evaluating the group process, and making suggestions for future group activities. Many of the members exchange telephone numbers and e-mails. The therapist does not encourage or discourage this practice.

CONCLUSION

Marsha Linehan's DBT was a huge advance in the treatment of clients with BPD. EMDR, ego-state therapies, resource installation, and attention to trauma are the next leap forward. Since I've been using EMDR and other trauma techniques in my groups, the hospitalization rate of group members has gone from three or four within every group period to one for the past 2 years. With a combination of individual and group sessions, focussing on skills, awareness, and trauma, I have developed a unique and effective approach to therapy with trauma and abuse survivors.

During the first half of the group sessions we concentrate on education, acceptance of oneself, skill development, and homework. The focus is on developing a commitment to the group, normalizing experiences of the members, setting effective limits, eliminating self-defeating behaviors, and empowering women. The therapist combines techniques of DBT, cognitive therapy, solution focus, crisis intervention, EMDR, and whatever else may be needed and useful at the time.

During the second half of the group we work on reeducating the brain physiology related to traumas and facilitate corrective emotional experiences. We use many methods, including but not limited to EMDR and adjunct therapies, interactive exercises, metaphors, stories, role-play, videos, and movies, to accomplish the goal of maximum recovery for each member. The use of EMDR within the group has decreased members' self report profiles of borderline, PTS, and PTSD symptoms by almost 30%.

SINCERE GRATITUDE

I am grateful for all of the scholars and pioneers in the field who have provided the tools to effectively do the work. I am most of all in awe and humbly grateful to the women who have trusted me, shared their lives, and allowed me to practice the profession for which I feel tremendous passion.

REFERENCES

Burns, D. (1992). *The feel good workbook*. New York: Avon.

Burns, D. (1993). *Ten days to self esteem*. New York: Avon.

Kiessling, R. (2002, October). *Integrating resource installation strategies into your EMDR practice*. Training workshop, Nashville, TN.

Linehan, M. (1993). *Skills training manual for treating borderline personality disorder*. New York: Guilford Press.

Rothschild, B. (2000). *The body remembers: the psychophysiology of trauma and trauma treatment*. New York: Norton.

Schmidt, S. J. (2002). *Developmental needs meeting strategy for EMDR therapists*. San Antonio, TX: Schmidt Press.

van der Kolk, B. A. (2002). In terror's grip: Healing the ravages of trauma. *Cerebrum, 4* (1), 34–50.

Wilson, D., & Foster, L. (2002). *Strengthening the ego, pre and post EMDR relaxation scripts*. Ashland, OR: Personal Development Press.

Chapter 13

Using EMDR in Couples Therapy

Robin Shapiro

WHY WOULD YOU DO EMDR, A DECIDEDLY INDIVIDUAL THERAPY, WITH couples? How do you decide with whom to use EMDR? And is there anything besides trauma processing that EMDR brings to conjoint couples therapy?

In 8 out of 10 couples sessions, I use the Standard Protocol to clear trauma from inside and outside the relationship and from before and after the couple met. The partners envision and practice new behaviors with the Future Template. Dual Attention Stimulus (DAS) can enhance self-soothing. Additionally, when a partner sees the other partner do EMDR or is seen doing EMDR, differentiation is enhanced in each.

Of course, I practice other modalities. EMDR by itself can't solve every relationship issue. From the "lenses" of Schnarch (1997), and Bader & Pearson (1988), I attend to the level of differentiation in the couple. Differentiation is the ability to be seen as one is and to clearly see one's partner as the partner is, with tolerance and understanding. Differentiated couples can "stick to their guns" when necessary and yield appropriately, without loss of self. Differentiated partners have enough affect tolerance to "self-soothe" or "partner-soothe" when the going gets rough. From Gottman's (1994) research, I teach couples communication skills, "bids" for connection, and "repair" after injuries. It's helpful to mention Gottman and tell clients that research shows that when men accept influence from their wives, both partners are happier in the marriage, and the marriage lasts longer. Even the most belligerent partner can't argue with research!

READINESS FOR EMDR

When I see that trauma or habitual triggers need to be cleared, I wonder if the couple is ready for EMDR. Then I ask myself these questions:

- Is there enough safety in the relationship for partners to move through issues and pain in the presence of each other?

  - Will either use the information gleaned from the session as a weapon in an argument?
  - Will both be able hold back from editorial comments during the processing?

- Is there enough base differentiation or characterological basis for learning differentiation for each to allow the other his or her own process?
- Are they capable of mutual support?
- Is each capable of self-soothing?
- Would the traumatic material of one client (for instance, sexual abuse) be too distressing for the other to bear?
- Are the issues developmental or normative or do they arise from personality disorders?
- As in individual therapy, is there enough containment in the therapy relationship to do EMDR?
- Have both clients been informed about EMDR and have both given their consent?

If the clients are able to "hold on to themselves" while the other works, are able to provide support and not attack the other with the content of the EMDR session, and are dealing with either solely traumatic or solely developmental issues, they could be good candidates for conjoint EMDR sessions. If they can't do these things but are on their way, EMDR could be a good teacher of these skills. If they aren't even close, think about working separately with each partner.

CLEARING TRAUMA

Trauma clearing is the most obvious use of EMDR. With couples, you can target the traumas that occurred inside the relationship, including fights, bad sex, abuse, and real or imagined betrayal or abandonment or snubs. Historical traumas from the client's family of origin or past relationships make great targets. The Two-Hand Interweave (Chapter 6) can help differentiate between a current distress and its historical antecedent, and the Standard Protocol can clear the bad history.

Client: He's just like my dad!
Therapist: *How old do you feel when he's just like your dad?*
Client: Five.
Therapist: *Put your husband in one hand and your dad when you were 5 in the other. [DAS] What's coming up?*
Client: They're exactly the same. I feel powerless with both of them.
Therapist: *Think about your dad when you were 5. Do you have a picture of the scene? Where do you feel it in your body? How true is it that you feel powerful? How distressed do you feel when you hold that picture of your dad in your mind; you feel it in your solar plexus and you're telling yourself that you are powerless?* [Standard Protocol] When the trauma is cleared the therapist can try the Two-Hand Interweave again. *So, now put your dad in one hand and your husband in the other. (DAS.) What do you notice?*
Client: They're way different people. I guess my kid stuff has been making me see my husband differently.
Therapist: *Go with that. (DAS.)*

EMDR can be used to clear the traumas that occurred before the relationship. Many clients clear abuse from parents, siblings, or prior relationships. When the EMDR client's partner gets to witness the clearing of the prerelationship trauma, he or she builds differentiation, understanding ("It's not about me!"), and, in most cases, less reactivity toward a reactive spouse.

Maureen Kitchur starts couples therapy with the focus on past trauma. She uses her Strategic Developmental Model on each client, separately. When the individual work is done, she finds that the relationship problems have often "miraculously" disappeared (see Chapter 1).

OTHER TARGETS FOR EMDR

Here are some other common processing targets that arise in conjoint therapy.

- Grief or rage

  - That one's partner will not fulfill all of one's needs
  - About past hurts or betrayals in the relationship
  - About former losses
  - About the loss of the fantasy of the ideal relationship

- Generational and cultural issues (Chapter 10) (When these are deconstructed it's much easier for partners to know, "It's not about me.")
- Self-soothing in the session: *Notice the distress you're feeling when you see his anger. Where do you feel that? What are you saying to yourself about yourself?* [Standard Protocol] At one time you might have one person processing a trauma or a recurrent feeling and the other partner processing his reaction to the first. Often couples will incorporate the butterfly hug (hugging oneself and tapping oneself alternately on each shoulder; Boel, personal communication, 1997) into their conflicts, in the session, and then at home.
- "Hugging to Relax" is a couples exercise described in *Passionate Marriage*, David Schnarch's (1997) groundbreaking book about differentiation and hot sex. A couple will stand and hug each other for up to 20 minutes. Each partner will allow whatever feelings and thoughts that arise to float through their awareness. Each person stays in the clinch even if anxiety arises. Each will self-soothe through grounding, breathing, or calming self-statements. The point of the exercise is to learn how to stay in contact no matter what one is feeling. EMDR clients often use some sort of DAS, such as alternating lifting fingers or eye movements, to self-soothe during this exercise. It works wonderfully.
- Future templates, bringing change to the future

  - *How would you like to act differently when she does that thing again?* (DAS.)

- ○ *Imagine soothing yourself the next time that happens.*
- ○ *Imagine what you would do if you did deserve having your needs met.*
- ○ *Imagine what it would take for you to change or get through this block.*

- ○ Before: *Imagine reaching your bottom line on this issue. What would that look like? What would that feel like? Let's do EMDR on that feeling.* (Standard Protocol.)
- ○ *Imagine staying in your oldest wisest adult when your partner shifts into that "scary" state* (Golston, personal communication, 2003).
- ○ After: *Imagine standing firm on that bottom line when the situation arises.* (Future Template.)

- Fear of differentiation itself: *Imagine that you notice the full range of differences between you and your partner.* (This often brings up fear.) *What are you saying to yourself about yourself? Where do you feel it in the body?* (Standard Protocol.)
- Regression and ego states: Lifespan Integration (Pace, 2003) or any of the EMDR-related ego-state treatments can assist a regressed partner to "grow up" in the session, and relate from their adult perspective.
- Fear of attaching to, then losing, one's partner. A good positive cognition (PC) in this case is "I'm willing to tolerate potential loss in order to have love now."

AFFAIRS

Affairs create tremendous trauma and many productive targets for EMDR. The first targets may be the shock, grief, and rage of the non-cheating partner. When the affair is recent, the Recent Events Protocol (Shapiro, 2001) is quite useful. The most disturbing aspect, usually when the client found out about the affair, is targeted first. The rest of the narrative of the event is targeted in chronological order. Often more affect or new aspects of the trauma arise for weeks or even months after the initial processing is complete.

Sometimes, the distressed affect alone may be the best first target. Expect to spend many sessions working on emotions. You may also target when and how the client heard about the affair, the realization of all the lies he or she has swallowed, and the client's sense of worth. ("How could I not have known?" or "How was I not enough to keep my partner home?" or simply: "I'm not lovable.") The straying partner often carries crippling shame and guilt. Schnarch (1997) stated that the majority of people who have affairs do so because they are afraid to be wholly seen by their partner at home. They take a part of themselves elsewhere. By the time they have the affair, they are used to lying about themselves. The shame begins before the affair starts. Focusing on the offending client's sense of worth can be extremely fruitful. The non-straying client gains differentiation ("It's really not about me!"). Both gain a clearer sense of the strayer's motivations through the negative cognitions: "I need to seduce everyone to prove I'm enough" versus "I'm enough as I am." "I can't ask for what I want at home. It will drive away my spouse if she knows me" versus "I can ask for what I want and can tolerate being seen as I am."

After affairs, fears for the future are enormous in each partner. Generally, the partners don't come to therapy unless they both are highly invested in the relationship. The strayer fears being dumped or never being forgiven. The nonstrayer fears another round of betrayal. Nonstrayers fear the consequences of trust. A useful positive cognition is "I can trust myself to survive the consequences of trusting my partner."

I tend to do all the therapy with both partners in the room, unless the "strayer" is a sex addict, a psychopath, or an unremitting narcissistic and needs individual therapy. A typical therapy in the aftermath of an affair lasts 4 to 8 months. Here are steps in a post-affair therapy:

1. Get the whole story from each partner, including the history of their relationship and the history of the affair (sometimes using continual or intermittent DAS to contain affect in either or both partners while the story unfolds).
2. Get a commitment that the affair is over. (It's usually, but not always, a "done deal" by they time they come in.) If the affair is not over, that's the issue until it is over.
3. Do the Recent Events Protocol with the nonstraying partner, possibly starting with affect rather than an event.
4. Do the Recent Events Protocol with the straying partner.

5. Work on shame and guilt issues with each partner. For the strayer, the focus is often on the betrayal. (Positive cognitions could include, "I've learned from my experience." "I can take responsibility for my actions." For the nonstrayer, the focus is often on worth. PCs could include: "I'm lovable." "I wasn't stupid to trust my partner."

6. Exploring what happened inside the relationship and or inside the individuals that created the affair. At this point, I attempt to get the clients to read *Passionate Marriage* (Schnarch, 1997). If they aren't readers, or can't get through the dense prose, I begin to introduce the ideas of differentiation and toleration of self and other. I teach self-soothing techniques. It may take one session (after reading the book) or many sessions (with hugely undifferentiated clients) for these ideas to take hold. When they "get" the concepts, we work with the issues of culpability and what went wrong. This is the most painful, the richest, and the most healing part of the therapy. When partners can truly speak to each other and hear each other on these issues, they can reach a depth of intimacy that they may never have experienced before. EMDR can target the fear of differentiation, the fear of reconnecting with the offending partner, and the fear of betrayal. Good PCs include: "I can survive being known." "I can survive being betrayed." And Schnarch's: "I can hold on to myself."

7. Forgiving or acceptance is the next step. The Buddha said that to understand is to forgive. Forgiveness may have spontaneously taken place during the exploration phase. If not, a good EMDR question can be *Think about forgiving your partner, remembering that forgiveness does not equal saying it was okay. Where do you feel the blocks in your body?* (Standard Protocol.) or *What would happen if you forgave yourself? What stands in the way of forgiving yourself, accepting what you did and guarding against future affairs? Think of that.* (DAS.) Be careful to not shame clients for not being ready or able to forgive. Explore with them where they are, not where you or anyone thinks they should be.

8. At this point in therapy, things are often much better. The partners may have resumed their sex lives (after a round of sexually transmitted diseases [STD] testing, for some of them). They may be more intimate than they have ever been before. The discussion

turns to the future and to prevention of other incidents. We talk about "affair-proofing" the marriage by sticking to the truth, showing oneself to one's partner "warts and all," and self-soothing. We discuss future temptations, avoiding "occasions of sin," and do Future Templates: *Imagine that a beautiful young person at the EMDR International Association (EMDRIA) conference invites you up to her room to discuss a new body-based technique. How do you plan to respond?* (DAS.)

SEX THERAPY

EMDR is of great use in the two major relational barriers to good sex: past trauma and current lack of differentiation. Send people to their physicians for the other barrier, physical inability. Then have them return to process their grief about it, if necessary, and plan ways to connect anyway. Use the Standard Protocol on past trauma targets including sexual abuse, rape, bad sex, sexual harassment, and having had sex when they didn't want to or when they didn't let their needs be known. Often, clearing the past trauma is sufficient to solve any problems with the current partner. Sometimes the Two-Hand Interweave can be used at the end of the trauma processing: *Put the man who raped you in one hand and your sweet boyfriend in the other.* (DAS.) If the two people still feel like the same guy, more trauma processing is in order. My favorite phone message occurred after the third EMDR session targeting childhood sexual abuse: "I just had wonderful sex with my husband [of 10 years]. For the first time ever, my grandfather wasn't in the room."

Many sexual issues arise from partners' inabilities to say what they want and don't want. Clients who can't say no when they don't want to have sex and who "go along with it" tend to tune out at the time and to resent future sexual overtures. With support from my rule, "Without a no, there's no true yes," a not-yet-assertive partner can imagine turning down their honey. Use the Standard Protocol to clear out the anxiety that arises when they think of saying no. "It's okay to say no" or "I deserve to have a no" are possible PCs. Imagine all possible and impossible responses and clear out all the anxiety. Then use the Future Template: *Imagine saying no.* (DAS, as many rounds as necessary.) *Good, now imagine saying yes when you do want to and showing up 100% for the experience.* (DAS, as many rounds as necessary.)

Some partners are poorly attached, capable of only "part-object" relations, and don't notice or care about their partners' pleasure or interest in sex. I often appeal directly to their most selfish interest. *Have you ever had truly connected sex? You don't know what that is? Well, it's about 20 times more intense than what you've been getting. Let me tell you how to create this with your partner.* We call this psychoeducation. *First, you need to make sure that she really wants to do it. Then you have to connect with her. It'll really turn you on, when she's really turned on. Don't you remember that from the beginning of the relationship? Don't you miss that? I'll tell you how to get back to that.*

DIFFERENTIATION

Work directly on the content of differentiation. With all of the below, clear the anxiety about doing the behavior with the Standard Protocol, and then use the Future Template to bring the experience into the person's brain.

- *Imagine saying what you want to do or have done to you. Imagine your partner's possible responses.*
- *Imagine saying what you don't want. Imagine your partner's possible responses.*
- *Imagine climbing over that wall that's been between you and making a sexual move on your partner. Imagine your partner says yes. Imagine your partner says no.*
- *Imagine you being exactly who you are, wanting exactly what you want, and making sure you get it.* (Don't use this one with the before-mentioned jerks.)
- *Imagine being seen exactly as you are and staying connected to your partner in that sexual situation (with your big hips/little penis/fat belly/wrinkles/cellulite/funny noises/ aging body/not knowing what to do next/not always feeling "on").* These issues can be discovered with the Two-Hand Interweave. *In one hand put the way you should be/look. In the other hand put the way you actually are.* (DAS.)
- *Imagine being truly connected to your partner (without being swallowed up, disappearing, or overpowering your partner).*

- *Imagine becoming disconnected during sex and then reconnecting with your partner.*
- *Imagine coming too soon/not coming as fast you think you should.* (Standard Protocol.) *Now imagine recovering from that and reconnecting with your partner.*
- *Imagine letting your partner "do" you.*
- *Imagine trying that new thing your partner wants you to do.*
- *Imagine sticking to your guns and saying, "No way!"*
- *Imagine "wanting to want" your partner.* (Schnarch, 1997).
- *Imagine telling your partner that if he wants you he needs to seduce you and then telling him how.*
- For sex addicts: *Imagine how you'll self-soothe instead of demanding sex when you begin to feel anxious. Imagine noticing the real feeling underneath the compulsion to have sex.*

Now can you imagine the experience of the partners witnessing their honeys moving through any of these issues? Can you imagine the differentiation that might arise in the witnesses? Can you imagine the behavioral changes that could occur before anyone says anything in bed?

REFERENCES

Bader, E., & Pearson, P. (1988). *In quest of the mythical mate.* Florence, KY: Brunner-Mazel.

Gottman, J. (1994). *Why marriages succeed or fail: What you can learn from the breakthrough research to make your marriage work.* New York: Fireside.

Pace, P. (2003, June). *Likespan integration.* Workshop at the EMDR International Association Conference, Denver, CO.

Schnarch, D. (1997). *Passionate marriage.* New York: Norton.

Shapiro, F. (2001). *Eye movement desensitization and reprocessing* (2nd edition). New York: Guilford Press.

Chapter 14

EMDR with Clients with Mental Disability

Andrew Seubert

UNTIL RECENT TIMES THOSE WITH THE DUAL DIAGNOSIS OF MENTAL retardation and mental health issues were deemed inappropriate candidates for counseling or psychotherapy. Dysfunctional behaviors and emotional displays generated by mood disorders, grief, or trauma were often written off as part of the mental disability, in what has come to be known as diagnostic overshadowing. Time, experience, and compassion have changed this. Counseling and psychotherapy have been shown to be "feasible and successful" (Fletcher, 1993, p. 328) with this population. Most effective are approaches that utilize and integrate concrete, experiential, and behavioral aspects of the treatment. The task and responsibility of the therapist is to follow the client's internal and interpersonal process as it reveals itself and find the ways, means, and language to facilitate this organic movement toward well-being,

INTRODUCTION

Persons with mental disabilities will often display all or many of the following characteristics: subnormal IQ and poor abstract thinking, passivity and dependence, self-absorption, restricted affect range, novelty avoidance (fear of change), developmental delays, and vulnerability to abuse. Consequently, treatment plans include normal therapeutic goals

and goals that for the nondisabled person are part of normal developmental growth. Among these goals are self-awareness, affect awareness
and expression, self-sufficiency and autonomy, interpersonal connection
and contact, reduction of the fear of change, boundary setting, shame and
grief processing related to the disability, and the resolution of trauma.

Even with a common therapeutic goal, for example, affect awareness, the therapist and client will spend more time on that goal due to
developmental lag. Consequently, it is particularly important to recall
that trauma processing is only one of a number of phases in trauma
treatment.

The transforming of traumatic memory (be it Judith Herman's
remembrance/mourning [1992], EMDR's phases from assessment
through closure, or Ricky Greenwald's "slaying the dragon" [in press])
is embedded in a larger framework that prepares and supports the
client before, during, and after the desensitization of painful memory.
This larger therapeutic map must be kept in the foreground at all times.

Therefore, while holding the basic protocol as our reference point and
employing it first as it has been developed and researched, it becomes a
primary task to creatively adapt the protocol when necessary to support
the healing of clients with mental handicaps. This is similar to ways in
which one would work with children (Greenwald, 1999; Lovett, 1999;
Tinker & Wilson, 1999). We enter the world of the disabled, not insisting
they speak our language, but finding the communicative channels that
can bring us together in a common journey (Seubert, 1999).

The following pages will focus on clients with mental health issues
and developmental disabilities (dually diagnosed [DD]) who are verbal and score in the mild (IQ level 50–55 to approximately 70) to moderate range (35–40 to 50–55) of disability (APA, 1994). This chapter will
employ the 8-phase protocol of Francine Shapiro (2001) as a point of
reference while making suggestions for extensions and adaptations of
that protocol. It will include points of information regarding clients
with mental disabilities and offer general principles as well as specific
strategies to guide therapeutic choices with this population.

PHASE 1: HISTORY AND TREATMENT PLANNING

The evaluation phase of the work and the development of therapeutic
rapport integrate over the course of many weeks. Two factors

differentiate evaluation and trauma history with this population. The first factor is that the clients are by nature of their disability more dependent on caregivers and are often not able to provide objective reporting. This requires thoroughly interviewing parents, family, teachers, direct care staff, and other service providers in order to re-create the story of the clients' lives, thereby making sense of the clients' symptoms, what Greenwald calls "solution behaviors" (Greenwald, in press).

A second factor is that the word *trauma* needs to take on a much broader meaning with this population, even more so than with nondisabled clients who may not experience big "T" or major trauma, but small "t" events that have wounded them and have been dysfunctionally stored. Given their psychosocial and cognitive deficits, clients with developmental disabilities are inherently more vulnerable to standard forms of trauma and experience as well many other forms of injury, particularly when they approach developmental milestones (graduations, driving cars, dating) and realize that they are not able to keep up with nondisabled peers or with younger siblings (Levitas & Gilson, 1994).

If possible, a meeting with all caregivers is tremendously helpful and necessary during this phase in order to clarify case formulation and treatment goals. Due to the frequent absence of subjective reporting, this is the place for compassionate (yet informed) guesswork or symptom translation. With the client's history in mind, as well as affective and behavioral symptoms, the team must explore what might be at the heart of the client's disturbance. Michael's background serves as a good example.

Michael scores in the mild range of mental retardation. He is 17 years old and has been mainstreamed into the local high school. He loves to play his harmonica while listening to the sound track of *Chicago* on his Walkman and, with his playful humor and active imagination, can steal your heart in a second. A primary goal in his treatment is for him to feel better about being Michael, Down syndrome and all. Yet, the closer a person's mental handicap is to the normal range of intellectual functioning, the stronger is the belief awareness that "something about me isn't right, and I can't change it." Feelings of shame, loss, and anxiety, consequently, became common experiences for Michael. Without affect awareness or the ability to communicate emotionally, he often simply withdrew or acted out his hurt and fear.

Most of his caregivers were in the habit of "protecting him" from his emotions, rather than exploring the possible connection between feelings and behaviors. Awareness of hurt, sadness, and shame was clouded by statement such as: "Oh, don't pay any attention to that!" or

"You're just fine!" Diversion was also employed, taking Michael's attention too quickly from frustration and disappointment to anything but that painful moment.

It became crucial then for me to meet with Michael's parents, teachers, aides, and job support people to elicit cooperation in encouraging him to notice feelings, particularly as they manifested as body sensations, name them, and then express them appropriately. Understanding what drove his behaviors (case formulation) as well as affective goals (goal setting and treatment contract) had been missing for major players on the team.

PHASE 2: PREPARATION

As in the previous phase, preparation must involve the client and the caregivers. All must understand the goals of treatment as well as what to expect whenever trauma processing takes place. Everyone must learn affect awareness and management. Everyone must be included in case management for safety and support. The therapist is working with an extremely interdependent system, and often it is the therapist who must coordinate the team. It becomes evident that EMDR, or any trauma resolution strategy, must be part of a larger trauma treatment model.

COMMUNICATIVE LANGUAGE

The parameters of communicative language must often be expanded beyond the representational and the abstract. Establishing the language(s)—verbal, facial, body-centered, movement, posture, art, music—that can facilitate communication between client and therapist is a prerequisite for therapeutic rapport and progress. The client has the clues and the cues to communication pathways, so the therapist's task is to observe follow, observe, and follow. This is an ongoing process in which the therapist and client discover the words, sounds, body postures, movement, and expressive channels (art, music, drama, sand trays, storytelling) that allow for communication (Seubert, 1999, pp. 92–93). Here, again, we see parallels with child and adolescent therapeutic approaches.

Dual Attention Stimulus (DAS) is often useful in practicing and reinforcing the success of appropriate communication, particularly with visualized skill rehearsal (positive template). Instead of hitting someone or screaming when anxiety arises, a client can be taught the skill of communicating the anxiety through words or gestures to a support person. Clients are then guided to imagine themselves in an anxiety-provoking situation and handling the disturbance with their newly acquired skill while the therapist applies DAS (eye movements, acoustic or tactile stimulation). After a positive imagined (and, later, in vivo) rehearsal, the success can be installed as a positive resource.

Therapist: *Now that you know what it's like to handle your nervousness this way, how does that feel?*
Client: Good!
Therapist: *And where is that "good" feeling in your body?*
Client: In my stomach.
Therapist: *So go with that.* (Applying DAS.)

PRETHERAPY

Prouty (1976) noticed that mentally handicapped clients were typically deficient in both relating (to self and others) and experiencing (the world). He developed a methodology using various forms of reflection to develop these impaired psychological functions in his clients so that therapeutic contact might take place. For instance, he employed facial, body, and word-for-word mirroring to enhance self- and other-awareness in clients, subsequently leading to more interactive functions and behaviors.

Additionally, clients will need to develop more of a sense of "inside and outside." Thoughts, feelings, body sensations, desires, and images all belong to the clients' "inside" world, whereas events, objects of desire or fear, people and things that stimulate the senses are "outside." The notion of a boundary, an abstract concept the nonhandicapped often take for granted, can be a challenge for clients with disabilities. In one group I facilitated, members of an "awareness and communication" group needed to walk toward and near one another holding a hula hoop around themselves to create the concrete sense of boundary and differentiation. The therapist must avoid taking for granted many of the concepts and interactive capacities typically belonging to a nonhandicapped world.

In all of this preparation, I use DAS whenever possible to facilitate the developmental learning in a sequence I call the "sandwich effect," in that the learning occurs between a calming and a reinforcing segment. I will precede the learning by applying DAS to some soothing, calming resource and follow any learning success with: *How does it feel to have learned what you just did?* If the answer is "Good!" this is followed with DAS in order to create a resource of each and every success. For example, in Michael's process of learning to be aware of (make contact with) others, I will use DAS to establish a calm state, then practice noticing the facial and body signals from myself or from anyone else participating in the session, and, finally, strengthen his awareness of his accomplishment. This success memory becomes an organically developed resource, and a sense of mastery is accomplished through "sandwiching" the exploratory and rehearsal use of DAS between a calming resource and a reinforced awareness of success.

AFFECT EDUCATION

In working with this population, the therapist must make everything as concrete and specific as possible and never take yes for an answer. Individuals with developmental disabilities can often be compliant and emotionally limited, not necessarily due to the disability, but often because of the conditioning and overprotectiveness of caregivers. Emotional education needs to involve the very basic elements of emotion recognition, as well as tolerance, management, and expression. Feelings need to be drawn, located in the body, and noticed in videos, photos, and stories. Clients with mental disability need to be taught to notice feelings when they arise. DAS can be very helpful in jump-starting as well as heightening this awareness. DAS can then be used in practicing management (verbalizing awareness, breathing positive affect states in and disturbing states out) and, at times, expression (verbalizing, sounding, drawing, role playing) of those feelings. This is some of the "psychological contact" with self of which Prouty (1976) wrote.

Michael and I are exploring his moody and somewhat belligerent attitude at a local pizza shop where he is learning job skills with the assistance of an aide. His attitude at times triggers a negative response from his manager, which, in turn, works against his agreed-upon goal of feeling better about himself.

In the following session excerpt, one can observe the focus on affect development, the use of the "sandwich" strategy, and the presence of an aide to provide feedback and observations (more evaluation and potential reevaluation).

AS: *Michael, the other day at work, Laurie* (aide) *tells us that you started to talk out loud to Jumbo* (his imaginary friend and internal critic). *Do you remember what you were feeling?*

Michael: No.

AS: *Do you remember what you were doing?*

Michael: No! I don't want to talk about it.

AS: *Would you be willing to explore that a bit so you don't get in trouble at work?*

Michael: Well . . . [He pauses.] Uh, well, okay.

AS: (putting headphones on Michael with tones shifting back and forth bilaterally) *Michael, start by taking that deep breath into your belly, just like we've been practicing, then remember one person who makes you feel good.* (pause) *Got it?*

Michael: Yep.

AS: *Great! Now imagine yourself back at work the other day. What are you doing?*

Michael: They want me to fold the pizza boxes different. I don't know how to do it!

AS: *Good. Now pay attention to those signals in your body that we talked about. When you don't know how to do this job, what happens inside?*

Michael: My stomach feels funny . . . (presently felt).

AS: *Does that funny feeling have a name?*

Michael: Kinda like . . . nervous.

AS: *Great, Michael. Now imagine telling Lisa how nervous you are instead of talking to Jumbo.*

Awareness is primary. It then becomes easier to develop a strategy for Michael to deal with his anxiety and fear of change by communicating this awareness to his job aide or someone else, than by talking out loud to an imaginary Jumbo, something that tends to interrupt the digestive process of customers. Later, we practice the new awareness and skill using continual audio DAS with a Future Template and, finally, reinforce how good it feels to be able to handle such situations more adaptively.

Michael's typical strategy of talking out loud to what we might call an internal ego state might be written off by some as due to the mental disability (diagnostic overshadowing), but the reality is that most of us employ similar coping methods but in a subtler manner. Mentally disabled clients use the same internal mechanisms and defenses as do nondisabled. They're just more transparent.

First use eye movements when establishing Future Templates. If this is not effective, then experiment with eyes closed (using taps or acoustic stimulation) or with continual DAS. The client is always the ultimate expert on what works.

Visualization is often effective. At other times, due to an inability to abstract and generalize, some mentally handicapped clients need to work with a very concrete, here-and-now reality. Gail, a 57-year-old client (mild mental retardation [MR]), couldn't believe me when I suggested that her reactions sounded as if there was something like a "younger part" of her being hurt. "Andrew, that's crazy! You mean like a little kid running around inside?" So much for ego state! Yet 43-year-old Carol (moderate MR), when asked what she needed to feel strong, said: "I need . . . Popeye! Eating spinach right inside my heart!"And Popeye became her resource as she learned to deal with the deaths of family members and friends.

RESOURCE DEVELOPMENT

For clients with mental disability, Resource Development will target and enhance aspects of developmental growth. Given the varying capacities to abstract and generalize among these clients, possible resources are (a) physical: photos, pictures, client drawings, physical objects; (b) representational: memories, imagery, creative visualizations; and (c) body-located: *Where in your body do you have this feeling or can you store that image?* The greater the variety and number of resources, the more options are available to jump-start stuck processing.

The letter *m* can also be useful as a mnemonic device in recalling the various kinds of representational resources: Memories, Mirrors, Models, iMaginings. A client's memory of experiencing a helpful emotion or internal resource is always more impactful than something imagined.

A mirror is someone who has seen that quality in clients and has reflected it back to them when they couldn't notice it without feedback. A model is someone who embodies that quality and then catalyzes and inspires it in the client (the model doesn't give us anything we don't already have).The imagined resource, whether from literature, movies, cartoons, or the client's own imagination, is called upon when all else fails.

With Michael, I was able to use a variety of resources before we began the assessment and desensitization phases. I coached him to focus on photos of resource people in his life (actual friends, family, and caregivers), newspaper clippings of his successes in bowling and Special Olympics, and his own drawings of positive emotional states, typically using DAS with headphones employing either bilateral music or any device that makes any music bilateral.

Since Michael is able to work with some abstraction, I guided him to develop the image of a "resource place" (I find this more open-ended than "safe place," particularly since for some clients there is no "safe place"). Within that place, we developed the image of a circle (an adaptation of the neurolinguistic programming "circle of excellence" [Collingwood & Collingwood, 2001]), a clearing in the woods, within which he placed all of the resources we had established in a more concrete fashion. From here I had him locate the entire scene in his body (*as if you took a picture of all of this, with all of the people, the good memories, and the good feelings, and planted it somewhere in your body that feels relaxed to you right now*). Then I had him choose a cue word or phrase that went along with the image ("happy," "calm," and "peachy," which was Michael's favorite). Finally he breathed in and out of that place in his body. The resource is now anchored via image, emotion, cognition, body sensation, body location, and breath. When practiced enough, a breath into that place in the body or repeating the cue word will connect Michael with the needed resource.

DAS is usually employed to reinforce the moment when the client experiences the positive emotion or body sensation, typically with auditory stimulus or at times by tapping the client's hands, shoulders, or knees.

DAS is also helpful as the client is learning how to release and modulate strong affect. For this task, I employ the word "LIDS" as an acronym to outline the steps for the client:

"L"—locate the feeling in your body

"I"—determine the intensity of the feeling on a scale of 0–10

(I take two measures: one of the present disturbance and one for the level the client wants to achieve).

"D"—describe the feeling (does it have color, shape, size, temperature?)

"S"—breathe into the feeling and send the emotional energy with the out breath into the universe to disperse or transform or send it into a previously visualized container of the client's creation (jar, milk can, safe, box) to put it on hold until a more appropriate time. Do this until the desired level of intensity is reached. Once the first three steps are completed, DAS accompanies the last stage of emotional release or moderation.

PHASE 3: ASSESSMENT

The primary purpose of the assessment phase is to gain access to the dysfunctionally stored material. One must employ as many of the elements of the standard assessment as possible. When not feasible, go with whatever the client can relate to and whatever seems to access the dysfunctional information, particularly in its emotional and somatic forms. This often requires a great deal of adaptation. Not once in working with this population have I been able to complete the formal assessment and not once have I had to. With the elements of the assessment in mind (image, negative cognition [NC], positive cognition [PC], Validity of Cognition Scale [VOC], feelings, sensations, Subjective Units of Distress Scale [SUDS]), I gather as much information as possible. Some of this information is obtained at different times (for example, during the evaluation or preparation phases, when we might briefly touch on the target), then brought together before processing.

Clients who are DD may be unable or reluctant to recall the target image. Sometimes an image of the worst moment is possible, but often a drawing representing the event or a person involved in the event is more concrete and more effective.

NCs and PCs are often difficult to obtain, and insisting on them will usually close down the client's somatic, emotional movement that may well already be activated. Some clients can pick a cognition from a list. If that fails, the therapist often can discover the imbedded cognition during the processing via compassionate guesswork and feed it back to the client, ideally by asking a question that gives the client space for discovery. Given the fact that we often have to be more directive with clients who are handicapped, it is important to be aware of their compliant tendencies and not automatically take yes for an answer.

The therapist typically combines the target image and the PC to determine the felt truthfulness of the positive belief in the present, then asks the client to combine the image with the NC in order to access affective and somatic information. During the phases of installation and body scan, holding two things in awareness simultaneously can be troublesome for clients with disabilities. Asking them to focus on a past event while assessing a presently held belief can be very confusing. Here we have to creatively punt, go with the client's abilities, gather what information we can, and focus on any affective or somatic movement. When a client shows that a feeling or body sensation is present, I typically will say, *Go with that!*

Sometimes the recognition of emotions can work, depending on how well affect training has proceeded. Naming feelings can, however, be an insidious act of abstraction, an area of typical weakness for clients such as Michael and Carol.

At times I will skip naming feelings and simply ask the client to focus on body sensations. At times it may be necessary to name areas of the body where feelings might be held, moving from more independent response to greater guidance, as necessary, to foster body awareness and contact.

As with children, we often have to create our own VOC and SUDSs. Two different scales proved to be confusing for Michael, so we created a "one scale fits all." *Zero to ten, Michael,* I suggested. *Zero is the pits and 10 is super-peachy!* This worked well, allowing him to indicate the strength of a negative emotional state by evaluating it somewhere between 0 and 5, 0 being the worst. As negativity dissolves and positive feelings grow, the numbers climb to 10. When he can think of a negative experience and still say he feels like a "10!" and can do this twice, the desensitization is complete. This scale proved to be effective in subsequent sessions when we checked on the staying power of the processing. At other times, having him spread my hands apart or closer to indicate more or less disturbance has been helpful.

PHASE 4: DESENSITIZATION

As in all other phases, if the Standard Protocol works, just do it. Very common with this population, however, is difficulty with affect tolerance (even with a great deal of preparation) and not being able to make sense of the need at all for trauma processing (even after goals have been determined). After all, "It just hurts. Why bother?" This is also where the therapist's own doubts in the client's ability to tolerate the desensitization can play a countertransferential role. Given possible fears in both client and therapist, it is in this phase that the door to healing has often remained closed.

It's like making soup, I tell clients. *If you swallow the ingredients* (trauma) *too soon, they'll make you sick. So you've got all of these raw ingredients; you add things at the start and sometimes more things as you go along to make it thicker, thinner, spicier, smoother* (resources), *and you slowly cook it until it's the way you like it* (processing). *At the end, instead of things you just can't digest, you have a wonderful soup.*

For DD clients many resources should be interwoven through the desensitization phase. Because these clients may not be able to generalize a resource from one event to another and because of occasional, persistent difficulties in managing affect, you may need to use more resources more often. Most of them should be established in advance, while the exigencies of processing may well require the development of a new resource during the desensitization itself.

Particularly if a client is looping or is still pain avoidant, a continuous resource interweave will often facilitate a successful resolution. Instead of either waiting for the client to spontaneously discover a resource or occasionally directing the client to a previously or presently created resource, the client's attention frequently can be directed to resources developed in the preparation phase, typically a short set focused on the target followed by a short set of resource attention. At times, the resource can be kept as a constant, the larger container within which the difficult material is briefly introduced and then allowed to recede from awareness. For example, I might suggest, *Stay in that safe place (or in that circle with the people who care about you) and just think about (or look at the picture of) _____ for a moment (pause) . . . now make it go away. . . .* This titrates the processing and simultaneously gives the sense of mastery over disturbing internal experience.

Peter Levine's (1997) notion of "pendulating"—going back and forth between target and resource—has given clients the courage to face what might otherwise be too intimidating. We must, however, eventually return to the target memory as originally experienced in order to determine whether desensitization is complete or not.

A second departure from standard processing is the frequent return to the target or image and a greater use of rating scales (e.g., SUDS, "one scale fits all,") due to the limited attention span of DD clients. Despite the often rapid processing of the chosen target, separate processing of similar events may be necessary given the fact that these clients often do not generalize their learning as well as the nondisabled. We will examine this more closely in the reevaluation phase.

The following clinical anecdote reveals the ongoing need for creative adaptation, particularly during the desensitization phase of treatment.

Michael had recently been suspended from school for threatening to get a gun and shoot people. He never would have done this, but post-Columbine reality prevailed. Michael had apparently become very upset about two things. First, he had fallen in love after one dance with a nondisabled high school girl, was convinced that she was his "girlfriend," and became angry and jealous when he now saw her with her current boyfriend. Around the same time his best friend, Josh, another boy with Down syndrome, wasn't returning his phone calls. This friend was like a brother to him, and Michael was finding this aggravating and hurtful.

In the session following his suspension, Michael put on the earphones to work with bilateral music, but noticed that he wasn't hearing well out of his left ear. He exploded immediately.

Michael: I hate this ear! I hate my life! People hate me!
AS: *Okay, Michael, just take off the earphones and take a few breaths with me.*

(At this point we were both sitting on the floor with two groups of pictures laid out in front of him: a group of his own drawings of faces representing various emotions and a handful of photos of people and events that are positive resources for him. He cooperated with my suggestion, breathed, and then pointed to the angry and hurt faces.)

AS: *A lot of hard things going on for you, huh?*
Michael: Yeah. Too much. (He pouts a bit.)
AS: *Seeing that girl in school, then Jeremy, now your ear.*
Michael: There's always something wrong!
AS: *Wrong with people, wrong with you?*
Michael: Wrong with me!

Organically we have arrived at the NC, one that underlies much of the difficulty experienced by those with a mental handicap who are also intelligent enough to know that something isn't right with them. Michael agrees to try something to help him feel better. I stand behind him, alternately tapping his shoulders, while instructing him to look first at the drawings of hurt and angry for several seconds and then shifting his attention to the resource photos. This is repeated with a quick SUDS assessment after each round. Within minutes, on the one scale of 0–10, Michael's mood shifts from low on the scale to a 6, and, finally, to a 10, as good as it gets on the "one scale fits all."

From the brightened look on his face and his increased energy and engagement, I could tell that he wasn't trying to please me with a 10. The ability of a client with disability to release negative emotion is very similar to what is often experienced with children. The lack of attachment to heavy "baggage" as well as an ability to return to the present moment may be the reasons for such a rapid emotional shift.

In the following two sessions, Michael chooses to use the bilateral music.

AS: *Michael, let's see how much all of those things, you know, the girl, Jeremy, your left ear . . . how much they're bothering you. You okay with that?*

My instinct is to lump them all together rather than focusing on any one in particular. A "general disturbance" is at times easier for Michael, who tends to avoid specific painful images or events.

Michael: Not really. But . . . all right.
AS: (Bilateral music is now played continuously.) *Start with your eyes closed and think of that circle in the woods, you know, with all your favorite animals and favorite people. Now, open your eyes and look at those happy photos* (about 10 seconds) *. . . Now look over at*

the angry, hurt, and something's-wrong-with-me faces (5–10 seconds depending on what his facial and body language tells me.) Zero to 10, *how does that feel?*
Michael: A 2.
AS: *Okay, once again. Start with the happy photos . . . now the pictures . . . 0 to 10?*
Michael: 2

Now, given the apparent looping, I simply add some eye movements while allowing the music to continue. With his love of music, Michael originally chose auditory stimulus as a processing modality. Previously, however, there was the need to use taps, and now, standard eye movements in order to move the desensitization forward.

AS: *Okay, Michael, look at those feelings and then just follow my hand back and forth [about 10 round-trips of eye movements]. Now focus on the happy photos . . . now back to the drawings. Zero to 10?*
Michael: 10!

He's beaming, and I'm wondering if he has actually cleared the target or does he just want me to get off his back with this painful stuff. We repeat the process several times and the 10 holds. The following week we continue on the same track, but now focusing more specifically on his left ear (10, no disturbance), the lost "girlfriend" (10, no disturbance), the girl's new boyfriend (10, no disturbance). Subsequent sessions reveal the same results and now, over a year later, Michael has never again brought up any disturbance regarding his ear or his unrequited love.

PHASES 5–6: INSTALLATION AND BODY SCAN

Dually diagnosed clients cannot always do installation of the positive cognition and the body scan because they can't always hold two things simultaneously in awareness: either two abstractions (memory and PC, then a VOC) or an abstraction plus body awareness (memory and PC and body scan). I have had even nondisabled clients experience difficulty with these tasks. The client with a handicap often finds this task too difficult, and it can dissipate the positive and successful experience of the processing by following a success with a perceived failure.

Usually I will have clients recall the original target and the NC, then guide them through a body scan without insisting that they hold them both in simultaneous awareness. I might, however, during the body scan, briefly make some mention of the target and NC and then continue on with the scan.

PHASES 7–8: CLOSURE AND REEVALUATION

As mentioned earlier, these phases with a DD client require more extensive involvement of the client's network of caregivers. Without team carryover, the client might flounder with spontaneous processing, not knowing what to make of it, and at times be penalized for "inappropriate behaviors" and reactivity.

In a community-based situation, family, direct caregivers, psychiatrists, and other mental health professionals all need to be informed of possible aftereffects of processing sessions to prevent misinterpretation of behaviors and to educate staff about how to deal with the occasional ripple effects of treatment. A client who shows increase in mood shifts, sleep disturbances, yelling, or aggressive behaviors may not need a medication increase or a behavioral program but a compassionate reminder that this is what was discussed in session and that it will pass. In an institutional setting, this coordination must be present among all team members, particularly the direct care staff who do most of the behavioral tracking of and interacting with clients.

A final point to recall is the difficulty a client with mental disability often has in generalizing learning from one event to others of a similar nature. Carol's case in particular demonstrates the importance of processing individual present triggers as well as Future Templates of successful behaviors.

In her early 40s, Carol, who tested in the moderate range of MR, had been acting out aggressively after the death of a close friend of the family. During our first session, with her case manager present, she informed me of a string of deaths in her family and network of friends over the past year. Not knowing how to handle this, and afraid of possible future losses, particularly her parents, she lashes out whenever any of her peers ask her how she is feeling or whether someone has died.

Blessed (some staff would say cursed) with a vivid imagination, Carol was able to create visual resources. I asked her to draw representations of various feelings, particularly sadness and fear. "I can't handle it!" emerged from our dialogue as her probable NC.

AS: *Carol, with all of these people dying on you, it sounds as if you don't believe you can handle one more.*
Carol: Right, I just can't handle it!

With a combination of eye movements and bilateral music, she developed resources and processed her losses and her anxiety surrounding the possibility of future loss. Shortly thereafter she received a phone call from her parents telling her of the death of one of their college friends. When I heard of this, I immediately regretted not having involved her parents more adequately in the preparation phase. Carol began acting out again, but one session eliminated the disturbance caused by the phone call. We spent the last two sessions creating resources out of her success in therapy, desensitizing her reactivity to being questioned by her peers, and practicing assertive skills ("I'd really rather not talk about that").

CONCLUSION

Clients with MR and their families have enough difficulty accessing services without being denied therapeutic treatment that could make their lives more tolerable. These services must include attention to a client's trauma history, an area of therapy that has been largely overlooked in the treatment of clients with mental disability. And these services must be delivered with compassion and creativity.

Disabled or not, we all experience heartache as well as happiness. We are all created with an innate healing system that impels us toward a state of equilibrium and well-being. We all yearn for the same emotional freedom and human connection. The clinician working with handicapped individuals faces the challenge and experiences the joy of creatively guiding the client toward a more fully authentic life based on awareness, choice, and freedom from dehumanizing history.

As Carol began to develop the resource she would need (courage) to deal with her losses, she spontaneously created a solution that could liberate anyone, disabled or not, from suffering.

AS: *So who could help you to be strong?*
Carol: Hm-m-m, I know, Popeye! Popeye eating spinach!
AS: *Great! And where would you keep him?*
Carol: In my heart.
AS: *And then what would you do?*
Carol: He would be in my heart, and then there would be a door in my heart, and I would just have to open the door and let all the sadness out!

And that is just what she did.

RESOURCES

An excellent format for multifaceted information gathering is the "biographical timeline" of Beth Barol (Barol, 2001).

See the work of Andrew Leeds (Leeds & Shapiro, 2000) for an in-depth treatment of resource development.

The National Association for the Dually Diagnosed (NADD) is a primary resource for conferences, contacts, tapes, and published materials regarding treatment for this population. Phone: (845) 331-4336. Web site: www.thenadd.org.

My previous article (pre-EMDR), "Becoming known: Awareness and connection with the dually diagnosed," as well as anecdotal case reports of clinical success using EMDR with DD clients, can be found on our Web site: http://www.clearpathhealingarts.com.

REFERENCES

American Psychiatric Association (1994). *Diagnostic and statistical manual of mental disorders* (4th ed.). Washington, DC: Author.

Barol, B. (2001). Learning from a person's biography: An introduction to the biographical timeline process. *Pennsylvania Journal on Positive Approaches, 3*(4), 20–29.

Collingwood, J. J. P., & Collingwood, C. R. J. (2001). *The NLP field guide: Part 1. A reference manual of practitioner level patterns.* Sydney, Australia: Emergent Publications.

Fletcher, R. (1993). Individual psychotherapy for persons with mental retardation. In R. Fletcher & A. Dosen (Eds.), *Mental health aspects of mental retardation* (pp. 327–349). Lexington, MA: Lexington Books.

Greenwald, R. (1999). *Eye movement desensitization and reprocessing (EMDR) in child and adolescent psychotherapy.* Northvale, NJ: Jason Aronson.

Greenwald, R. (in press). *Child trauma handbook: A guide for helping trauma-exposed children and adolescents.* New York: Haworth.

Herman, J. (1992). *Trauma and recovery.* New York: Basic.

Leeds, A. M., & Shapiro, F. (2000). EMDR and resource installation: Principles and and procedures for enhancing current functioning and resolving traumatic experiences. In J. Carlson and L. Sperry (Eds.), *Brief therapy strategies with individuals and couples* (pp. 469–534). Phoenix, AZ: Zeig/Tucker.

Levine, P. (1997). *Waking the tiger: Healing trauma.* Berkeley, CA: North Atlantic Books.

Levitas, A., & Gilson, S. F. (1994). Psychosocial development of children and adolescents with mild mental retardation. In N. Bouras (Ed.), *Mental health in mental retardation: Recent advances and practices* (pp. 34–45). Cambridge, UK: Cambridge University Press.

Lovett, J. (1999). *Small wonders: Healing childhood trauma with EMDR.* New York: Free Press.

Prouty, G. (1976). Pre-therapy: A theoretical evolution in the person-centered/experiential psychotherapy of schizophrenia and retardation. In G. Lietaer, J. Rombauts, & R. Van Balen (Eds.), *Client-centered and experiential psychotherapy in the nineties* (pp. 645–658). Leuven, Belgium: Leuven University Press.

Seubert, A. (1999). Becoming known: Awareness and connection with the dually diagnosed. *The NADD Bulletin, (2)5,* 88–96. Available at http://www.clearpathhealingarts.com

Tinker, R., & Wilson, S. (1999). *Through the eyes of a child: EMDR with children.* New York: Norton.

Chapter 15

Treating Anxiety
Disorders with EMDR

Robin Shapiro

EVERYONE NEEDS ANXIETY. ANXIETY CAN BE AN EFFECTIVE EARLY WARN-ing that something is awry: that you've just left your wallet on the dresser or that the car ahead of you is swerving erratically. WATCH OUT! According to Daniel Siegel (2003), our bodies respond to fear-producing symptoms before we can name what's happening. Our lower brain gets our body ready to move; then our brain tells us what to do. Anxiety can serve as a social control. (When's the last time you picked your nose in public?) It can be a course corrector and the best kind of safety monitor. Gavin de Becker, in *The Gift of Fear* (1997), wrote that for most people, paying attention to our anxiety keeps us safe.

For other people, anxiety is paralyzing. Panic attacks may storm through their bodies, creating racing hearts, tingling hands, hyperventilation, copious sweat, shaking, perceptual distortions, fears of dying, impending doom, and the next horrible panic attack. Generalized anxiety creates worriers in constant states of high arousal saying: "What if? What if? What if?" Social phobia, often linked with shyness, can make every public or social situation uncomfortable or unbearable. Obsessive-compulsive people are often crippled by their repeated rituals. Phobics know that their reactions are unfounded or out of proportion, yet are compelled to avoid the objects of their fears. None of these people are stupid; they're simply terrified.

EMDR clears posttraumatic stress disorder (PTSD). It eradicates the anxiety that accompanies PTSD. How do you use it with anxiety that isn't pure PTSD?

First, you need to know what kind of a client you have. Since you've done a complete case and family history, you know if the client has a genetic or cultural history of anxiety. You've found out if anyone else in the family had phobias or anxiety attacks or was a worrier. If the clients came from a long line of nervous people, if Aunt Bess never left the house and Dad was ritualistically compulsive, you have a clue about the origins of their anxiety. If the client, for instance, reported that his family underwent pogroms in Poland before almost being wiped out in the concentration camps, you might surmise that there is family legacy of trauma and concurrent high arousal that may or may not be complicated by genetic factors. If clients say that everything has always been great, their life was wonderful, and 2 months ago, for no good reason, the panic started, you might surmise that physiology is running the show.

Whether trauma or biology started the anxiety disorder, by the time a client reaches your office, you have to treat both. Anxiety is an intensely physical experience, and the experience of an out-of-control body is traumatic.

ASSESSING ANXIETY

Get to know their anxiety in the context of a complete assessment. I use Kitchur's Strategic Developmental Model (Chapter 1) and colorcode the anxious family members, symptoms and events on the genogram.

- When did it start? When does it happen? Are there triggers? Does it happen all the time or some of the time?
- Have they always been "high strung"? Are they able to tolerate much stimulation (noise, crowds, intense people) and hold on to their equilibrium?
- What's it like? Get them to be behaviorally and somatically explicit about the experience.
- Is the anxiety really a symptom of something else? (mania? psychosis? PTSD? an attachment disorder? dissociative identity disorder [DID]?)
- Do other people in the family experience the same thing?

- What's the family history?
- How do the people around them treat them when they're anxious? (supportive? shaming? ignoring?)
- How do they treat themselves when they're anxious? (self-shaming? guilty? soothing? feeling worthless? feeling hopeless?)
- What, if anything, works to calm them down? What have they tried? What didn't work? (medication? relaxation training? running? drinking? recreational drugs? petting the dog? snuggling? computer games?)
- Will anything bad happen if they let down their guard or if the symptoms went away?

NORMALIZE THE ANXIETY RESPONSE

People who have anxiety disorders often feel crazy or stupid. Let them know that they aren't with the following interventions:

- Share information about the physiology of anxiety. Explain what's happening in the body and the brain.
- Explain the positive uses of anxiety (see first paragraph) and that their brains and bodies are overdoing it.
- Tell them that they're not stupid for being anxious. Make sure that they believe that you believe that they're not stupid or crazy, even if they still feel that way.
- Talk about how repeated experiences of anxiety can create a whole neural network that responds to triggers that create arousal and then chaos in the body.
- Explain behavior chains: An internal or external event happens, then they feel scared, then they explain to themselves why they're scared ("something must be threatening me"), then they get more scared.
- For worriers and obsessive-compulsive types, explain that FEELINGS DO NOT EQUAL DANGER and that their brains and bodies have been lying to them about it. (I have a white board in my office with the trauma response, behavior chains, and "Feelings ≠ Danger" and "Fear Won't Kill You.")
- There are people who can't tolerate much external stimulus, are exhausted by arousal, seem to have long, bushy antennae that

pick up every vibration in their vicinity, and thus crave quiet time. They may not have anxiety disorders, but they're likely to. Have them read Elaine Aron's *The Highly Sensitive Person* (1997). It is marvelously validating and full of good advice for the highly sensitive people (HSPs) of the world. You should read it too.

GET READY FOR PROCESSING

If anxiety in an otherwise calm person is caused strictly by PTSD, go ahead and start EMDR processing. If your client has physiological or attachment bases for anxiety, try some of these interventions before you proceed with EMDR.

- If and only if clients endorse having ever felt "safe," install a Safe Place. Some anxious people can't go there. Sometimes a name change works. It could be a "comfortable place," a "relaxing place," or a "place where you can let down your guard with no bad consequences." Obsessive-compulsive disorder (OCD) types may need to build bigger and better fortifications around their "places." Let them. Many anxious people build guardians into their Safe Place. I've seen them use eagles, wolves, and Samurai warriors in this role.
- Do relaxation training. Possibilities include: progressive muscle relaxation (tensing and relaxing muscle groups, starting from the head and going down), self-hypnosis, Mark Grant's *Calm and Confident with EMDR* (1997), other relaxation tapes, grounding and breathing, and mindfulness meditation. I may try several of these techniques with clients to see what fits the best. Any positive experience of being "embodied" is good. Most anxious people see their bodies as "the enemy." Bodies are the places that feel all that anxiety!
- Go back to *What calms you down?* and install several experiences of being calmed. For instance: *Think of a time when you were really wired and your husband put his arms around you and you calmed down.* (Dual Attention Stimulation [DAS].) *Can you feel it now?* (DAS.) *Feel him holding you, notice your body loosen.* (DAS.) *That's right.* (DAS.) *Breathe that feeling through your whole body.* (DAS.) *That's right.* (DAS.) *Feel the sense of safety.* (DAS.) *Is that good feeling*

all the way through you? Does any part need an extra dose? Now, think of a time in the future when you'll need to calm yourself down. Imagine bringing the feel of your husband's presence into that time. (DAS.) *Keep going.* (DAS.) *That's right.*

- For people with attachment issues, April Steele's *Developing a Secure Self* procedures (2004) are wonderfully helpful.
- Roy Kiessling's Conference Room (Chapter 2) can be a helpful installation. I've seen anxious people install lions and Arnold Schwarznegger on their teams.
- Any affect tolerance training is helpful. Most obsessive-compulsive behavior, at root, is avoidance of affect. Other anxious people may avoid affect because they feel it so intensely. Feelings increase arousal and arousal often increases anxiety. Have people "hang out" with little bits of any feeling, supplemented with little bits of DAS (two or three eye movements or taps). Gradually increase the length of the sets. Congratulate them on the tiniest increase in tolerance. Do this in every session for weeks. When they've got a handle on regular affect, you can have them think about the objects of their greatest anxiety, obsession, or compulsion and have them stay with that affect for increasing lengths of time. Marcia Whisman is the reigning expert in using EMDR with OCD. If you have OCD clients, get the tapes of her 1999 or 2001 EMDR International Association (EMDRIA) presentations.
- Stop or slow down panic attacks by having the clients:

  o Do "negative breathing" by exhaling all the way, and breathing in halfway for at least 10 breaths. (An unknown workshop participant suggested this to me while I was teaching a workshop on EMDR and anxiety in 1998.)
  o Run in place, thus tricking the overactive "fight or flight" response into thinking that clients have "escaped."
  o Do the butterfly hug (J. Boel, personal communication, Sept 10, 1997). Tell clients to stop immediately if the tapping increases discomfort.
  o Challenge the irrational thoughts that go with panic by saying, for instance,

    — I'm going to survive this.
    — This is my body overreacting. It's panic, not death.

— I'm sane; my body is just having a fit.
— This will be over in 5 minutes (or however long their attacks last).

CHOOSE EMDR PROCESSING TARGETS

Francine Shapiro stated that "for current anxiety and behavior the clinician assists the client to specify the anxiety to be treated, the initial cause and memory (if available) and the desired response. . . . The targets are reprocessed in the following order: 1. Initial or earliest memory; 2. Most recent or most representative example of a present situation that causes anxiety; and 3. Future projection of a desired emotional and behavioral response" (2001, p. 224). In many cases, this is sufficient. Other potential targets include:

- Anxiety triggers:

  o External triggers include phobia objects, anxiety-producing social situations, or "demand" situations like test-taking.
  o Internal triggers include.

    — thoughts: "What if the worst thing that could happen did happen? The plane will crash; I'll choke on lunch and die; I'll make a fool of myself and die of embarrassment."
    — sensations, including heart rate, a tight chest, muscle-tightening, and rapid breathing.
    — emotions (for OCD people, any emotion might be overwhelming and trigger the ritual thoughts or behavior)

- Irrational thoughts are perfect negative cognitions. Find the positive cognitions, set up the rest of the Standard Protocol, and you're on your way. I sometimes use the Two-Hand Interweave to help delineate the issue and (hopefully) connect the right neural nets:

  o *In one hand put the thought that you'll die if you walk over that bridge. In the other hand put the actual level of danger that you'll be in on that bridge.* (DAS.)

○ *In one hand hold your fear of the embarrassment you might feel if you go to that party. In the other, hold the number of people you know who have died of embarrassment.* (DAS.)

- Panic attacks and extreme incidents of anxiety create PTSD. With the Standard Protocol, I target the first one, the last one, and the worst one. Occasionally, the processing doesn't generalize, and we have to process almost every attack. Anxiety cognitions are often about survival. Sometimes, a small Cognitive Interweave of *Did you survive it?* speeds up the processing.
- Other cognitions are about the shame of being out of control. I target the shame itself: *Notice where you feel the shame in your body. What image comes to mind?* (often an early shaming incident). I set up the rest of the protocol, and we go for it. The shame generally doesn't return, even if the person has another panic attack. Somehow, this lessens the severity of the attacks. It may be that the person is more ready to go through it.
- For people with OCD, after a lot of relationship and affect-tolerance building, target a story of being unable to avoid that which they most want to avoid (Whisman, 1999). With a germ phobe, for example, use a story about touching something unclean (like a dollar bill) and having no way and no place to wash up. Embellish the story (there's no water in the whole town, all the stores are closed, and the hand cleanser has dried up.) Set up the Standard Protocol and go. Other examples include not having the obsessive thought, not checking that they turned off the stove or locked the door.
- Clearing cultural and generational traumas can give relief to some clients (Chapter 10).
- Grief becomes a target for many anxious clients. For some, it comes when you have gotten the anxiety under control. They grieve all the "lost time" they spent being anxious or avoiding situations or potential emotions. Others grieve that they may always be a "skinny nervous person" or a "highly sensitive person." After processing, comes more acceptance. Good positive cognitions (PCs) could be, "Even though I'm nervous, I completely accept myself." "I have anxiety, and I don't let it stop me." "I'm sensitive, and I'm okay."

- EMDR's Future Template is wonderful for rehearsal of coping skills.

  o *Imagine a situation when you would normally start obsessing.* Set up Standard Protocol for that situation, then process it. If the (SUDS) doesn't go to 0: *Now imagine putting up that big red STOP sign, while silently saying, "STOP!" if the obsessive thoughts come on.* (DAS.)
  o *Imagine being in that new social situation and using your grounding, breathing, and relaxing skills.*
  o *Imagine walking over that bridge.*
  o *Imagine beginning to obsess/worry/ruminate and then switching to planning/practicing what you need to do.* (DAS.)
  o *Imagine surviving and even thriving in that triggering situation.* (DAS.)

CLEARING THE ANXIETY OF A
DISSOCIATED PART

Often, hypervigilance is connected to an early trauma involving abandonment or the fear of annihilation. If the client remembers the trauma or can "float back" to it, use the Standard Protocol and integration will occur naturally. If the client can't remember the situation or is too fragile or dissociated for EMDR processing, you can find other ways to connect the young, terrified neural network (ego state) to the older, wiser network.

Here's an example of a way to bring the neural nets together. I often use DAS throughout this induction after each direction or question.

Get in touch with your oldest, wisest part, the one who does your job and takes care of your children. Good. Find that terrified part of you that has to be so vigilant. Good. How old is that child? Just a baby! Get her attention. Can you pick her up? Good! Let her know who you are. Show her around your life. Are you tall enough to touch the top of that shelf? Is that taller than she is? How much? Can that baby drive? Can you? How old are you? How old is she? Which of you would be better at assessing current situations and deciding if there's danger present? Good! Right answer! Can you tell that baby that you'll be in charge of noticing if there's danger? Can you tell her that she doesn't have to be on guard anymore? Great! How's the baby doing now? She's falling asleep? Wonderful. She's been holding off sleep until she knew that you were there. Can that baby live inside of you? Where? Your heart. Is she there yet? Bring her in. Let her know that she will always have an adult handy, you!

If the client begins to remember what happened, you can build in appropriate interweaves: *So did Mommy ever leave for good? Did she always come back? Did your dad ever really kill you? Did you survive?* If these are stumpers, or you get a really wrong answer, ask, *What does your older/wiser self say about this?* When the questions have been answered (and don't ask them unless you know the answers), proceed with the rest of the process.

When the lifelong anxiety is based in an early trauma, the symptoms can completely disappear after standard EMDR processing, Kitchur's First Order Processing (Chapter 1), Kiessling's Conference Room of Resources (Chapter 2), April Steele's (2004) secure self work, or other ego-state interventions.

"SKINNY NERVOUS PEOPLE," "HSPS," AND PEOPLE "WIRED THAT WAY"

Some people are born to be more reactive or responsive to their environment. They may come from good families, have good attachment, and have no history of big "T" traumas. However, for them, seemingly small traumas resonate like big ones. After successful trauma processing, they may be easily retriggered into the same old fear. Their unpleasant experiences may convert to phobias. They have a low tolerance for arousal. Many, but not all, are introverts. The good news, according to Elaine Aron (1997), is that people wired to be sensitive are often the most creative and responsive people you know. The bad news is that anxiety can permeate their lives. They are more prone to anxiety disorders. Their PTSD is worse and more easily triggered. Some can develop debilitating panic disorder, barely containable by medication. EMDR won't cure their physiology. However, EMDR targets for this group of people include:

- Sadistic older brothers, junior high school peers, and other people who most enjoyed getting a rise out of a sensitive soul
- The constant humiliation of being "out of control" or being "different"

- The grief and anger over having a body that reacts so strongly to everything
- The use of the Future Template to practice self-management skills
- The fear of taking medication
- The Future Template focused on the assertiveness necessary for good self-care

  o *Imagine that you tell your partner that you need a half hour to your-self when you come home. Imagine your partner doesn't like that.*
  o *Imagine that you tell your friends that you want to skip the Metal-lica concert.*
  o *Imagine that you ask your hiking partner for help to get over that narrow log across the stream.*
  o *Imagine saying that you'll be "fit company" after your run, and then imagine going running.*

CASE 1

Sylvia was a petite, extremely athletic, brilliant, artistic, middle-aged woman, married 10 years, who came to me for sports performance en-hancement. She said that she'd had tons of therapy already and wanted to focus solely on sports. Her history, at first, sounded fairly benign, but every time we targeted a performance issue, trauma popped up. Each time, we cleared the trauma with the Standard Protocol and her performance improved drastically. This 5-foot-3-inch woman was playing sports with mixed teams of mixed ages. She'd broken bones in various sports, but still wanted to become more aggressive in rushing people who were a foot taller than she.

The anxieties came forward slowly. Sylvia was terrified of being alone in the house, checking the doors constantly. Upon leaving her car, she would go back to check her locked car doors three or four times. She obsessed about the signs of aging, her appearance, and her breath. Due to Sylvia's perceptual problems, we did tapping. Before she would let me tap, she pulled out a tube of toothpaste and dabbed some on her tongue. She worried her breath would disgust me. (Her breath was fine.) She obsessed about smelling bad while playing sports. (Doesn't everyone?) She taught classes for a living. By all reports, she was an exceptional teacher, with waiting lists for every class. People tended to reenroll in these classes for years. If one person left, for any reason, Sylvia would ruminate about the classes falling apart. The phone ringing was cause for terror. A knock on the door, in her benign neighborhood, felt dangerous.

Sylvia portrayed a mix of hypervigilance and dissociation. The real history, which came out over a long time, included a tremendous amount of trauma, both Sylvia's and generational trauma. Sylvia's parents were both orphaned and had had unstable and poorly parented upbringings. Her mother could have won the "checked-out narcissistic parenting" award. Mom was obsessed about appearance and aging. Any physical contact came from her father, who was seductive and eventually molested her. Her older sister was bipolar, from an early age. She committed suicide when Sylvia was in her early 20s. Her father died in his 70s. Sylvia believes it was suicide tied to his disgust at looking old.

Treatment included me giving her information about anxiety and OCD, lots of EMDR for clearing, and thought field therapy (TFT) for affect reduction. We used an ever-more-complex Safe Place for dissociated parts that arose in the EMDR work. Sylvia was on a high rev and couldn't tolerate many kinds of bilateral stimulation. We settled on knee or hand tapping, one tap every 4 seconds. At her insistence, we usually started with a present concern, for instance, anxiety about the phone ringing. In the EMDR process we discovered the underlying terror. With the phone, it was two things. She learned about her sister's death on the phone. And her parents were both frightened of the phone, expecting the worst news at all times. We spent many EMDR sessions on her response to her sister's death, first processing through trauma, then grief. We spent several more sessions targeting her parents' fears of bad news or bad events. In EMDR sessions, we sent all the generational anxieties back to her ancestors: the oppression, the rapes, "the knock at the door." (*Locate the fear of your parents' generation that is in you. It's not yours. Pull it out of you and give it back to them. Imagine your grandparents' fear. Imagine the fear of every ancestor in all the generations of oppression. Pull it out of you. Send it back. It's not yours.*) Many of her anxieties and her compulsive behaviors fell away after this work. She was able to understand that she'd been stuck in "waiting" for the phone call about her sister for years. With cognitive interweaves in EMDR, she understood that it had already happened. It was over. She didn't have to wait for it. Sylvia said that she felt let out of prison. She no longer checks her car or front door myriad times. She no longer locks her bedroom door. She doesn't tense when the phone rings.

Other EMDR targets included the molestation by her father and her internalization of her mother's fears and societal obsessions with appearance and youth. *(Pull it out and send it back to her.)* While doing EMDR about her fears about enrollment in her classes, we found a terrified child whose mother had left her alone and never responded adequately to her. We developed a wonderful room in the Safe Place for her with an adoring presence with whom to bond. Then we did a resource installation of the many people who currently adored her. Sylvia no longer connects enrollment in her classes with abandonment of her child. She's fine with it and simply allows people from the waiting list to enroll.

We completed work after 3 years of weekly, then monthly, contact. Sylvia remains a "highly sensitive person." She has let go of generations of trauma that have shaped her life. She has grieved her sister. She has integrated and healed the small, terrified, hypervigilant child that knew she was abandoned because she wasn't good enough. Distressing anxieties and compulsive behaviors are gone. Sylvia now understands that she can be afraid on the ball field and that it's okay to protect herself. Her game has improved by many points. Five years after the end of therapy, she reports that the anxiety has never returned.

CASE 2

Patsy was slender, tall, agitated, and 23 years old. She'd always been "high strung," easily embarrassed, and a worrier. She avoided crowds, scary movies, and loud rock and roll. She enjoyed hiking and having friends to dinner. Running and other aerobic exercise calmed her down. She came from a great family, recalled no major trauma, and was happily married to her college sweetheart. Her father was a bit obsessive, a "neat freak" who would straighten out crooked pictures in anyone's living room. The first panic attack happened on her way to a job interview. She thought she was dying. First she called the interviewer, then drove herself to the Emergency Room. She'd had an attack once or twice a month since then, each time feeling that she was dying or going crazy. Her attacks were increasing in frequency. She lived in terror of "the next one." Her doctor had offered her SSRIs, which she refused. The doctor referred her to me.

We connected right away. After a thorough intake, including an extensive description of her anxiety and panic symptoms, I explained the physiology of anxiety and panic. I told her that she wasn't crazy. (I used my role as a "trained professional" to tell her this many times throughout the therapy.) In the first session, 90 minutes long, I taught her ways to deal with the panic attack: *When your brain mistakenly thinks you're under attack, it tells you that you need more oxygen in order to fight or flee. That's why you start hyperventilating. Since you're not fighting or running, your body overdoses on the oxygen. It actually changes the pH of your entire body. To change that, try breathing this way: Exhale all the way, all the way out. Breathe in halfway. Exhale all the way, all the way out. Breathe in halfway. Let's do that 10 times. Good. You feel more relaxed? Great! You just changed the way your body acts.*

When you have attacks, you tell yourself that you're going crazy and dying. I want you to imagine that you're having an attack, start doing the negative breathing now, and chant the mantra, "It's just adrenaline making my body rev up. I'm sane and healthy and having a panic attack." With her permission, I tapped her knees in sets of six taps.

In the next two sessions, I taught her progressive relaxation, grounding, and mindfulness meditation. Her general anxiety was a bit lowered, and she felt a little more in control. I told her that she was part of the tribe of "skinny nervous people," one of my favorite flavors of people. I asked her to read *The Highly Sensitive Person* (Aron, 1997). She identified with the book and began to do some its self-care exercises.

She was still terrified of panic attacks and had had two since the beginning of therapy. The "panic management techniques" had worked to lessen the intensity and duration of the attacks. I introduced EMDR, and we targeted the last attack, the first attack, and what she thought of as the worst one. I warned her that EMDR might trigger an attack and that we could then work on it in session. She had no attacks during processing. The EMDR cleared a lot, but not all, of her trauma. Her next attack was a week later; it was less intense and less distressing. When she reported it, we installed, "I can handle this." Since tapping didn't trigger attacks, she added the Butterfly Hug to her panic-reducing arsenal. We both laughed as we installed running in place, tapping, negative breathing, and "I'm sane, healthy, and can get through this," in her Future Template for future attacks. (She did it all. It worked well.)

We worked on her close-to-obsessional worrying. I told her that she had a bad case of the "what-ifs." With the Standard Protocol we targeted "What if the worst thing happened?" about job interviews, social gatherings, earthquakes, air travel, learning to skin-dive, and being home alone. Ridiculous worries disappeared with brief Two-Hand Interweaves: *Put the thought that you are going to forget how to talk in one hand and what your smartest self knows in the other hand.* In two rounds of 10 taps, she laughed and said, "That's just another unlikely 'what if.' I'm over it now." She learned to use the Two-Hand Interweave to compare worries to probable realities, away from the office.

Near the end of therapy, we used the Standard Protocol to clear the grief and shame that she had the nervous system she had. The PCs included "I am lovable," "I accept myself the way I am," and "I don't let anxiety stop me." Therapy lasted 4 months. When she left, her panic attacks were less frequent, less severe, and less upsetting. She had a handle on her worrying and was more accepting of herself as a highly sensitive, skinny, nervous person.

CONCLUSION

EMDR is not the cure for every anxiety disorder. Medication, exercise, relaxation and cognitive behavioral techniques, and affect tolerance training are helpful for many anxious people. EMDR is an effective tool to clear the traumas that can cause or exacerbate anxiety disorders. It can be used to build affect tolerance and self-acceptance, clear OCD ritual behaviors, and support self-care and fear-defying actions.

RESOURCES

These are just a few of the many good Web sites, books, and workshops about treating anxiety.

Web Sites

The Anxiety Panic Internet Resource: http://www.algy.com/anxiety/files/barlow.html

Health Beat: http://www.hsilib.washington.edu/your_health/hbeat/hb9404 26.html

Books

Aron, E. N. (1997). *The highly sensitive person.* New York: Broadway Books.

Girodo, M. (1978). *Shy? (You don't have to be!)* New York: Pocket Books.

Levine, P. A. (1997). *Waking the tiger.* Berkeley, CA: North Atlantic Books 1997.

Workshops

Whisman, M., & Keller, M. (1999). *Integrating EMDR into the treatment of obsessive compulsive disorder.* Paper presented at the EMDRIA Conference, Las Vegas, NV.

Whisman, M., de Jongh, A. (2001). *Panic/phobias: Diagnoses and treatment with EMDR.* (2001), Paper presented at the EMDRIA Conference, Houston, TK. Available at http://www.soundontape.com

REFERENCES

Aron, E. (1997). *The highly sensitive person.* New York: Broadway Books.

de Becker, Gavin. (1997). *The gift of fear.* New York: Dell.

Shapiro, F. (2001). *Eye movement desensitization and reprocessing: Basic principles, protocols and procedures.* (2nd ed.). New York: Guilford Press, page 224.

Shapiro, R. (1998, September). *Using EMDR with anxiety disorders.* Paper presented at Northwest Regional EMDRIA Conference, Seattle, WA.

Siegel, D. (2003, March). *Transforming adult authorized.* Presented at the New Developments in Attachment Theory Conference, UCLA, Los Angeles.

Grant, M. (1997). *Calm and confident with EMDR* [audiotape]. Oakland, CA: New Harbinger Publications Inc.

Steele, A. (2004). *Developing a secure self: A handbook for EMDR therapists.* Gabriola Island, BC: Author.

Whisman, M. (1999, June). *Integrating EMDR into the treatment of obsessive compulsive disorder.* Paper presented at the EMDRIA Conference, Las Vegas, NV.

Chapter 16

Affect Regulation for Children Through Art, Play, and Storytelling

Elizabeth Turner

THE MOST COMMON PROBLEM THAT I HEAR FROM CONSULTEES USING EMDR with kids and adolescents is that the kids "just won't do it anymore."

When this happens, we have moved too fast. EMDR is so powerful, and the suffering of these kids so great, that we feel compelled to rush through preparation and skip quickly to trauma processing. Instead of healing, we may retraumatize, reinforce a tendency to dissociate, and cause children and adolescents to refuse further EMDR treatment.

As Judith Hermann warned, "No intervention that takes power away from the survivor can possibly foster her recovery, no matter how much it appears to be in her immediate best interest" (Herman, 1992, p. 133).

Because of the very nature of childhood and development, it's more difficult to give power to children than to adults. Children are still developing verbal and cognitive capacity. Adolescent minds are in a state of rapid change with emotional systems that are overactive. Reasoning and planning functions are in fledgling states. Children and adolescents rarely have the power to make the decision to come to therapy to be treated, but are usually brought to therapy because the adults in their lives are having a problem with the kids' behaviors. Children do

not have the power to leave or change the systems that have abandoned or traumatized them: their families, their schools, their neigh-
borhoods, their medical providers, their foster homes, their residential
treatment centers.

Also, many children and adolescents arrive in a therapist's office
with complex histories: neonatal difficulties, severe illnesses in infancy
or early childhood, repeated physical or emotional abuse, maternal depression or separation. Early experiences such as these have been
shown to influence brain development and result in fewer neural networks to regulate affect. The experience of almost any emotion for
these children may evoke a massive tidal wave of affect.

With these children, it is all too easy to overshoot the therapeutic
window with the Standard Protocol. They need skills and practice in
identifying and building tolerance for the spectrum of affect: from en-
joyment/joy to anxiety/fear. When children are engaged in play—
their native tongue—and EMDR principles are integrated into the play,
the learning is safe, fun, and rapid.

The following are favorite activities for the preparation stage of the
protocol that interweaves EMDR principles into art, play, and storytelling to build safety, develop affect tolerance, and engage children in
their own healing. Therapists who work with children and adolescents
will use these ideas as a springboard to developing their own toolbox
of preparation activities.

THE COLOR OF FEELINGS

This simple exercise, which pairs emotions and colors, helps children
and adolescents access emotion safely. It targets nonverbal, right-mode
processing, which is dominant in emotions. It helps a child whose emotional experience feels global and undifferentiated to bring in elements
of left-mode processing, which can name, organize, and separate out
components of experience, transforming them from overwhelming to
manageable. Since the exercise is concrete, it is developmentally easier
for children to grasp than having them "just think about it." Since it
does not require a child to draw realistically, it avoids performance
anxiety and seems to help a child get to the emotional core of experience more quickly. It introduces bilateral stimulation to calm the body
and help process emotion. Many adults also find this exercise helpful

in learning how to deconstruct, understand, and tolerate emotions. Throughout the process, the therapist must be curious and interested in the child's experience, letting the child know that everybody's internal experience is different, that there is no "wrong" way to do this.

STEP 1: SETUP

With the child, make a list of emotion-words, such as angry, sad, proud, happy, excited, nervous, afraid, ashamed, hurt, calm. Most children will start to come up with feeling words of their own: freaked out, bummed, wasted. Oftentimes, they will come up with words and phrases that must eventually be further deconstructed. Children may talk about the feeling of not good enough, not needed, invisible, rejected, and similar phrases. These are actually negative cognitions (NCs) that can be broken down into several strands of affect: sadness, anger, hurt, shame. Start with a fairly short list of words and let kids know that feelings can always be added as needed.

STEP 2: POSITIVE AFFECT

Starting with concrete, positive experiences helps build neural networks for positive affect and allows a child to start exploring emotion in a safe, nonthreatening manner. Have the child think of an experience that you know is enjoyable for him: hitting a baseball, petting the kitty, singing in choir, drawing a picture, getting a goodnight hug. Avoid installing electronic experiences such as playing video games and watching television, since many children and adolescents are overly dependent on these media for self-soothing, which detracts from activities that encourage interpersonal relationships. Have them notice and talk about how they feel in the body when they think of the positive experience, then have them pick colors that "go with" the experience. Each kid will express this in different ways—from neat little boxes or lines of color to actual figures or faces to great swirling abstracts. The colors will be individual too: one child in my experience picked black for happy and used it very appropriately.

A single experience will generally have several feelings attached to it. Winning an award, for instance, may contain yellow, pink, and orange, which may translate into the words *happy, excited,* and *proud.* Have the child identify the location of each feeling in the body and "tap in" or "wave in" the good feeling with a few (6–8) bilateral taps or eye movements. (Too many taps can lead to diffusion of the good feeling or association to something that might be distressing. At this stage, the goal is simply to identify and amplify positive affects.) After each feeling has been tapped in, the therapist can have the child remember the experience and feel all the associated feelings: happy, excited, and proud. Positive cognitions such as "I try hard," "I can succeed," "I am loveable," may be suggested for younger kids and elicited from older kids and adolescents. These cognitions are paired with the color, the experience, the emotion, and body sensation with Dual Attention Stimulation (DAS).

Have the child color the experience again. Notice if the colors are bigger, the strokes are bolder, or the child more animated, and reflect this back to the child. Repeat this exercise several times, with different experiences, as long as the child is interested.

STEP 3: MINI TARGET

Have the child think of an experience that wasn't so great but wasn't horrible. We are looking for a target at about a 5 or less Subjective Units of Distress Scale (SUDS) level with which to practice. For some kids, this can be a challenge since all their negative emotions may come packaged in huge, global masses of overwhelming affect. The therapist may need to use clinical judgment to choose a target most likely to evoke a manageable level of affect: not getting the ice-cream cone, brother getting the front seat today, stubbing a toe, breaking a toy.

Again, have the child notice what it feels like in the body to have this experience, then pick out colors that go with the experience and then draw them on the paper. This time, a SUDS level can be added by drawing a line on the bottom of the paper, marking off 10 units, and asking the child to show how bad it feels on this line with 10 being the very worst and 0 being no problem at all. Actually drawing the SUDS line seems to make judging the intensity of affect more concrete and containing for children than thinking about it or pointing to a chart. If the child has picked out three emotion colors—angry, sad, embarrassed—ask the child which one he or she wants to work with first. Then ask: *Where do you feel that anger in your body? Good! Notice where it is and let's tap* (or move eyes or drum). After a few sets, ask the child to put a mark on the SUDS line and show you with colors what it feels like inside now when they think of that experience. Many older children and adolescents will associate naturally to other emotions. (Child: "Now it feels more like sad.") Younger children will tend to need cues to move to the next emotion. (Therapist: *So the anger is all gone now? Where does the sad feeling hang out?*) Continue to process and color until the experience feels neutral or positive to the child.

As time and the child's interest level allow, repeat this for several low SUDS events until it seems that child is really getting the hang of it.

STEP 4: CONTAINMENT AND RESOURCING

At the end of the exercise, put any unfinished difficult feelings in an imaginary container (the child may want to draw this). Then return to the positive memories. Let the child choose the favorite experience he wants to remember. Using the positive words and colors and body sensations the child connected to this experience, install this memory state with bilateral stimulation, using few (6–8) taps or passes at a time to prevent association into negative material.

SUMMARY

The purpose of this exercise is to titrate the protocol in steps. You are teaching the child in small, controllable bites how to identify emotion and affect, and you're breaking a global feeling into components that can be seen on paper, felt in the body, and named. The bilateral stimulation helps amplify positive affect and reduce negative affect. The child learns how to name, structure, and contain his experience and is able to handle increasing levels of disturbing experience.

By using this incremental approach, the therapist can more accurately assess whether the child is likely to feel overwhelmed by affect and dissociate. Even when the child has adequate ability for handling affect, this method increases awareness, understanding, and skill.

THE VOLCANO

The volcano is an excellent teaching metaphor for children who are experiencing rages. These kids generally have a low awareness of affect building in the body. This exercise improves body awareness and affect control.

Begin by introducing the metaphor of anger being similar to a volcano, showing children how lava is always underground and how it builds up before it erupts:

It's like this. Say a kid doesn't sleep too well and when his alarm goes off, he's already crabby, and the lava is beginning to swirl around in his ankles. Then his mom yells at him because he's not dressed yet, and the lava moves up to his calves. He makes his way to the kitchen and finds out that his favorite cereal is all gone and there's only his mom's stuff that tastes like dead twigs. He's hungry and frustrated, thinking nobody cares about what he wants and the lava moves up even further, maybe to his knees. Then the kid remembers some math that he should have finished last night, and he gets a big shot of lava in the belly. By this time, he's really cranky, but he's holding it together. His mom nags some more about how slow he is, and the lava moves up to his shoulders. Then, his brother gets the front seat of the car. He always gets the front seat of the car, and Mom won't listen. That does it! The lava fills up his face, shoots out the top of his skull, and he has a meltdown: he's kicking and yelling and hitting his mom and won't go to school.

We're going to make a volcano and figure out what happened to your lava in that explosion with your mom. So, tell me the story of what happened to you on Thursday.

The object is to get enough of the story or enough of the events of the day so the child can notice points where he was handling the affect and realize how it was building up with cumulative experiences. Then the child draws a volcano and together the therapist and child write down the incidents that bumped the affect up a notch and mark the level of "lava" or affect at each step. At each step, the therapist has the child notice where the lava is in the body and uses a few taps or other DAS to "bookmark" that level in the body. As the child goes through this exercise, he begins to be more in touch with his body and to distinguish subtler degrees of affect. He also begins to recognize how much affect he has been able to handle throughout the day, and he receives affirmation from the therapist for this. The therapist then asks the child to pick the level at which he'd like to begin noticing the lava so he can vent it safely.

Kid: It's not so bad until it gets up around my knees.

ET: *So let's make a list of what you can do when it gets up around your knees. (You can jump on the trampoline, take a shower, tell Mom, color it out, butterfly hug, breathe into it, blow bubbles, throw spongy balls, listen to music, drum.)*

Therapist: *Let's try one of these. Now think about the things that happened on Thursday until the lava gets up around the knees and try breathing into it while I tap. Tell me when you're ready. Okay.* (About a dozen taps) *How is it now?*

Kid: It's down to here. (calves)

ET: *Great, let's go again.* (A dozen taps) *So how was that?*

Kid: It's down to my toes—it's all gone.

The therapist helps the child practice a Future Template by imagining checking into the lava level at various trigger points in the child's life—brother taking control of the TV, homework time—and is instructed to go home and do lava checks throughout the week, seeing if he can "catch it" and do self-soothing activities before it gets up to the knees. The parents are also informed about the volcano metaphor and told the child will be monitoring lava levels throughout the week.

HEART RATE MONITOR

This is a simple biofeedback exercise that shows kids how much control they have over their affect. It can be used in conjunction with the volcano metaphor. The child is asked to think of something that makes him really, really mad—blows the top off the volcano. Then he looks at their heart rate on the monitor. (The small index finger monitors sold by the Gottman Institute, www.gottmaninstitute.com, work well.)

ET: *Where do you feel that in your body? Good, breathe into it while I tap.*

Child: Hey, I'm making it come down!

ET: *Great, let's keep going.*

Child: I got it down more.

ET: *Let's see if we can get it down even lower. We have to be really quiet.*

Children, even with attention-deficit/hyperactive disorder (ADHD), are quite capable of achieving meditative-type states through concentration, breathing, and the therapist tapping in this easy exercise. They usually enjoy the process and ask to repeat it on various targets over and over again. Unlike reward charts, which rely on external motivators to get a child to practice breathing and relaxation, this approach relies on children's natural curiosity and interest in their own internal workings. With this method, children find managing affect fun and challenging and want to master it.

The bilateral stimulation here helps the SUDS go down, and it also enhances the learning process so the child will associate breathing with calming and become rapidly skilled at self-soothing.

MOTIVATIONAL INTERVIEWING

Kids and adolescents are usually not invested in changing their behaviors when they arrive in the therapist's office. In fact, many, if not most, have their heels dug in and challenge the therapist to make them change. The following exercise is based on the tenets of Motivational Interviewing (Miller, Rollnick, & Conforti, 2002) and embedded in Robin Shapiro's Two-Hand Interweave technique (Chapter 6).

I first used this in a session with a 12-year-old boy with severe Crohn's disease. He came into my office thin, weak, and lethargic but also extremely angry, defiant, and uncooperative. The boy, whom I will call Chris, had been referred to me with a report by a psychiatrist who described him as one of the most severely depressed kids she had seen in years. Chris was refusing to take antidepressants or medications for Crohn's and refusing to do any homework or chores. He was intellectually gifted but flunking all of his classes. Chris lived with his father, who had tried to motivate Chris by adding more and more restrictions and taking away more and more privileges. His TV, music, Magic Cards, and video games had all been taken away, but Chris simply did less and less. He slouched into my office, slumped down on the couch, and pulled his hat down over his eyes.

I started the conversation by telling him that I was impressed with how powerful he was—how no restriction could change his behaviors and how helpless that made the adults in his life feel. This caught his interest. The conversation moved to his flunking all of his classes.

ET: *Let's just look at all the good things about flunking. Put all the good things about flunking in one hand and think about them while I tap on your knees.*
Chris: It feels good. My dad can't make me do anything. He's taken away everything and I just don't care.
ET: *What else is good about flunking?*
Chris: I can be more like my friend Joe. The teachers are all down on him because he doesn't do his work. I can be like him and we're a team together and that's good.
ET: *Great. What else is good about flunking?*
Chris: I can get back at the teachers. They can't make me do anything either.
ET: *Great. Is there anything not so good about flunking? Put the not so good things in the other hand.*
Chris: (suddenly and quickly) No college, no job, no life.
ET: *Anything else?*
Chris: I'm not hurting my dad so much. I'm hurting me.
ET: *Anything else?*
Chris: I'm *really* not hurting the teachers. They couldn't care less.
ET: *Anything else?*
Chris: Why would I want to be like Joe?

This 5-minute intervention was a critical turning point for Chris. He decided to take care of himself and his future. He became engaged in therapy. His depression turned around quickly without medication. He went back to studying immediately, ending second semester with an A average. His Crohn's abated, and within a year he was an award-winning swimmer and musician and an honors student. Four years later, he uses music, meditation, breathing, and boundaries to keep a good handle on stress levels. He is doing well with occasional, but manageable, Crohn's symptoms.

Motivational Interviewing is a very valuable skill for working with children and adolescents and is exceptionally powerful in working with addictive behaviors. More EMDR interventions based on these principles can be found in *EMDR with Children and Adolescents* by Ricky Greenwald (1999).

GAMES AND PLAY

All games and play have the potential to be therapeutic. When children are in a playing mode, they are likely to feel safe and in a state of flow; their minds are more flexible, and they are able to learn more easily and process emotions safely. A therapist used to working with children knows how to assess the quality of a child's play, noting if it is rigid, anxious, competitive, or defensive, if it has the compulsively repetitive pattern of traumatic play or if it has the easy rhythms of interest, enjoyment, and excitement.

An EMDR therapist will find that the principles of EMDR can be applied in almost any play situation to process negative affect and beliefs and enhance positive affect and beliefs. The following are some suggestions of how to apply EMDR thinking to games and play, but skilled therapists will quickly adapt these principles to their own favorite therapeutic activities. The activities aren't meant to replace Standard Protocol trauma processing but to enhance relationship, safety, and affect tolerance.

MECHANICS OF BILATERAL STIMULATION DURING PLAY

Using bilateral stimulation during play can be tricky. The therapist and the child may be moving around the room or have a board game between them. The bilateral stimulation in this stage should *not get in the way of the play* and should only be used when it feels right and comfortable. Using the principle of mirroring, I assume that bilateral stimulation on myself will have a resonating effect in the child. I will often tap on myself when the child is in an awkward position for me to reach to tap on, or eye movement isn't comfortable. Some children like to listen to Biolateral tapes (http://www.biolateral.com) or other bilateral audio sounds while they play. Shoulders and knees can be tapped on. Drumsticks can be great tools. The therapist can rock from side to side. Toys and puppets can fly back and forth or hop from one knee to the other. Children 5 and under have difficulty crossing the midline with eye movements and seem to do better with alternative bilateral stimulation (Tinker & Wilson, 1999).

GAMES OF FRUSTRATION

Games such as Candyland (Milton Bradley, Hasbro), Chutes and Ladders (Milton Bradley), and Sorry (Parker Brothers) are perennial favorites for children. They have in common the fact that a player can suddenly shoot way ahead or fall tragically behind. There is little or no skill involved and the player's fortune is determined by blind luck. The therapist assesses affect tolerance by noticing how the child is handling frustration. If the child resorts to cheating, it's an indication that the child is incapable of withstanding the emotions that come up around setbacks. This gives an in vivo opportunity to use EMDR to moderate distress. When the child has difficulty handling frustration, the therapist can do one of the following:

1. The therapist can model dealing with the frustration.

   Therapist: *Oh no! I got the big slide. I'm going all the way down to the bottom. I'm never going to win. Feels like a big lump in my stomach.* (Therapist taps or pounds on her own knees) *I can handle it. It's okay. It's no big deal. I'll have another chance.*

   The therapist can join and lead, reflecting how the child is dealing with the frustration and shape progress toward frustration tolerance.

   Wow! That's a bummer. Looks like it's hard for you. How bad do you hate it when that happens? You hate that a 10? Well, you're dealing with a 10 pretty well. Where do you feel that 10? Do you want to drum that down or tap that out?

2. If child is cheating, the therapist can say:

   Getting a 6 would have sent you down to the bottom. Ouch, that would have really hurt. (Therapist taps her own knees.) There is no need to label what the child did as cheating, give an ethical lecture, or take back the move. This will only add shame and decrease trust. The treatment is to give the child empathy, awareness, and tools to deal with the distress so she won't feel compelled to cheat.

   Hey, that slide didn't bother you so much that time—let's tap that in. Think about how you are learning to handle that.

You can handle going down that big slide really well already. Boy, you learned that fast. You look proud of yourself. Let's tap that in. Think about how you can handle that.

3. The therapist also notices and reinforces positive affect when the child is simply having fun or is excited about coming up from behind or getting close to the finish.

And she's gaining! She's coming up from behind. Yes! Therapist joins in enthusiasm with voice and body and taps on her own knees or on the child's shoulders or knees if they are easily available.

GAMES OF SKILL

Games that require physical skill or dexterity such as a hockey game like Rebound (Tyco, Mattel), magnetic darts, pick-up sticks, or Jenga (Milton Bradley) present excellent opportunities for building frustration tolerance as in the previous games, plus they also provide opportunities to build focus, concentration, determination, and pride. This can be particularly useful for children with learning disabilities and attentional difficulties as the therapist can help the child bridge the skills learned in play to school and other environments.

The therapist first must be able to genuinely join in the fun of the game. The sense of play takes the edge off performance anxiety and allows the child to begin to get into the flow of practicing a skill. As the child begins to show focus and concentration, the therapist can comment on it and from time to time use bilateral stimulation to "nail in" the mood state that accompanies these experiences of competence.

Wow, you've got a steady hand with those pick-up sticks. That takes focus and patience. Notice what that focus feels like. Let's tap that in.

You went for a really tough one. You can handle challenges, can't you? Let's tap in what that feels like.

If the child is not mastering the activity but is floundering, process as above for games of frustration.

If the child wants to bring more focus and concentration to schoolwork, sports, music, or other activities, the experiences of mastering play can be used as resources for improved performance in those arenas.

Remember the feeling of focusing on the Jenga blocks? Get that in your body. Let's tap that in. Now, think of doing math with that feeling in your body. (A few more taps.) *How was that for you?*

Positive experiences like these build relationship and resources that will lay the groundwork for Standard Protocol trauma processing.

STORYTELLING

Storytelling is one of the most ancient and beautiful therapies humans have developed for processing difficult experiences and learning new behaviors. Creative therapists began early on to integrate EMDR principles with storytelling for children. In *Small Wonders: Healing Childhood Trauma with EMDR* (1999), Joan Lovett presented an excellent protocol for having parents write and tell a therapeutic story for a child with bilateral stimulation to process trauma. Debra Wesselman has developed a beautiful protocol for having parents write and tell stories to children to develop secure attachment (Wesselman, 2001).

I have found that metaphorical stories, combined with puppets and toys to provide bilateral stimulation, can be very powerful for children who are overwhelmed by, resistant to, or shamed by hearing a story they can identify as their own. Stories can be made up by the therapist, using animals, magical creatures, and situations that are just enough different from the real situation so that the child can relate to the imaginary character's issues but have enough distance so that they are not overwhelmed. Nancy Davis (1991, 1996) offers a wealth of stories written for trauma and other therapeutic issues.

The story the therapist finds or writes needs to outline a problem or conflict, talk about the trauma or problem, and illustrate the difficult feelings, beliefs, and behaviors the protagonist is having. The protagonist may receive wise instruction or help (from a character who provides bilateral stimulation by flying back and forth, hopping from hand to hand or knee to knee, or by waving a magic wand), but the protagonist still must struggle to overcome the problem through action if the story is to be really effective. The story ends by installing the positive feelings, beliefs, and behaviors the protagonist developed by meeting the challenge.

Storytelling is a profound art. A well-told story is a multidimensional performance that stimulates the entire mind and interweaves many elements of the Standard Protocol. Through tone of voice, rhythm, and movement, the teller and audience are united in an empathic moment in which they are resonating with the character's affect in a safe manner. The story line provides a coherent narrative that helps make sense of the character's emotions and beliefs. The character's heroic journey brings the listener into new territory that opens up possibilities for healthier beliefs and behaviors. Therapists who work with children would greatly benefit from joining a local storytellers' guild or listening to tapes on the art of storytelling to refine this skill.

The following was inspired by the Nancy Davis story, *The Siamese Twins* (1991). I have been surprised by the popularity and the power of this seemingly simple and innocuous tale. The dogs going away and coming back are a natural opportunity to incorporate eye movement into the story. I added the element of the wizard flying back and forth to reinforce positive cognitions.

I first used this story with a 6-year-old boy who was refusing to go to school without his mother and, in fact, would not even let go of her at school so she could go to the bathroom alone. He came into my office, clinging to his mother and burying his face behind her back. He refused my offer to look at the toys in the room, buried his head deeper behind his mother, and kept pulling at her insistently, whining: "Let's go. Let's go now." I began to tell this story, and he spat out: "I'm not listening!" and covered his ears. I told him that he didn't have to listen, I'd just tell the story to his mom. As the story went on, his body relaxed and his head began to peep out from behind his mother. At the end, he said: "Tell that story again." After the second telling, he got up and started investigating the toys in the room. Before he left the office, he said: "Mom, I'm ready to take the bus to school now." I've used this story with children of borderline mothers, kids who suffered from extreme separation anxiety, and kids who are struggling with differentiation in normal development. I've even told this story to groups of adult women who found it helped them get a perspective on some less-than-healthy aspects of their relationships. (Adults love to hear kid stories. One simply has to preface the telling with the words: "This reminds me of a story that I tell to kids.")

Remember, in order to make this, or any, story come alive, it should be performed, rather than simply read.

BIG DOG, LITTLE DOG: A TALE OF
DIFFERENTIATION

Once upon a time there were twin dogs. (Hold up two dog puppets or toys, one considerably bigger than the other, holding them so they appear "stuck" together.) *These were very unusual twin dogs: one, they were born stuck together, and two, one dog was much bigger than the other. And this caused a lot of trouble.*

Every time the big dog wanted to go somewhere, the little dog had to go too. When the big dog wanted to go play, the little dog had to go play. (Illustrate the big dog pulling the little to one side to play, then to the other side to eat.) *When the big dog wanted to go eat, the little dog had to go eat. When the big dog wanted to flop over to sleep, the little dog had to flop over to sleep too.* (The big dog flops over, pulling the little dog along with him.)

This went on for a long time and after a while, the little dog started getting tired of doing everything that the big dog wanted to do. He got more and more frustrated and more and more angry. Finally, the little dog got SO mad that he started yelling "NO, NO, NO, NO. I want to play and I want to play NOW!" (Little dog puppet beats on big dog puppet's head.) *and "NO, NO, NO, NO, I want to eat and I want to eat NOW!" Well, the big dog didn't want the little dog to be upset, so he started eating when little dog ate, and playing when little dog played, and sleeping when little dog slept.*

You know what happened next? That's right. Big Dog got tired and frustrated and upset and angry. He started yelling: "NO, NO, NO, NO, NO!" (Big Dog jumps up and down.) *"You can't do everything you want! You're going to do things my way from now on."*

Well, this went on and on. These were two very unhappy puppies, and they were stuck together. But one day, as they were fighting, a wise wizard happened upon them, studied them carefully, and came up with an idea for them. (Therapist brings in a puppet or toy that represents wisdom.)

"Hey guys," the wizard said. "You don't have to be this miserable. I can separate you and then you each can do whatever you want and need to do without dragging the other one with you."

The two dogs looked at the wizard suspiciously. They weren't so sure they liked this idea.

"I don't know," said Little Dog, "I'd be scared to be all alone without Big Dog."

"I don't know," said Big Dog, "I'd be worried if Little Dog went off without me."

"Well," said the wizard, "you sleep on it and in the morning you will know what to do."

That night, Big Dog and Little Dog curled up and went to sleep and they *both* had the same dream. The wizard flew back and forth over them, back and forth, back and forth (Wizard puppet or figure flies back and forth in front of the child's eyes) *and each time the wizard went by, he said:* (in smooth, rhythmic tones) *"You'll be safe." "It's okay, you'll be safe." "You'll be safe."*

When Big Dog and Little Dog woke up the next morning, they felt much calmer and clearer. They were still a little nervous, but they decided to go ahead and let the wizard separate them. The wizard had them go to sleep and then, gently, gently he separated the two pups.

When they woke up, they were lying side by side, so very close, but they weren't attached!

"I don't know," said Big Dog, "This is weird. I don't know if I like this."

"It's really weird," said Little Dog. "I'm not so sure either."

"Well, let's try it out," said Big Dog. "Why don't you go get that bone over there."

Little Dog ran and got the bone, and he came right back. (The puppet moves away to fetch the bone and comes back.)

"Whew, that worked okay." Then Little Dog said, a little uncertainly, "I think I'll go play with that ball over there."

So Little Dog went and played and came back, he played and came back, he played and came back. (Little dog puppet is moving back and forth across the child's visual field.) *Each time he went away and came back, he felt stronger and stronger and stronger.*

Then Big Dog decided to try it. He went away and came back, went away and came back, went away and came back, and each time he felt stronger and stronger and stronger. (Big dog puppet is moving back and forth across the child's visual field.)

Now those two dogs are very happy dogs. They play together and eat together but they can also go away and come back, go away and come back (one puppet moving away and coming back) *and they can each do the things that make them happy.* (Puppets come together in middle and cuddle.)

EXTENDING THE STORY

The child often wants to step into a story by becoming one of the characters, extending the story, or directing the play. Whenever this happens, let go of the need to "tell the story," encourage the child's process, and improvise along with the child. The therapist keeps remembering and integrating the basic tenets of EMDR: to process the difficult feelings and beliefs and to install the positive feelings, beliefs, and behaviors.

Sometimes the story will be told and acted out with different iterations over a period of weeks. Parents can be given or can create stories that they tell their child at bedtime while the child listens to bilateral tones or receives bilateral taps, or gentle foot squeezes.

SUMMARY

Therapists who work with children tend to be creative and playful by nature. These qualities alone help children feel safe and allow them the venue to process trauma and learn healthier beliefs and behaviors. However, when a child therapist intentionally integrates the principles of EMDR into the early stages of therapy, relationship and safety become established quickly and soundly, allowing the child to develop the capacity to manage affect and proceed safely to trauma processing with the Standard Protocol.

REFERENCES

Davis, N. (1991). *Therapeutic stories to heal abused children* (revised ed.). Burke, VA: Author.

Davis, N. (1996). *Therapeutic stories that teach and heal.* Burke, VA: Self-published.

Greenwald, R. (1999). *Eye movement desensitization and reprocessing (EMDR) in child and adolescent psychotherapy.* New York: Jason Aronson.

Herman, J. L. (1992). *Trauma and recovery.* New York: Basics.

Lovett, J. (1999). *Small wonders: Healing childhood trauma with EMDR.* New York: Free Press.

Miller, W., Rollnick, S., & Conforti, K. (2002). *Motivational interviewing: Preparing people for change* (2nd edition). New York: Guilford Press.

Perry, B., Pollard, R., Blakley, T., Baler, W., & Vigilante, D. (1995). Childhood trauma, the neurobiology of adaptation, and "use-dependent" development of the brain: How "states" become "traits." *Infant Mental Health Journal, 16,* 271–290.

Shapiro, F. (2001). *Eye movement desensitization and reprocessing: Basic principles, protocols and procedures* (2nd edition). New York: Guilford Press.

Shore, A.N. (1994). *Affect regulation and the origin of self: The neurobiology of emotional development.* Hillsdale, NJ: Erlbaum.

Siegel, D.J. (1999). *The developing mind: Toward a neurobiology of interpersonal experience.* New York: Guildford Press.

Tinker, R.H., & Wilson, S.A. (1999). *Through the eyes of a child: EMDR with children,* New York: Norton.

Wesselman, Debra (2001, June). *Treating Core Attachment Issues in Adults and Children.* Paper presented at EMDRIA Conference, 2001.

RESOURCES

Association for Play Therapy, 1350 M Street, Fresno, CA 93857

Play Therapy Bibliography, Center for Play Therapy, University of North Texas, P.O. Box 310829, Denton, TX 76203-0829

Glossary

Adaptive Information Processing Model The theoretical model of EMDR that refers to the innate tendency of the brain to process disturbing life experiences to an adaptive resolution.

Bilateral Stimulation (BLS) *see* Dual Attention Stimulus (DAS)

Blocking Belief A cognition that stops EMDR processing—for example, "I'll never get over this."

Body Scan Phase six of the Standard Protocol, in which, after the bulk of the processing is complete, clients are asked to think about the disturbing event and notice their bodily sensations. Any sensations are targeted with DAS.

Butterfly Hug A self-administered bilateral stimulation technique in which the client places their hands on the opposite shoulders or crossed on the chest, tapping alternately. The butterfly hug is often used in groups, or for self-soothing outside of sessions.

Calm Place *see* Safe Place

Dual Attention Stimulus (DAS) As EMDR has responded to research, the name of the *Eye Movement, Tapping, and Audio* tones has changed at least three times. First we had *Eye Movements*, now *Bilateral Stimulation* or *Dual Attention Stimulus* best describes the effect of the eye movements or other stimulation that accompanies processing in EMDR.

Desensitization Phase four of the Standard Protocol, in which DAS is used to process the distressing event.

Future Template Part of EMDR's Three-Pronged Protocol, in which attention is brought to the past, the present and the future components of a particular processing target.

Healing Place *see* Safe Place

Looping A form of blocked response in which the client is cycling through the same sensations, emotions, images or thoughts, rather than processing them through to an adaptive resolution.

Negative Cognition (NC) The old, currently illogical, thought about self that is connected to a disturbing event.

Positive Cognition (PC) The currently true thought about self that clients strive for in EMDR processing. PC's are measured with the seven-point Validity of Cognition scale (VOC).

Resource Development/Resource Installation (RDI) A Preparation Phase procedure of front-loading remembered or imaginary positive strengths, experiences, attributes, or (less often) external support. RDI is used for clients who cannot tolerate regular EMDR processing, and is not usually necessary for clients with good affect tolerance.

Safe Place Introduced in the Preparation Phase, the imaginary safe place is used as resting place during prolonged reprocessing, a method of reducing distress at the end of an incomplete session, and a self-care method between sessions.

Standard Protocol

- Phase One: Client History, including client readiness, client safety factors, and dissociation screening
- Phase Two: Preparation, includes creating bond with the client, setting expectations, creating a safe place and testing the eye movements or Dual Attention Stimulus

- Phase Three: Assessment, includes selecting the picture or disturbing event, identifying the Negative Cognition (NC), developing a Positive Cognition (PC), rating the Validity of Cognition (VoC or VOC), naming the emotion, estimating the Subjective Units of Disturbance (SUD or SUDS) and Identifying Body Sensations.
- Phase Four: Desensitization includes reprocessing the memory, using DAS.
- Phase Five: Installing the Positive Cognition, while holding the memory in mind
- Phase Six: Body Scan, searching for any bodily disturbance
- Phase Seven Closure, includes homework, expectations, and , if needed, bringing the client to a state of emotional equilibrium
- Phase Eight: Reevaluation includes checking in at the next session to see if the client requires new processing for associated material

SUDS Subjective Units of Disturbance Scale, a 0–10 scale that measures the intensity of negative affect

VOC Validity of Cognition Scale, a subjective 1–7 scale that measures the believability of a suggested positive cognition

Index